D1460062

A Handbook of
Vascular Disease Management

A Handbook of
Vascular Disease Management

Wesley S Moore • Juan Carlos Jimenez

University of California, Los Angeles, USA

Editors

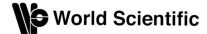

NEW JERSEY · LONDON · SINGAPORE · BEIJING · SHANGHAI · HONG KONG · TAIPEI · CHENNAI

Published by

World Scientific Publishing Co. Pte. Ltd.

5 Toh Tuck Link, Singapore 596224

USA office: 27 Warren Street, Suite 401-402, Hackensack, NJ 07601

UK office: 57 Shelton Street, Covent Garden, London WC2H 9HE

British Library Cataloguing-in-Publication Data
A catalogue record for this book is available from the British Library.

A HANDBOOK OF VASCULAR DISEASE MANAGEMENT

ISBN-13 978-981-4317-77-1
ISBN-10 981-4317-77-2

Typeset by Stallion Press
Email: enquiries@stallionpress.com

Printed in Singapore by Mainland Press Pte Ltd.

Contents

Contributors

Ali Alktaifi
Research Fellow
Division of Vascular Surgery
David Geffen School of Medicine at UCLA

Jonathan Bath
Vascular Surgery Resident
David Geffen School of Medicine at UCLA

J. Dennis Baker
Professor of Surgery
Division of Vascular Surgery
David Geffen School of Medicine at UCLA

Ankur Chandra
Assistant Professor
Division of Vascular Surgery
University of Rochester Medical Center

Jessica O'Connell
Assistant Professor
Division of Vascular Surgery
David Geffen School of Medicine at UCLA

Gavin Davis
Vascular Surgery Resident
David Geffen School of Medicine at UCLA

Brian G. Derubertis
Assistant Professor
Division of Vascular Surgery
David Geffen School of Medicine at UCLA

Steven Farley
Assistant Professor
Division of Vascular Surgery
David Geffen School of Medicine at UCLA

Hugh A. Gelabert
Professor of Surgery
Division of Vascular Surgery
David Geffen School of Medicine at UCLA

Carolyn Glass
Vascular Surgery Resident
Division of Vascular Surgery
University of Rochester Medical Center

Juan Carlos Jimenez
Assistant Professor
Division of Vascular Surgery
David Geffen School of Medicine at UCLA

Peter F. Lawrence
Professor and Chief
Division of Vascular Surgery
David Geffen School of Medicine at UCLA

Wesley S. Moore
Professor Emeritus
Division of Vascular Surgery
David Geffen School of Medicine at UCLA

William J. Quinones-Baldrich
Professor of Surgery
Division of Vascular Surgery
David Geffen School of Medicine at UCLA

David A. Rigberg
Associate Professor
Division of Vascular Surgery
David Geffen School of Medicine at UCLA

Darin J. Saltzman
Assistant Professor
Division of General Surgery
David Geffen School of Medicine at UCLA

Allan Tulloch
Vascular Surgery Resident
Division of Vascular Surgery
David Geffen School of Medicine at UCLA

Chapter 1

Atherosclerosis: Basic Principles and Medical Management

Jessica O'Connell and Jonathan Bath

———

Learning Objectives

- Understand the pathogenesis of atherosclerosis.
- Describe the progression of atherosclerotic lesions by histologic findings and classification.
- Understand the role of specific cells in atherosclerosis.
- Describe the theories of atherogenesis.
- Understand the various risk factors for atherosclerosis.
- Understand the mechanisms of injury for the main risk factors for atherosclerosis.
- Describe the risk factor modifications that can slow the progression of atherosclerosis.
- Describe the medical management of atherosclerosis.

1. Introduction

Arterial disease is the leading cause of death and significant morbidity in the United States and throughout the world. The American Heart Association estimates that 80 million (36.3%) Americans have cardiovascular disease, leading to 864,500 deaths annually. Patients with peripheral arterial disease (PAD) make up a significant proportion of this group, including 795,000 Americans who will have strokes each year. Stroke itself is the third leading cause of death in the Unites States with an estimated 143,600 patients dying each year. Those who do survive often have significant neurologic deficits that can become major social and economic burdens to the patients and their families.

Atherosclerosis, or "hardening of the arteries", is a disease process that leads to plaque formation in the arteries. Over time, these plaques can become hemodynamically significant leading to decreased oxygenation of tissues distal to the disease, or unstable plaques that can rupture and cause thrombosis, embolization, and acute ischemia. Atherosclerosis is a systemic disease that can affect arteries throughout the body from the carotid arteries, to the coronary arteries, to the lower extremity arteries. This not only can result in transient ischemic attacks, angina, and claudication, but also can lead to significant morbidity from major strokes, myocardial infarctions (MIs), and extremity gangrene and amputation.

PAD is a significant public health issue requiring extensive long-term care for patients with these serious disabilities, but also because atherosclerosis, and, therefore, PAD is largely preventable or diminishable by avoiding tobacco, fatty foods, and taking medications regularly to control hypertension, diabetes, and hyperlipidemia. Though we now have excellent diagnostic modalities that can help identify patients at risk for atherosclerosis, along with well-planned preventative strategies, patients are often still reluctant to make the necessary lifestyle modifications. It is estimated that for 2009, the total direct and indirect cost of cardiovascular diseases and stroke in the United States was $475.3 billion.

In this chapter, we will discuss the pathogenesis of atherosclerosis, risk factors for development of atherosclerosis the clinical relevance of the disease and discuss preventative modalities and evolving medical treatments.

2. Pathogenesis of Atherosclerosis

2.1 *Normal arterial anatomy*

In order to understand the process that occurs within the arterial wall that leads to atherosclerosis, one must first begin with the normal anatomy. Arteries are made of three distinct layers that are designed to withstand a lifetime of stress from pulsatile blood flow. These three layers or tunics are the *tunica intima*, the *tunica media*, and the *tunica adventitia*.

The *tunica intima*, or the endothelium, is the innermost layer of an arterial wall. It consists of a monolayer of endothelial cells with a thick underlying matrix of elastic fibers and collagen. The intimal endothelial cells are responsible for a variety of functions including the regulation of vessel tone and the initiation and formation of thrombus as a response to endothelial injury. The intima receives its blood supply directly by diffusion from the flowing blood within the arterial lumen. An internal elastic membrane, or lamina, separates the intima from the next layer, the media.

The *tunica media* is the thick middle layer of the arterial wall. It is composed of varying amounts of collagen, elastic fibers, and smooth muscle. The amount of elastin found within the media of an artery decreases progressively from the "elastic" thoracic aorta to the peripheral medium-sized "muscular" arteries, such as the femoral or carotid arteries, to the small high-resistance peripheral vessels. The media provides structure to the vessel and is involved in maintaining vessel tone by responding to signals from the intimal endothelial cells. It is here in the media where the atherosclerotic process begins and proliferates. The media receives oxygen and nutrition not only from diffusion of the circulating luminal blood, but also from small vessels (vasa vasorum) that penetrate the outer arterial wall. The media and the adventitia are separated by an external elastic membrane.

The *tunica adventitia* is the outermost layer of an artery. The adventitia appears fragile and thin; however, its strong collagen and elastic structure make it one of the key components in the overall strength of an artery. The adventitia is composed of collagen, autonomic nerves, and the vasa vasorum that course along and through the adventitia. This layer must be included in a vascular anastomosis in order to prevent future anastomotic breakdown and pseudoaneurysm formation.

2.2 *Etiology and progression of disease*

The term atherosclerosis comes from the words *atheroma* and *sclerosis*. *Atheroma* is derived from the Greek *athere*, means "gruel" or "porridge," and *sclerosis*, means "hardening" or "induration." Arteriosclerosis is a general term that refers to any hardening of the arteries or loss of elasticity, and though the two words are often used interchangeably, technically atherosclerosis is a type of arteriosclerosis. Atherosclerosis describes changes in the arterial wall causing thickening of the vessel wall due to focal accumulation of lipids, fibrous tissue, hemorrhage, and calcium deposits. Atherosclerosis is a complex process that is linked to a combination of factors. These include genetic predisposition (*e.g.* familial hyperlipidemia and diabetes), mechanical factors (*e.g.* hypertension and shear stress), environmental factors (*e.g.* tobacco and fatty food intake), and a robust immune response.

2.2.1 *Intimal thickening*

Intimal thickening may represent one of the earliest indications of atherosclerotic disease. Intimal thickening is thought to be either an adaptive response, possibly acting to reduce the diameter of the lumen in reaction to chronically reduced blood flow, or a response designed to increase arterial wall thickness secondary to chronically increased wall tensile stress. Focal intimal thickenings have been noted at or near branch points very early in life in the arteries of infants and even in fetuses. However, diffuse fibrocellular intimal thickening can also been seen in a more generalized fashion without clear relation to branches. This results in a diffusely thickened intima that can be even thicker than the media. Lipids do not appear to accumulate in these areas of intimal thickening though they do tend to occur in similar locations as atherosclerotic lesions. Initial work was hopeful that intimal medial thickness, particularly in the carotid artery, would be a simple and useful predictor of atherosclerotic disease, and has been shown to correlate with future cardiovascular risk for stroke and MI. However, there are several limitations to measurements of carotid intimal medial thickness (CIMT). The common carotid artery is the vessel generally sampled, whereas atherosclerosis is much more common in the distal internal carotid artery or carotid bulb. There are other contributors to intimal thickening that are not necessarily related to atherosclerosis, including age and hypertension. The measurement of CIMT is highly dependent on the ultrasound equipment, technique, and operator. One of the primary limitations is the inability to distinguish lesions with a necrotic core, which is felt to be a better predictor of atherosclerosis. Future work and improved ultrasound technology may improve results in the area of measuring intimal medial thickness as a predictor of atherosclerotic disease.

2.2.2 Fatty streaks

Atherosclerosis begins in the earliest years of life and tends to affect primarily the large- and medium-sized elastic and muscular arteries. The earliest lesions, the so-called "fatty streaks" are found in young children and even infants. Fatty streaks are yellow and slightly raised lesions often found in the aorta of infants and children. This is a purely inflammatory lesion and is composed of lipid-laden macrophages (foam cells) and T lymphocytes. Cholesterols, specifically low-density lipoproteins (LDL), are the main lipids found in these early lesions, and once oxidized they are engulfed by monocyte-derived macrophages and become foam cells. Stary *et al.* classified these early lesions into Types I–III (see Classification of Vascular Lesions). Cigarette smoking greatly accelerates the formation of these fatty streaks by increasing the oxidation of LDL and their phagocytosis by macrophages. There is evidence that with exercise, modification of risks factors, and statin medications, these early lesions can stabilize or regress.

2.2.3 Fibrofatty lesions/gelatinous plaques

Another type of early atheroma precursor is the fibrofatty lesion or gelatinous plaque. These lesions were first noted by Virchow in 1856, thought they have been less studied than other lesions. Plasma proteins, particularly the hemostatic components, are thought to be the source of these lesions. These gelatinous plaques are described as translucent and neutral in color, with central gray or opaque areas. They have finely dispersed lipid with collagen strands around the lesions and have a low lipid content and high fluid content. Grossly, they are soft with the gelatinous material separating easily from the arterial wall.

2.2.4 Fibrous plaques

Fibrous plaques appear later in life and are a more permanent lesion. Often found at arterial bifurcations, fibrous plaques are comprised of a lipid core surrounded by a capsule made of collagenous and elastic tissue. These lesions are termed Type IV plaques (see Classification of Vascular Lesions), and are composed of large numbers of smooth muscle cells and connective tissue that forms a fibrous cap over an inner yellow core. This soft yellow core contains the highly irritating and inflammatory cholesterol esters and cholesterol oxysterols likely derived from disrupted foam cells. A large number of macrophages are also present. These plaques protrude into the arterial lumen, and in the beginning arterial enlargement compensates for atheroma growth. However, with continued growth, symptomatic stenoses occur along with ulceration, rupture, or overlying thrombosis leading to arterial luminal compromise.

2.2.5 *Complicated lesions*

Complicated lesions (Types V and VI, see Classification of Vascular Lesions) develop from the fibrous plaque through several potential processes including necrosis, ulceration of the surface of the plaque, calcification, or intraplaque hemorrhage. These are the pathologic developments that lead to the clinical complications of MI, stroke, and gangrene. Ulcerated plaque is thrombogenic and causes platelet aggregation and thrombus formation. Intraplaque hemorrhage can lead to plaque instability and rupture. With the development of a complicated lesion, the elasticity of the arterial wall is lost and the vessel can become narrow leading to stenosis, or degenerate leading to dilation of the arterial wall and aneurysm formation.

2.3 *Classification of vascular lesions*

In the mid-1990s, Stary and colleagues reported for the American Heart Association Committee on Vascular Lesions. They classified atherosclerotic lesions into six types (Types I–VI). Type I lesions are not visible, but represent the first atherosclerotic changes, including increasing numbers of intimal macrophages and the appearance of foam cells. Type II lesions are the fatty streak lesions, the first grossly visible lesions, which contain layers of macrophage foam cells and lipid droplets within intimal smooth muscle cells (Fig. 1). Types I and II are generally the only lesion types that found in infants and children, although they may also occur later in adulthood. The Type III lesion is the intermediate stage between Type II and Type IV (atheroma, a lesion that can be potentially symptomatic). Type III lesions not only include all the components of Type II lesions, but also contain scattered pools of extracellular lipid droplets and particles that disrupt the coherence of some intimal smooth muscle cells. This extracellular lipid is the precursor to the large, confluent, and more troublesome core of extracellular lipid seen in Type IV lesions (Fig. 2). Beginning around the fourth decade of life, lesions with a lipid core often will have thick layers of fibrous connective tissue or a fibrous cap (Type V lesion). Largely

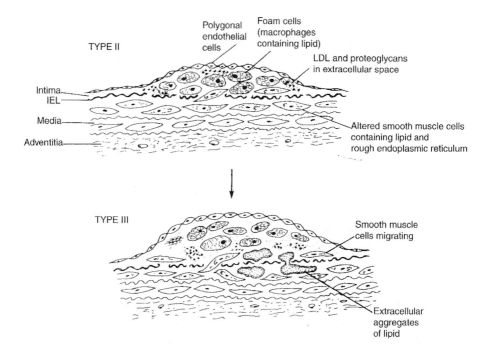

Fig. 1. Type II and III Lesions. Type II lesions are fatty streaks containing foam cells. The lesion is also comprised of low-density lipoprotein (LDL) particles in the matrix and altered smooth muscle cells. With development of a Type III lesion there are now extracellular aggregates or pools of lipid in the intima and extending into the media. IEL, internal elastic lamina. (From DePalma RG: Atherosclerosis: Pathology, Pathogenesis, and Medical Management. In Moore, WS [ed]: Vascular and Endovascular Surgery: A Comprehensive Review, 7th Edition. Philadelphia, Elsevier Saunders, 2006, p. 93.)

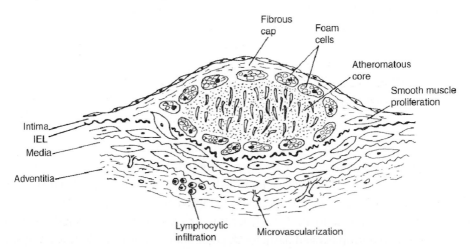

Fig. 2. Type IV Atheroma. With this degree of maturation of the atheroma there is a fibrous cap, central lipid core, macrophage accumulation and zone of active smooth muscle proliferation at the edge of the core. IEL, internal elastic lamina. (From DePalma RG: Atherosclerosis: Pathology, Pathogenesis, and Medical Management. In Moore, WS [ed]: Vascular and Endovascular Surgery: A Comprehensive Review, 7th Edition. Philadelphia, Elsevier Saunders, 2006, p. 92.)

calcified lesions are termed Type Vb, and mainly fibrous lesions with significant connective tissue and little or no lipid or calcium are deemed Type Vc lesions. Once a lesion becomes fissured, develops a hematoma or thrombus, it is deemed a Type VI lesion.

2.4 *Atherosclerosis at the cellular level*

2.4.1 *Endothelium*

In early atherosclerosis, including in fatty streaks, endothelial cells in animal and human studies become altered, showing signs of endothelial dysfunction. They begin to be oriented away from the direction of arterial blood flow, show evidence of increased proliferation, become rounded or polyhedral, and increase the formation of multinucleated cells and cilia. This increased cell turnover leads to increased cell death, exposure of subendothelial foam cells, and permeability. As the endothelium becomes more permeable to macromolecules, there is increased mural thrombus formation and tissue factor expression. There is also increased leukocyte adherence with increased expression of VCAM-1 a monocyte adhesion molecule. Increased vasoconstriction of the vessel occurs with decreasing levels of endothelium-derived relaxing factor, nitric oxide, and prostacyclin.

2.4.2 *Smooth muscle cells*

Experimental models of early atherosclerosis have shown a variety of changes that occur in smooth muscle cells. There is increased expression of dermatan sulfate, stromelysins, proteoglycan, and both Type I and III collagens. Smooth muscles cells are induced to produce a variety of cytokines, such as tumor necrosis factor (TNF), macrophage colony-stimulating factor, and monocyte chemoattractant protein-1. These smooth muscle cells ingest and accumulate native and modified lipoproteins by standard receptor pathways and nonspecific phagocytosis. These smooth muscle cells also express increased lipoprotein lipase activity and experimentally display a scavenger receptor like foam cells.

2.4.3 *Macrophages*

In early atherosclerosis, macrophages proliferate and express a variety of factors that induce further proliferation and uptake of normal and oxidized cholesterols. These include monocyte chemoattractant protein-1, macrophage colony-stimulating factor, TNF, intraleukin-1, platelet-derived growth factor, immune antigens, and tissue factor. Plaque macrophages contain increased free and esterified choles-terol and increased acetyl coenzyme A, cholesterol acyltransferase, and acid cholesterol ester hydrolase. These abnormal cells also express the scavenger receptor

15-lipoxygenase and exhibit increased lipoprotein oxidation products in both animal and humans models.

3. Theories of Atherogenesis

3.1 *Response to injury hypothesis*

There have been several theories of atherogenesis over the decades of study in this area. The most comprehensive and inclusive theory with the most current support is the response to injury hypothesis.

Healthy endothelium provides a smooth and nonadherent surface over which blood can flow. However, this normal endothelial surface can be disrupted or injured by a variety of stressors. Normal healing leads to rapid regeneration of the endothelium. However, if the injury is extensive, the healing response may be accompanied by an influx of inflammatory agents including smooth muscle cells, which causes intimal thickening, or in some sense "scar tissue" formation. According to the response to injury hypotheses, endothelial injury may be caused by a variety of factors including mechanical forces (*e.g.* hypertension and arterial wall shear stress), circulating metabolites (*e.g.* oxidized lipids, cigarette smoke), immunologic reactions, and exposure to vasoactive agents. Endothelial injury leads to endothelial dysfunction that results in altered responses to the normal homeostatic properties of the endothelium.

Once the endothelium is desquamated, the subendothelial tissues are exposed leading to T cells, monocytes, and platelets adhering to the injured area in an attempt to repair damaged endothelium. However, in areas of chronic injury, the intimal permeability is altered and there is increased activity leading to an immune-directed inflammatory response involving these monocytes, T cells, and macrophages. All of these, which secrete cytokines, induce cell migration into the medial layer of the vessel. Smooth muscle cells become altered in function increasing the production of extracellular matrix and calcium, and macrophages engulf oxidized lipids and become foam cells. This leads to early atherosclerotic lesions and eventually calcium deposition between vessel layers forming the fibrous cap of atheromas, finally leading to mature plaque formation.

Atheromas not only cause a continued local inflammatory and proliferative response, they can also extend into the arterial lumen causing luminal compromise. The atheroma can then become "unstable" and open or rupture, inducing local thrombosis or releasing thrombogenic debris into the bloodstream and causing embolization.

The local inflammatory response is due to the secretion of cytokines, which leads to a state called "vascular remodeling." Remodeling is a process where smooth muscle cell proliferation activates matrix metalloproteinases (MMPs). A few specific MMPs are able to destroy the structural proteins in the media and adventitia resulting in a weakened and dilated arterial segment. This dilation initially compensates for the stenosis, but can also lead to arterial aneurysm formation if unchecked.

3.2 *Lipid hypothesis*

Lipids have been thought to be an important factor in atherosclerosis since the time of Virchow. Oxidized lipids are a major component of foam cells, and as such the lipid hypothesis is a sub-set of the response to injury hypothesis. Patients with elevated circulating cholesterol have been noted for decades to have a higher prevalence of atherosclerotic lesions. Patients with familial hypercholesterolemias provide convincing evidence to support this. These autosomal dominant conditions have been linked to at least 12 different molecular defects of the LDL receptors. They occur in approximately 1 in 500 live births. Homozygotes usually die in their mid-20s due to severe advanced atherosclerosis, and heterozygotes often have total cholesterol levels ranging up to 350 mg/dL and have severe atherosclerotic disease as they age.

3.3 *Thrombogenic hypothesis*

This theory hypothesizes that degenerated blood proteins deposit fibrinous substances on the intimal arterial surface. These deposits in turn could become atheromatous masses comprised of cholesterol crystals and goblets. This may also be the process by which gelatinous plaques are formed.

3.4 *Mesenchymal hypothesis*

The mesenchymal hypothesis of atherosclerosis explores why physical factors such as vasoactive agents, shear stress, and repetitive injuries induce a similar sequence of events in the vessel wall that appears to lead to atherosclerosis. Hauss *et al.* postulated that smooth muscle cells migrate from the media to the intima, where they proliferate and produce connective tissue. Furthermore, they felt that this is a nonspecific arterial reaction to any injury and that atherosclerosis reflects a normal arterial response.

3.5 *Monoclonal hypothesis*

Benditt and Benditt noted that in atherosclerotic lesions, smooth muscle cells are derived from one or a few smooth muscle cells and, like tumor cells, proliferate in an unchecked fashion. This is based on the finding of only one allele for glucose-6-phosphate dehydrogenase in lesions from heterozygotes. In addition, in other studies, it has been noted that the presence of transforming growth factor-beta receptors in human atherosclerosis provides evidence of an acquired resistance to apoptosis, which can also lead to unchecked cellular proliferation.

4. Lesion Arrest and Regression — Plaque Modification

The potential for lesion arrest and regression is crucial to treatment options for patients with atherosclerotic disease. Regression of these lesions, because of a low cholesterol state, has been seen in autopsy studies of starved humans circa World War I. Similar results have been seen in animal models and in human trials of smoking cessation and lipid reduction. The exact mechanism of lesion regression is not completely understood, but this occurs with a clear decrease in the volume of the intimal plaque. It is thought to be related to an efflux or resorption of lipids or extracellular matrix, cell death, and cell migration out of the plaque. Evidence of regression in rhesus monkeys has been shown in studies of serial observations of decreased plaque bulk, decreased luminal encroachment on sequential angiography, decreased plaque lipid, and altered fibrous protein content measured histologically and chemically. Many of these findings were also confirmed on autopsy or surgical observation and biopsy. With lengthy and extensive reduction in blood cholesterol for 42 months in rhesus monkeys, microscopic evidence of regression included the disappearance of macrophages, foam cells, lymphocytes, and extracellular lipids. However, there was no change in the arterial wall calcium deposits. This finding is not surprising and points to calcification as a significantly limiting factor in atherosclerotic lesions. In some cases, fibrous protein increases during regression and may also limit regression; however, this process converts a soft plaque to a fibrous, more stable, and less thrombogenic lesion. Lipid levels must be aggressively reduced in order to induce regression of atherosclerotic plaques.

5. Mechanism of Injury

5.1 *Tobacco*

Cigarette smoking is an extremely strong inducer of atherosclerosis even in the setting of normal circulating lipids. It is directly related to high mortality from ischemic heart disease, failure of aortic and femoropopliteal bypasses, and limb amputation. The exact mechanisms by which cigarette smoking contributes to atherosclerosis and graft thrombosis are not fully understood. However, it is known that cigarette smoke is a powerful oxidizing agent that leads to lipid oxidation, vessel spasm, and vasoconstriction. The main component of cigarette smoke is nicotine, which is a strong pro-inflammatory agent, significantly contributes to endothelial dysfunction by initiating the adhesion cascade and stimulating inflammatory events to induce atherosclerosis and hypertension. Carbon monoxide predisposes to arterial wall injury, producing increased endothelial permeability and influx of LDL and other proteins. Cigarette smoking also causes increased platelet reactivity and lowered HDL levels.

5.2 *Hypertension*

Prospective studies have shown that premature atherosclerotic disease is independently associated with hypertension. In experimental animals, hyperlipidemia-associated atherosclerosis is accelerated by chronic hypertension. Patients with hypertension often have elevated levels of angiotensin II, the main product of the renin-angiotensin system. Angiotensin II is a potent vasoconstrictor and also stimulates the growth of smooth muscle and increases intracellular calcium concentrations and smooth muscle hypertrophy. Angiotensin II also can increase inflammation and oxidation of LDL by smooth muscle lipoxygenase activity. Hypertension itself also has proinflammatory actions increasing the formation of plasma hydrogen peroxide and other free radicals such as superoxide anion and hydroxyl radicals. These free radicals reduce endothelial formation of nitric oxide, increase leukocyte adhesion, and increase peripheral resistance.

5.3 *Shear forces*

Advanced atherosclerotic plaques commonly occur at arterial branch points. This finding suggests that local shear stress related to turbulent flow at these branch points may also act as an atherosclerotic accelerating factor. Experimental and clinical observations also have noted that early endothelial injury is more likely to occur in areas of blood flow separation and low shear stress. This is seen clearly in models of the carotid artery bulb (Fig. 3). The layer of blood flowing along the intima is termed the boundary layer. Flow in the middle of the arterial lumen is laminar; however, the outer area of boundary layer separation has slower more disturbed currents. These are areas of low shear force ($<4\,\mathrm{dyne/cm^2}$) tend to occur at the outer walls of arterial branch points and have been shown to induce endothelial dysfunction.

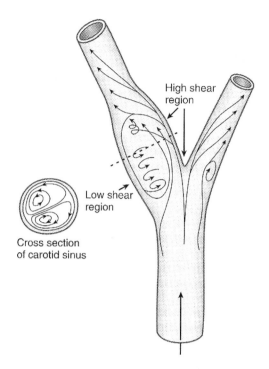

Fig. 3. Carotid artery bifurcation depicting an area of flow separation near the outer wall of the carotid bulb. High shear stress occurs in areas of rapid flow such as along the inner wall of the carotid bulb. Atherosclerotic lesions usually are located along the outer wall where there is slower flow and lower shear stress produced by the boundary layer separation. (From Zarins CK, Xu C, Glagov S: Artery Wall Pathology in Atherosclerosis. In Rutherford, RB [ed]: Vascular Surgery, 6th Edition. Philadelphia, Elsevier Saunders, 2005, p. 133.)

5.4 *Hyperlipidemia*

As has been previously discussed in detail in this chapter, elevated circulating lipids play a critical role in atherosclerosis. Patients with elevated circulating cholesterol have significantly higher risk of atherosclerotic lesions. Oxidized lipids are a major component of lipid-laden macrophages or foam cells, which are one of the main contributors to atherosclerotic plaque formation. Modified LDL itself is a chemo-tactic factor for other monocytes and propagates the inflammatory process within the plaque.

5.5 *Diabetes*

Diabetes is one of the most important and well-documented risk factors for atherosclerosis. Anatomically, diabetes is most often associated with severe tib-ial and coronary atherosclerosis. Enhanced atherogenesis in diabetes is likely due to abnormalities in apoproteins and lipoprotein particle distribution, particularly elevated levels of lipoprotein (a), which itself is an independent risk factor for atherosclerosis. Poorly controlled serum glucose leads to a procoagulant state with *in vitro* models showing accelerated platelet aggregation. Growth factors, hormones, smooth muscle cell proliferation, and increased foam cell formation are also thought to be further altered in diabetes mellitus leading to accelerated atherogenesis. Hyperinsulinemia and insulin resistance are associated with atherosclerosis, and both insulin and glucose stimulate smooth muscle cell proliferation in the infrageniculate location in diabetics.

5.6 *Infection*

Several viruses and bacteria have been shown to be associated (at some level) with atherosclerosis. These include *Chlamydia pneumoniae*, cytomegalovirus (CMV), *Helicobacter pylori*, herpesvirus, *Porphyromonas gingivalis*, and *Actinobacillus actinomycetemcomitans*. *C. pneumoniae* or its DNA has been intermittently found in atherosclerotic plaques. It is hypothesized that *C. pneumoniae*-infected macrophages enter the arterial intima and mediate inflammatory and autoimmune responses *via* chlamydial heat shock protein 60. Evidence of CMV in atherosclerotic plaques has been noted histologically and in culture. It has been noted that patients who are seropositive for CMV have a high incidence of restenosis after coronary atherectomy.

Periodontal disease has been shown epidemiologically to be related to atherosclerosis. It is thought that periodontal disease might increase circulating cytokine levels, promote a proatherogenic endothelium, and lead to endothelial dysfunction causing a prothrombotic state, cell proliferation, and vasoconstriction. A recent prospective study suggests that the exposure to periodontal pathogens or endotoxin induces systemic inflammation leading to increased risk for cardiovascular disease. The periodontal pathogens *Porphyromonas gingivalis* and *Actinobacillus actinomycetemcomitans* have been associated with coronary artery disease and *P. gingivalis* has been shown to increase IL-6 levels and accelerate atherosclerosis. Results of antibiotic trials as potential treatment for atherosclerotic lesions have been mixed. In a recent pilot study, long-term clarithromycin was noted to reduce recurrent cardiovascular events in subjects without periodontitis, but not in subjects with periodontitis. It was suggested that "periodontitis may overpower the beneficial effects of antibiotics."

6. Atherosclerosis Basic Principles and Medical Management

6.1 *Risk factors for atherosclerotic disease and modification strategies*

Many theories and causes of atherogenesis have been postulated and studied, and have lead to a handful of clear risk factors for atherosclerosis. These risk factors have

Table 1.   Risk factors for atherosclerotic cardiovascular disease.

Well-established:	Smoking
	Diabetes mellitus
	Hypertension
	Dyslipidemia
	Physical inactivity
	Advanced age
	Family history of early cardiovascular disease
Emerging:	High sensitivity C-reactive peptide
	Lipoprotein (a)
	Fibrinogen and fibrin-degradation products
	Homocysteine

long been recognized as the framework for a preventative strategy for cardiovascular diseases. The identification of specific cardiovascular risk factors that led to the concept of risk factor modification arose from the findings of the Framingham Heart Study of the 1960s. A risk factor can be simply defined as an entity that can be identified early in the disease course of an individual or group and confers an increased risk of disease development. An essential part of disease prevention in the context of identification of risk factors is the ability for modification of that specific risk factor, usually in the form of behavioral or pharmacologic manipulation.

Cardiovascular disease is increasingly recognized as the largest growing burden of disease for healthcare systems. Though progress in treatment regimens and surgical outcomes once atherosclerotic disease is established has improved morbidity and mortality from cardiovascular complications, there has been a shift in emphasis toward the development of effective clinical guidelines for prevention and modification at an earlier stage in the disease process. Table 1 lists the most common risk factors for atherosclerotic cardiovascular disease.

6.2 *Smoking*

Smoking is the greatest contributor to atherosclerotic cardiovascular disease and the number one cause of preventable deaths in the United States per year. There has been an increase in the number of smokers, despite extensive anti-smoking campaigns, and smoke-related deaths continue to rise particularly in the developing world.

A dose-related phenomenon has been described for cigarette-smoking that correlates with increased rates of coronary events, ischemic strokes, and peripheral vascular disorders. Despite this dose-effect, complete smoking cessation has been demonstrated to be the only significantly effective approach to reduce health-risks associated with smoking. Smoking cessation remains a pivotal part of cardiovascular disease prevention. However, initiatives aimed at improving public awareness of the deleterious effects of ischemic heart disease, peripheral vascular disease including amputation, and cerebrovascular events have met with limited success. As much as one-third of cardiovascular mortality can be prevented by abstinence from smoking, an effect that has not yet been realized by pharmaceutical risk-factor management. Effective holistic treatment plans exist for patients who are motivated to cease smoking such as nicotine replacement by transdermal patch or chewable gum, behavioral modification, and antidepressant therapy. However, many physicians do not routinely document smoking behavior or pursue smoking cessation at every clinical encounter, an endeavor that should form part of the standard of care for any patient who endorses an active or recent history of smoking.

6.3 *Diabetes mellitus*

Coronary artery disease is the principal cause of death in diabetic patients and rivals smoking in contribution to cardiovascular mortality. The rate of coronary and peripheral arterial disease approximately doubles in patients who carry a diagnosis of diabetes. The length of time and severity of diabetic control are strong predictors of atherosclerotic events and have been correlated with the degree of peripheral arterial disease experienced by patients. The microvascular complications of diabetes are beyond the scope of this chapter but diabetic nephropathy, heralded by microalbuminuria, exacerbates large vessel changes imposed by insulin resistance and hyperglycemia. Atherosclerosis can be shown experimentally to be induced by insulin resistance preceding the development of a clinical diagnosis of diabetes and has been diagnosed in adolescents and teenagers as part of the metabolic syndrome.

Significant improvements in the glycemic profile and reduction in diabetic complications with prolongation of life expectancy can be achieved through behavioral modification of diabetes. Level 1 data from large randomized national trials of monitored lifestyle modification demonstrates up to 30% reduction in frank diabetes with associated reduction in cardiovascular events. The addition of effective glycemic agents such as metformin, sulfonylureas, and thiazolidinediones further contribute to cardiovascular risk reduction. Current glucose targets for diabetic patients are listed in Table 2. A causal relationship has been described for long-term blood glucose control as assessed by the Hemoglobin AIc (HbA1c) in the national United Kingdom Prospective Diabetes Study (UKPDS) with an increase in the risk of adverse cardiovascular events for each percentage point above an HbA1c level of 6.2%. The UKPDS recommendations for metabolic control of diabetic patients also

Table 2.   Current target guidelines for diabetic patients.

Fasting blood glucose <110 mg/dL
Hemoglobin A1c <7%
Blood pressure <130/80 (combination HCTZ/ACE inhibitor as
    first-line therapy)
LDL <100 mg/dL (<70 mg/dL considered if established coronary
    artery disease)
Triglyceride level <150 mg/dL

Note: HCTZ = hydrochlorothiazide; ACEI = Angiotensin-converting enzyme;
LDL = low-density lipoprotein.

focus on other parameters that are known to interact deleteriously with diabetes to increase cardiovascular risk such as hypertension and hyperlipidemia. Physicians now recognize the need for aggressive management of patients with the constellation of diabetes, hypertriglyceridemia, hypertension, and obesity, some of which will fit the definition of the metabolic syndrome.

6.4 *Hypertension*

The prevalence of hypertension in the United States is estimated at one in three individuals and rising steadily. Part of the difficulty in managing hypertension is the racial disparity in prevalence, response to antihypertensive medications and associated exacerbating factors such as renal disease and diabetes. High risk groups include African-Americans, those over 60 years of age, and women. A dose phenomenon has been described for hypertension. In general, an elevation in blood pressure of 20 mm Hg systolic from a theorized normal of 120 mm Hg systolic confers a cardiovascular risk double that of the normotensive population. A working definition of hypertension is a systolic blood pressure greater than 140 mm Hg or a diastolic pressure greater than 90 mm Hg. Prehypertension can be defined further as blood pressure ranging between 120 and 139 mm Hg systolic and between 80 and 89 mm Hg diastolic. Traditional views of hypertension primarily focused on diastolic dysfunction and elevation as more significant than the systolic component; however, this perspective has been shifted with more recent data pointing to a greater risk for cardiovascular events and mortality in the face of systolic hypertension. Pulse pressure increases for a given systolic blood pressure have also received more attention as a marker of impairment of vascular receptive relaxation and predict coronary risk over normal controls. Although hypertension is an independent risk factor for the development of coronary disease, it should be noted that it is much more potent when considered alongside other commonly associated risk factors such as triglyc-eride profile, diabetes, and obesity. Almost two-thirds of patients with hypertension have at least one other risk factor for cardiovascular disease and thus treatment of hypertension should be ideally managed by using therapies that are multivariate in effect; for example, dietary modification or pharmacological agents with benefits for both triglyceride and blood pressure profile.

The 2003 Joint National Committee on Prevention, Detection, Evaluation and Treatment of High Blood Pressure (JNC-7) panel published guidelines that sum-marize management goals for the treatment of hypertension-associated risk factors. For example, hyperlipidemia may be more difficult to control when a combina-tion of diuretic and beta-blocking agents is used due to slight alterations in lipid metabolism as a side-effect of these medications. In the presence of diabetes, calcium-channel blockers, angiotensin-converting enzyme (ACE) inhibitors, and beta-blockers are recommended. Lifestyle modifications are clearly identified with the following JNC-7 guidelines: weight reduction/maintenance of BMI between 18.5 and 24.9 kg/m^2; DASH eating plan (dietary approaches to stop hypertension) consisting of a diet rich in fruits, vegetables, low-fat dairy products, low sodium (ideally less than 100 mmol or 6 gm of sodium chloride per day), reduced fat con-tent, moderate alcohol consumption with less than two drinks per day for men and one drink per day for women, and lighter weight individuals; and regular aerobic activity for at least 30 minutes most days of the week.

6.5 *Dyslipidemia*

LDL is firmly established in cardiovascular risk profiling as the major contributor to atherosclerotic disease and is found in abundance in atherosclerotic plaque. Higher serum levels of LDL correlate to a higher risk of cardiovascular disease; data borne out of clinical studies indicate LDL as the main risk factor for coronary disease. The post-coronary artery bypass graft (Post-CABG) trial examined this relationship further and attempted to define a threshold target level for LDL. The results supported a true risk reduction with intensive LDL treatment to a level lower than 100 mg/dl as evidenced by a favorable change in atherosclerotic plaque morphology (see Table 2).

Although LDL has been identified as a target for cardiovascular risk reduction, there are other lipid and lipoprotein abnormalities that have been recognized in con-tributing to the overall risk of atherosclerotic disease. Elevated levels of very low density lipoprotein (VLDL), apolipoprotein B, and decreased high density lipopro-tein (HDL) are adverse markers for cardiovascular risk. Clinical evidence for the involvement of these lipoproteins is found in the acceleration of atherosclerotic build-up seen in patients suffering from inherited forms of dyslipidemia such as familial hypercholesterolemia.

First-line therapies for reducing cholesterol, LDL, and VLDL and increasing HDL involve behavioral modification in the form of dietary changes. Animal fat including meats and egg yolk are significant sources of cholesterol and goal strategies focus on reduction of cholesterol-rich products by at least 50%. Simply reducing body weight toward goal body mass index will produce significant reductions in LDL levels and reduce the overall cardiovascular risk profile.

The main pharmacological modality employed to impair cholesterol metabolism is the hydroxymethylglutarate coenzyme A reductase inhibitors (HMG-CoA reductase inhibitors or "statin" medications). The mechanism of statin action occurs at the hepatocellular level to inhibit cholesterol synthesis in the liver. Statins are powerfully effective in reducing total body LDL levels (from 30% to 60% depending on dosage). Not surprisingly, these medications have become first-line drug therapy for patients with elevated lipid profiles in the absence of drug contraindications. Myopathy, heralded by a rise in creatine kinase, and transient elevation of hepatic aminotransferases are the most commonly quoted side-effects of statin use. These derangements usually resolve with discontinuation of the medication.

Four other medications deserve brief mention. Ezetimibe is a cholesterol transport inhibitor that acts primarily on the small intestine to reduce cholesterol absorption. Ezetimibe is most effective when combined with statin medications and has been shown to have a synergistic effect on lipid reduction in this setting. Niacin (nicotinic acid) has been demonstrated to be beneficial both in reducing VLDL and LDL and in increasing levels of HDL. Flushing, diarrhea, and a mild diabetogenic effect are all recognized side-effects of niacin use and form the majority of reasons for discontinuation of the medication. Fibric acid derivatives such as Gemfibrozil and Fenofibrate have limited applicability in the primary risk reduction strategy for dyslipidemia as their effect on LDL levels are marginal, however, are of marked benefit in patients with pancreatitis associated with hypertriglyceridemia due to their selective reduction in triglycerides. Bile acid sequestrants are weak cholesterol and LDL lowering medications and act by interrupting the enterohepatic recirculation of bile acids *via* inhibition of small intestinal bile acid reabsorption.

6.6 *Metabolic syndrome*

Over the past half-century, a constellation of metabolic derangements have been seen more frequently occurring in association. Hypertension, diabetes mellitus, obesity, and dyslipidemia are the four entities most commonly described as part of the metabolic syndrome or colloquially known as Syndrome X. According to the definition drawn up by the 2001 Adult Treatment Panel-III of the National Cholesterol Education Program, metabolic syndrome is diagnosed when three of the following criteria are present.

1. Central obesity (waist circumference >102 cm (M), >88 cm (F)).
2. Fasting plasma glucose >6.1 mmol/L.
3. Hypertension ≥135/85 mmHg or the presence of antihypertensive medications.
4. Dyslipidemia including triglycerides ≥1.7 mmol/L, HDL cholesterol < 1.0 mmol/L (M), <1.3 mmol/L (F).

The metabolic syndrome for many of the reasons highlighted earlier in the chapter is strongly associated with the development of cardiovascular disease portending an approximately 2.5 times risk of fatal cardiovascular events in the population. The single most effective treatment for the metabolic syndrome is loss of body weight either by nonsurgical or surgical means, which in almost all cases of dramatic weight loss leads to amelioration of all individual components.

6.7 *Emerging novel risk factors*

Although the above well-established risk factors have been strongly linked to the development of cardiovascular disease, there remains a significant proportion of the atherosclerotic population that does not possess these described risk factors. Searches for other contributing factors have focused on molecular biomarkers as diverse as homocysteine levels, high-sensitivity CRP (hs-CRP), fibrin-degradation products (FDP), and microalbuminuria.

Elevated plasma homocysteine levels have been cited as a defined risk factor for the development of atherosclerotic coronary arterial disease in epidemiological as well as clinical research studies. On a molecular basis, high levels of homocysteine have been demonstrated to occur with disruption of normal methionine metabolism. Homocysteine and related metabolites can be detected in abnormally high levels in the blood and have been linked to an increased risk of stroke, due to carotid plaque buildup, as well as cardiovascular disease. Endothelial damage in association with an alteration of the normal coagulation balance has led to the hypothesis that elevated homocysteine levels directly influence atherogenesis in large vessels. Therapeutic options for individuals diagnosed with homocysteinemia have centered on replacement of vitamin B12 and folic acid as a primary treatment with additional restriction of dietary intake of methionine in vitamin B12-insensitive patients. However, studies have not as of yet shown that lowering homocysteine levels decreases the risk of cardiovascular disease in these patients.

Inflammatory markers such as hs-CRP and FDP have been deemed cardiovascular disease risk-associated and, although originally thought to play a role as potential serum biomarkers of cardiovascular disease, have only been weakly associated with risk stratification and burden of atherosclerotic disease. The relative lack of specificity of these markers dilutes their clinical effect, as many unassociated noncardiovascular conditions can cause elevations of either marker. The clinical applicability of these markers has, therefore, been limited and their use in the setting of cardiovascular risk reduction is yet to be elucidated.

High-sensitivity CRP (hs-CRP) has recently been the subject of much attention with the results of the JUPITER trial — a large multinational and double-blind placebo-controlled trial of more than 17,000 people. The trial was designed to observe the effect that treatment with a statin (rosuvastatin) had upon individuals with normal lipid profiles but elevated hs-CRP levels. The study arose from the observation that statins have an anti-inflammatory property and decrease hs-CRP levels in an effect that is independent from their cholesterol-lowering ability. The JUPITER trial demonstrated a reduction in both LDL and hs-CRP levels to around half of pretreatment and was terminated prematurely based on this beneficial result. However, the benefit of a normal hs-CRP has not yet been firmly established as a treatment goal in cardiovascular risk profiling and is additionally confounded by the possible benefit of statin therapy in the face of normal lipid profile in certain populations. Nevertheless, hs-CRP remains an active and controversial area of cardiovascular risk-modification research and its clinical role yet to be formally determined.

Microalbuminuria is a sensitive predictor of mortality and highly associated with cardiovascular adverse events in specific. Diabetic and hypertensive nephropathy can be diagnosed reliably by evidence of proteinuria, which is also associated with an increase in cardiovascular risk profile. Microalbuminuria is similarly associated with an elevated risk of coronary disease, independent of proteinuria, and thus may have clinical utility in patients who do not carry a diagnosis of hypertension or diabetes as a screening tool for atherosclerotic disease. Treatment strategies based upon the detection of microalbuminuria are, therefore, likely to take the form of existing risk-reduction strategies for well-established cardiovascular risk factors.

6.8 *Surveillance and secondary prevention*

Given the focus on prevention of atherosclerotic disease, increased surveillance for the development of signs of atherosclerotic disease in those with established risk factors should be included in the routine health-care maintenance and follow-up of patients. Regular carotid duplex evaluation for older patients with one or more risk factors for atherosclerosis in addition to at least annual physical examinations is a relatively inexpensive and highly effective screening tool for carotid disease. Similarly, screening aortic ultrasonography, physical examination, and ankle-brachial pressure indices should be considered for at-risk patients in the primary care setting. Electrocardiography and two-dimensional and stress echocardiography are procedures that are best used as diagnostic rather than screening tools; however, their utility is as a prediction tool for those at the highest risk of cardiovascular disease and may act as the gateway to more invasive diagnostic and treatment options such as angiographic interventions or cardiac surgery.

For those patients who progress to severe or acute cardiovascular disease, secondary prevention guidelines are well documented and rigorously studied. Many cardiovascular centers have established protocols for treating patients with established disease. One such example is the University of California, Los Angeles CHAMP (Cardiovascular Hospitalization Atherosclerosis Management Program), which focuses on employing secondary prevention measures while patients are in the hospital in order to improve clinical outcomes. This program arose through the observation that although evidence-based guidelines for secondary risk prevention are widely disseminated, they are consistently underutilized. The CHAMP guidelines are summarized as follows.

1. Aspirin 81–162 mg daily should be initiated. In the presence of contraindications to aspirin, other platelet agents should be considered, for example, Clopidogrel. Combination therapy can be recommended in the setting of acute coronary syndromes (ACS) or post-revascularization therapy.
2. Statin therapy should be initiated in all patients in the absence of contraindications and in all diabetic patients regardless of their lipid profile. Target levels of LDL should be <70 mg/dL, HDL >40 mg/dL, and triglycerides <150 mg/dL.
3. Angiotensin-converting enzyme (ACE) inhibitors or angiotensin-receptor blockers (ARB) should be commenced in the absence of contraindication irrespective of the blood pressure or cardiac ejection fraction.
4. Beta blockade should be prescribed for all patients in the absence of contraindication.
5. Fish oil or omega-3 fatty acids should be commenced with dietary instruction for all patients.
6. Aerobic exercise programs that involve 30–60 minutes of moderately intense exercise at least five times a week should be prescribed.
7. Smoking cessation should be pursued including access to formal smoking cessation programs.
8. Before hospital discharge and at six week follow-up, cardiovascular lipid profile and liver enzymes should be checked and routinely thereafter at future follow-up appointments.

7. Conclusions

As the population ages and becomes more obese, there will be a rise in the number of patients with cardiovascular disease. Aggressive risk-factor modification can only occur if there is vigilance and attention to the detection and subsequent treatment of such conditions as diabetes, obesity, dyslipidemia, smoking, and renal disease. Although there are many effective strategies for risk reduction, once these conditions have been diagnosed, there is a growing body of epidemiological evidence that points toward greater health outcomes when the predisposing factors for these diseases are addressed early, prior to full blown disease diagnosis.

Preventing individuals from becoming smokers rather than focusing on smoking cessation and educating individuals about diet and exercise strategies to prevent obesity and modulation of cholesterol intake to reduce hyperlipidemia are all paradigms for reducing the exposure of the population to cardiovascular risk factors. Unfortunately, patients have not embraced these preventative strategies and public health measures have not been successful in a cost-effective and widespread manner at the present time.

Cardiovascular disease continues to be the most significant cause of mortality in the United States and similarly developed countries. The detection of modifiable risk factors for atherosclerosis continues to remain one of the most promising areas of research in the field of cardiovascular medicine. Despite advances in pharmacological treatment of identified risk factors, however, behavioral modification strategies that are effective are limited. Attitude toward health and cultivation of risk-factor avoidance has been difficult to implement; however, these attributes are most likely to reduce the burden of cardiovascular disease most significantly. These core health traits must be adopted by individuals themselves and supported by education and demonstration of identifiable health benefit before prevention of cardiovascular disease can be entertained at a population level.

References

Abdel-Maksoud MF, Hokanson JE. The complex role of triglycerides in cardiovascular disease, *Semin Vasc Med* 2002; **2**:325.

Ameli FM, Stein M, Prosser RJ, *et al.* Effects of cigarette smoking on outcome of femoral popliteal bypass for limb salvage, *J Cardiovasc Surg (Torino)* 1989; **30**(4):591–596.

Bajpai A, Goyal A, Sperling L. Should we measure C-reactive protein on earth or just on JUPITER? *Clin Cardiol* 2010; **33**(4):190–198.

Balakumar P, Kaur J. Is nicotine a key player or spectator in the induction and progression of cardiovascular disorders? *Pharmacol Res* 2009; **60**(5):361–368.

Cannon CP, Braunwald E, McCabe CH, *et al.* Intensive versus moderate lipid lowering with statins after acute coronary syndromes, *N Engl J Med* 2004; **350**:1495.

Chiuve SE, McCullough ML, Sacks FM, *et al.* Healthy life style factors in the primary prevention of coronary heart disease among men: Benefits among users and nonusers of lipid-lowering and antihypertensive medications, *Circulation* 2006; **114**:160.

Chobanian AV, Bakris GL, Black HR, *et al.* The Seventh Report of the Joint National Committee on Prevention, Detection, Evaluation, and Treatment of High Blood Pressure: The JNC 7 Report, *JAMA* 2003; **289**:2560.

Cook NR, Buring JE, Ridker PM. The effect of including C-reactive protein in cardiovascular risk prediction models for women, *Ann Intern Med* 2006; **145**:21.

Danesh J, Wheeler JG, Hirschfield GM, *et al.* C-reactive protein and other circulating markers of inflammation in the prediction of coronary heart disease, *N Engl J Med* 2004; **350**:1387.

DePalma RG. Atherosclerosis: pathology, pathogenesis, and medical management. In: Moore WS (Ed.), *Vascular and Endovascular Surgery*, 7th Edition, Philadelphia, 2006, pp. 93–94.

Eckel RH, Grundy SM, Zimmet PZ. The metabolic syndrome, *Lancet* 2005; **365**:1415.

Garrison RJ, Kannel WB, Feinleib M, *et al.* Cigarette smoking and HDL cholesterol: The Framingham offspring study, *Atherosclerosis* 1978; **30**(1):17–25.

Glagov S, Weisenberg E, Zarins CK, *et al.* Compensatory enlargement of human atherosclerotic coronary arteries, *N Engl J Med* 1987; **316**(22):1371–1375.

Glagov S, Zarins CK, Masawa N, *et al.* Mechanical functional role of non-atherosclerotic intimal thickening, *Front Med Biol Eng* 1993; **5**(1):37–43.

Hobeika MJ, Thompson RW, Muhs BE, *et al.* Matrix metalloproteinases in peripheral vascular disease, *J Vasc Surg* 2007; **45**(4):849–857.

Julius S, Nesbitt SD, Egan BM, *et al.* Feasibility of treating prehypertension with an angiotensin-receptor blocker, *N Engl J Med* 2006; **354**:1685.

Kannel WB, McGee DL. Diabetes and glucose tolerance as risk factors for cardiovascular disease. The Framingham Study, *Diabetes Care* 1979; **2**:120.

Khot UN, Khot MB, Bajzer CT, *et al.* Prevalence of conventional risk factors in patients with coronary heart disease, *JAMA* 2003; **290**:898–904.

LaRosa JC. Cholesterol lowering, low cholesterol, and mortality, *Am J Cardiol* 1993; **72**(11):776–786.

Lloyd-Jones DM, Wilson PWF, Larson MG, *et al.* Lifetime risk for coronary heart disease by cholesterol levels at selected ages, *Arch Intern Med* 2003; **163**:1966–1972.

Malek AM, Alper SL, Izumo S. Hemodynamic shear stress and its role in atherosclerosis, *JAMA* 1999; **282**(21):2035–2042.

Navas-Nacher EL, Colangelo L, Beam C, Greenland P. Risk factors for coronary heart disease in men 18 to 39 years of age, *Ann Intern Med* 2001; **134**:433–439.

Nicholls SC, Phillips DJ, Primozich JF, *et al.* Diagnostic significance of flow separation in the carotid bulb, *Stroke* 1989; **20**(2):175–182.

Nissen SE, Tuzcu EM, Schoenhagen P, *et al.* Statin therapy, LDL cholesterol, C-reactive protein, and coronary artery disease, *N Engl J Med* 2005; **352**:29.

Ogden CL, Carroll MD, Curtin LR, *et al.* Prevalence of overweight and obesity in the United States, 1999–2004, *JAMA* 2006; **295**:1549.

Pussinen PJ, Jousilahti P, Alfthan G, *et al.* Antibodies to periodontal pathogens are associated with coronary heart disease, *Arterioscler Thromb Vasc Biol* 2003; **23**(7):1250–1254.

Ross R. Atherosclerosis — An inflammatory disease, *N Engl J Med* 1999; **340**(2):115–126.

Stampfer MJ, Malinow MR, Willett WC, *et al.* A prospective study of plasma homocyst(e)ine and risk of myocardial infarction in US physicians, *JAMA* 1992; **268**:877–881.

Stary HC, Chandler AB, Glagov S, *et al.* A definition of initial, fatty streak, and intermediate lesions of atherosclerosis. A report from the Committee on Vascular Lesions of the Council on Arteriosclerosis, American Heart Association, *Arterioscler Thromb* 1994; **14**(5):840–856.

Third Report of the National Cholesterol Education Program (NCEP) Expert Panel on Detection, Evaluation, and Treatment of High Blood Cholesterol in Adults (Adult Treatment Panel III) Final Report, *Circulation* 2002; **106**:3143–3421.

Third Report of the National Cholesterol Education Program (NCEP) Expert Panel on Detection, Evaluation, and Treatment of High Blood Cholesterol in Adults (Adult Treatment Panel III) Final Report, *Circulation* 2002; **106**:3143–3421.

UCLA CHAMP, http://www.med.ucla.edu/champ/default.htm (accessed on April 13, 2010).

Wolf-Maier K, Cooper RS, Banegas JR, *et al.* Hypertension prevalence and blood pressure levels in 6 European countries, Canada, and the United States, *JAMA* 2003; **289**:2363.

World Health Organization. Definition, Diagnosis and Classification of Diabetes Mellitus and its Complications. Part 1: Diagnosis and Classification of Diabetes Mellitus. Report of a WHO Consultation. Geneva: World Health Organization, 1999.

Chapter 2

Physical Examination and Noninvasive Diagnosis of the Patient with Vascular Disease

J. Dennis Baker

Learning Objectives

- Learn to identify the associated signs and presenting symptoms of patients with vascular disease. Understand the common presentation of these disorders with respect to each anatomic region.
- Learn the specific techniques described in this chapter for the vascular physical examination with respect to each anatomic region.
- Understand the principles and the application of the noninvasive imaging techniques described in this chapter with respect to each anatomic region and disease process. Learn the benefits and limitations of the individual modalities described.

1. General Principles

1.1 *History*

The workup of a patient for vascular disease requires careful attention to both the history and the physical examination; subsequent tests that are ordered simply refine the initial impression. Many common vascular problems result from gradually evolving pathology so it is important to trace back any symptom to its initial onset and to follow its evolution over time. Onset may be insidious or acute. Patients may have trouble remembering when the problem first presented, but acute conditions have a clearly defined onset, usually well remembered. The specific answers to these questions often help to focus the differential diagnosis.

The risk factors for the specific patient are also an important part of the assessment. Both the prior medical history and family history need to be covered. Tobacco consumption (past and current), hypertension, hyperlipidemia, coronary artery disease, and diabetes must be reviewed in all patients with peripheral arterial disease.

1.2 Physical examination

1.2.1 Pulse palpation

Pulse palpation is a key part of the examination of patients with arterial disease. The examiner should always be in a relaxed position and should not stretch over the patient or attempt palpation through clothing. Different schemes have been proposed for describing the quality of pulses, but the most practical is to determine whether a pulse is normal, decreased, or absent. On occasion, the pulse may be more prominent (either more forceful or wider) than normal, due usually to aneurysmal dilation of the vessel. Decreased pulses often present a challenge, for sometimes what is palpated is the examiner's finger pulse. Whenever a weak pulse is palpated, the examiner should palpate his own radial or carotid pulse with the other hand to make sure that what is being detected is indeed the patient's pulse.

1.2.2 Auscultation for bruit

Bruits can be produced in the arterial system by conditions of turbulent flow. The most common is the disturbance produced by the high-velocity jet of blood going through a tight stenosis. The sound will be loudest just beyond the stenosis but can be transmitted down the vessel for many centimeters. Anytime a bruit is detected, the stethoscope should be moved up and down along the course of the underlying vessel in order to detect the site of the most prominent finding. The frequency and the duration of the bruit help give a qualitative indication of the severity of the stenosis. The higher the pitch and the longer the duration, the tighter is the narrowing. Other conditions producing high velocity or disturbed flow can also produce bruits. The high flow of an arteriovenous fistula can produce a systolic bruit, but in this case the sound may be transmitted up the vein. If the flow is sufficiently high, a palpable thrill is found. Occasionally an abdominal aortic aneurysm will have sufficient turbulence within the sac to produce a soft systolic bruit.

1.2.3 Documentation of inspection

Most patients with vascular disease have chronic conditions that will be followed for long periods. Many of the findings undergo slow or gradual improvement or deterioration. Whenever possible, general qualitative description should be avoided in favor of quantification. When an ulcer is found, it is not adequate to state that it is present; a measurement of long and short axis provides objective data for comparison of future examination. With venous insufficiency, severity of edema is a relevant parameter. Pitting edema should be noted. Measurement of limb circumference, usually at the calf and ankle, provides an objective baseline for follow-up.

2. Extracranial Cerebrovascular Disease

2.1 *History*

Patients with extracranial occlusive disease often present with intermittent symptoms known as transient ischemic attacks (TIA). Classically, a TIA is defined as a temporary neurologic deficit lasting less than 24 hours, but most of these episodes last a few minutes — rarely over an hour. Symptoms can include hemiparesis, hemiparesthesia, monocular vision changes, and altered speech. Documentation of frequency, duration, and specific distribution of symptoms should be performed. Amaurosis fugax (temporary blindness) of carotid disease may present with "graying out" of the entire vision in one eye, but more frequently involves just a portion of the visual field. Simultaneous bilateral symptoms indicate posterior circulation abnormalities. Patients with strokes have fixed deficits, although these may improve gradually with time. The history should include the severity of symptoms and the extent of recovery.

2.2 *Examination*

Palpation of arterial pulses in the neck requires special attention. Examination should be started low in the neck and each carotid artery followed up to the mandible. It is important that only gentle pressure be applied over the carotid artery, especially higher in the neck, adjacent to the carotid bifurcation. Excessive pressure on the bifurcation can cause hypotension and bradycardia, especially in people with abnormal carotid sinus sensitivity. In rare cases of extreme sensitivity, it is possible to induce cardiac arrest. Never palpate both sides simultaneously! One cannot determine the condition of the internal and external carotid branches by palpation, since it is not possible to palpate each branch separately. The presence of a normal carotid pulse simply indicates that at least one of the branches is open so as to maintain the patency of the common carotid artery. Temporal artery pulses are also part of the examination. Absence of this pulse can indicate severe stenosis or occlusion of the external carotid artery. Widening of the pulse in the mid neck suggests aneurysm formation at this level; however, carotid aneurysms are extremely rare. Palpation is completed by feeling the subclavian arteries. In geriatric patients, it is not uncommon to get the impression that the subclavian artery is bulging above the clavicle. This finding is most often associated with elongation and tortuosity of the vessel rather than development of an aneurysm.

Auscultation for arterial bruits should start at the heart and follow the carotids to the mandible. The examination is also carried out along the course of the axillo-subclavian system. When a bruit is detected, one needs to determine the point of the greatest intensity and to characterize the sound at this point. Both the pitch and the duration are indicators of the severity of the stenosis. However, a tight stenosis can exist without any detectable bruit. The most common scenario is where the lesion reduces the flow to such an extent that there is too low velocity to create sufficient turbulence to be heard. It is important to appreciate the extent to which vascular turbulence can be transmitted. It is common to hear a murmur originating from the aortic valve at the level of the carotid bifurcations. A tip-off that this is the case is the fact that the bruit will sound alike on both sides. Likewise, it is possible for innominate artery stenosis to produce a bruit heard high in the right neck. Side-to-side transmission is occasionally found, with a severe carotid stenosis producing a prominent bruit on the ipsilateral side and a softer bruit with similar pitch and duration on the contralateral side.

2.3 *Vascular laboratory*

The primary noninvasive test for carotid bifurcation disease is the duplex scan (see appendix). The examination is carried out from the low neck to the jaw and in most patients can provide satisfactory assessment of the carotid bifurcation together with the proximal portions of the internal and external carotid branches. Atherosclerotic plaque in the vessel shows up on the imaging modality. If significant stenosis is present, its effect is assessed by the alterations in flow pattern (increased velocity at the point of narrowing and turbulence beyond). Arterial occlusion is verified by a lack of flow signal in the involved segment. Diagnostic criteria are used to categorize the severity of stenosis, usually reported as the percent reduction of the lumen diameter compared with the normal portion of the internal carotid branch. The specific stenosis ranges for each category may differ by laboratory. Other arterial pathologies such as fibromuscular dysplasia or dissection can be determined from the imaging. A limitation of the duplex scan is that lesions in the distal-most portion of the internal carotid artery cannot be examined.

A carotid ultrasound scan is an essential part of the evaluation of patients for cerebrovascular problems. Because of its noninvasive nature, the test is well-suited for follow-up examinations and for screening of subjects at high risk for atherosclerotic disease. Most vascular surgeons obtain postoperative studies to look for recurrence at the operated site and to monitor for possible progression of disease on the non-operated side.

3. Arterial — Abdomen

3.1 *History*

Many patients with abdominal arterial problems are asymptomatic, with the condition detected during the workup for some other problem. There is a definite familial association with aortic aneurysm disease, so older patients should be queried about a family history of this condition. One type of abdominal arterial disease that is clearly symptomatic is mesenteric ischemia (intestinal angina). The condition requires severe stenosis or occlusion of the celiac and superior mesenteric artery branches. The classical history involves no pain when fasting, with severe mid-abdominal pain coming 30–45 minutes after a meal. The patient tries to adjust to the pain by eating smaller meals, with resulting weight loss.

3.2 *Physical examination*

The examination starts with routine palpation of the abdomen, with special attention to the aortic pulse. The most important objective is to determine the possible presence of an aortic aneurysm. (In patients with even moderate obesity it may not be possible to locate a pulse unless a large aneurysm is present.) If a pulse appears to be widened, examine with both hands and try to determine whether there is a lateral pulsation or whether the motion is only in the anterior–posterior direction. This latter can occur when a solid mass overlying the aorta transmits the pulse of the aorta. Examination of the aorta requires deep palpation, and many patients will have some tenderness. In the presence of an aneurysm, moderate tenderness should be noted but does not reflect an acute problem.

A vascular bruit in the abdomen is usually not specific as to the source, but auscultation should always be done. Bruits can originate in stenotic renal, mesenteric, or iliac arteries. Some aortic aneurysms may produce soft systolic bruits as a result of turbulent vortices in the sac. Many aneurysms do not produce bruits, even with large diameters, because laminated thrombus narrows the residual flow lumen so it is near normal diameter and little turbulence results.

3.3 *Vascular laboratory*

The duplex scan is the primary tool to study abdominal pathology. Imaging is used to search for aortic aneurysms, documenting the location and size. Visceral artery aneurysms can sometimes be documented, but these are a challenge due to the relatively small size and variable location of the aneurysm. Detection of abnormal flow signals in the aorta and its branches permits detection of significant stenosis. With atherosclerosis, the majority of the plaques are at the origins of the vessels off the aorta, making it easy to find the pathology. Bypass grafts in the abdomen can be examined to determine deterioration or malfunction. The combination of imaging and velocity studies can often document aortic dissection.

The abdomen provides a special challenge to obtaining satisfactory duplex scan because gas is a strong absorber of ultrasound energy, blocking penetration. Elective tests should be scheduled after overnight fasting to minimize bowel gas. This protocol is usually enough to obtain adequate studies for most patients. Emergency studies, where there is no overnight fast or where the patient may have an ileus, are often technically inadequate.

4. Arterial — Legs

4.1 *History*

Most patients with arterial problems in the legs present with complaints of pain. When dealing with pain as a symptom, there are five questions which should always be covered. (1) Where is the pain? (2) How is the pain characterized? (3) What brings on the pain or makes it worse? (4) What makes it better? (5) How has the pain pattern evolved over time? The specific answers help to focus on etiology. Arterial insufficiency in the legs typically presents with intermittent claudication (pain or cramping in the calf and occasionally thigh). Onset may have been gradual, almost unrecognized by the patients, but with progression the pattern becomes well-established. It is not uncommon for symptoms to progress for a period and then plateau. To determine the level of disability, patients should be asked how far they can push themselves when walking at a normal pace (maximum claudication distance). Many patients with arterial insufficiency also have long-standing diabetes, so it is important to question about neuropathy.

4.2 *Physical examination*

The majority of patients evaluated for peripheral arterial disease have a chronic condition, and the appearance of the legs gives information about the duration and severity. On the mild end of the spectrum, the patient only has complaints with walking (intermittent claudication), but the appearance of the legs is normal. With more severe flow limitation, a point is reached where there is decreased flow at rest leading to gradual atrophy of skin and skin appendages. Skin becomes thin and dry (loss of sweat glands) together with loss of hair and slow, irregular toenail growth that produces distorted nails. With very severe disease, there are chronic foot ulcers that are very painful and have little granulation. Changes in skin color can also provide an index of severity of vascular insufficiency. When examining the patient in the supine position, there is often no skin color abnormality in the feet, but abnormalities will appear with provocative maneuvers. In the patient with severe disease, elevating the legs to 45° will result in a blanching of the affected foot. When the legs are put in the dependent position, the abnormal foot rapidly turns red in a hyperemic response. This change is produced by the abnormal vasodilation caused by chronic hypoxemia. This finding is commonly referred to as "dependent rubor." An additional sign of severe disease is unilateral edema. In the presence of severe rest pain, the patient will keep the leg in the dependent position, even to the extent of sleeping with the leg hanging over the side of the bed.

Pulse palpation is the most important part of the lower extremity examination. Pulses should be evaluated at the common femoral, popliteal, dorsalis pedis, and posterior tibial arteries. Evaluation of the femoral pulse in obese patients provides a challenge, and one may not be able to tell whether a weak pulse is due to arterial disease or due to difficulty in examination. In most patients, the popliteal pulse is the most difficult to assess. This part of examination is best carried out with the knee in partial flexion and the leg completely relaxed. Palpation below the knee joint level is preferable, for the artery is not as deep and is more easily trapped against the bone than in the above knee position. With experience, one can make an accurate assessment of arterial stenoses. It is important to note abnormal widening of the pulse at the femoral or popliteal levels, for aneurysms can develop at these sites. Palpation of skin temperature along the full length of the leg is done to seek the presence of a temperature gradient. Bruits are sought at the femoral level but not lower, for these arteries are smaller and rarely produce sufficient turbulence to be heard.

4.3 *Vascular laboratory*

The most common test for arterial disease of the legs is the ankle-arm index (AAI). A normal extremity has a ratio of above 0.95 and may go as high as 1.4. Values down to 0.6 are typical of patients with moderate claudication, usually resulting from single-level occlusive disease. Values below 0.6 are usually associated with severe claudication, rest pain, or signs of limb threat. If pressure at the ankle is abnormal, additional information can be obtained by segmental testing at different levels of the leg. This expanded examination helps to confirm location(s) of significant pathology. In order to avoid problems with the artifact resulting from arterial wall stiffness, the pressure test is usually combined with either Doppler waveform recordings or pulse volume recording (see appendix). There is some day-to-day variation in the value for pressure index; a change in ratio of 0.15 is required for the change to be considered significant. These simple physiologic tests are useful not only for initial assessment but also for follow-up examinations, especially after an intervention.

Some patients with early occlusive disease may have typical symptoms of inter-mittent claudication but have normal pressure tests at rest. A more complete assess-ment can be obtained with an exercise test that will show an abnormal response after walking (see appendix). People with a normal response have no significant arterial occlusive disease. Exercise testing is not needed routinely but should be reserved for those patients who have (a) symptoms consistent with arterial insufficiency in the presence of a normal resting test or (b) atypical symptoms for which occlusive arterial disease is to be excluded.

A duplex ultrasound scan provides more detailed information about the anatomy of the occlusive disease. Such a test is not needed for routine initial evaluation but can be useful to formulate treatment options. The scan can show, in detail, specific sites of stenosis or occlusion. Scanning is also very helpful in identifying postoperative changes of deterioration in a bypass or stent that may lead to subsequent occlusion. It is the usual practice to carry out repeated scans of vein bypass grafts in the leg to detect the development of graft stenosis since this problem can occur in the absence of new symptoms.

5. Arterial — Arms

5.1 *History and physical examination*

Most upper extremity arterial problems present as arm claudication or hand ischemia. Patients may complain of increased pain and cramping in the affected arm when everyday activities are performed (lifting objects, brushing or drying hair, *etc.*). In the case of claudication, there may be no changes to be seen on examination; however, one must look for evidence of decreased muscle bulk or atrophy as an indicator of the extent of the occlusive disease. With hand ischemia problems, careful documentation of skin temperature, color, and the presence of skin breakdown is important.

Arterial pulse palpation includes examination at the axillary (or high brachial), brachial just above the elbow, radial, and ulnar sites. Although the ulnar artery is usually the dominant vessel in the forearm, this pulse is often harder to find than the radial due to its deeper position. In situations where alteration of the radial artery flow is anticipated, the Allen's test evaluates the integrity of the palmar arch. With the hand closed tightly, the radial and ulnar arteries are compressed at the wrist. The hand is then opened, leaving it in a relaxed position. Pressure is released for one of the arteries while observing for return of color to the palm. The second artery is then released. The maneuver is then repeated with initial release of the other artery. With normal palm arch circulation, the whole hand should fill from each artery. With an incomplete arch, only a portion of the palm fills from the first artery with filling of the remainder on release of the second artery. Another abnormal pattern is for one artery to fill the entire palm with little or no filling from the opposite side. This pattern indicates a significant inflow abnormality on the abnormal side. A pitfall in performing this test can occur if the patient hyperextends the hand, for there is overall delay in palmar filling. Measurement of brachial artery pressure in both arms is essential. One must never rely on the presence of a brachial pulse to exclude significant subclavian artery disease; it is possible to have a palpable pulse distal to a tight stenosis or occlusion.

5.2 *Noninvasive laboratory*

Measurement of Doppler pressures and recording waveforms in the upper and lower arm provides a good initial screen for occlusive disease. Any change between the upper and lower arm is abnormal and indicates significant disease between the sampling sites. Since occlusive disease in the arms is not usually bilateral, side-to-side comparisons can also be helpful. When disease below the wrist is suspected, Doppler velocity or pulse volume recordings can be made at the digital level. This test can provide objective documentation in patients with small vessel emboli or vasculitis.

Accurate visualization of arm arteries can be obtained with duplex scanning. The specific anatomy of occlusive disease can be mapped. The scan can be particularly helpful in identifying plaque and calcification in the distal arteries of diabetics. This can be an important determination about the suitability of a radial artery to create a dialysis fistula or as a conduit for coronary artery bypass grafting.

6. Venous

6.1 *History*

All patients being evaluated for venous disease should be queried about family history of similar conditions. In thrombotic disease, similar problem in relatives points to possible coagulation disorder. Patients with acute deep venous thrombosis frequently exhibit a rapid onset of extremity pain and/or swelling. Erythema and development of new venous varicosities may also occur. When dealing with either acute or chronic symptoms, a history of major trauma, leg surgery, or periods of immobilization all point to possible etiologies of thrombosis. Varicose vein disease has a strong familial association. Common symptoms associated with lower extremity venous insufficiency include: extremity pain or aching, burning, itching, and swelling. Patients should be asked about the presence of prior or active lower extremity ulceration.

6.2 *Physical examination*

Most commonly, venous disease affects the lower extremity. With acute deep venous thrombosis, the primary findings involve pain/tenderness and leg swelling. Palpation along the course of the deep veins of the leg reveals tenderness in the region of the acute thrombus. Testing for Homan's sign (the eliciting of posterior calf tenderness with passive dorsiflexion at the ankle) is often used; however, this clinical test has a low accuracy. The degree of swelling helps to define the extent of the process. In general, the swelling is below the level of thrombosis. In some cases of calf thrombosis swelling may not be pronounced. Whenever there is a question of venous disease, it is best to measure calf circumference in both the legs to document the actual size.

With isolated superficial vein thrombosis, there is often little or no swelling of the leg itself. There is swelling, tenderness, and erythema adjacent to the thrombosed segment. It is helpful to document the specific location and length of the involved vein. When there is thrombosis of the great saphenous vein in the thigh, document the distance between the top of the thrombus and the sapheno-femoral junction.

In the patient with chronic venous disease, there is no concern about active thrombosis and the emphasis changes to evaluation of reflux. Evaluation of swelling is still a key component, but the focus changes to documentation of skin changes. Skin thickening is firm and does not having the pitting characteristic of edema. The extent of brown pigmentation reflects the extent and duration of the underlying venous hypertension. Presence of active ulcers or scarring from healed lesions is documented.

Varicose veins can exist independent of thrombotic disease. A varicose vein consists of a section of superficial vein which is enlarged usually both in diameter and in length so that it presents with tortuous folds. Most frequently, these occur along the course of the great saphenous vein, but are usually branches of rather than on the saphenous itself. The varicosity may have some degree of tenderness and occasionally has surrounding erythema. This feature should be documented as a part of examination. Often the location of multiple lesions is most easily recorded on a diagram of the legs. The severity of varicose vein disease is aggravated in the presence of reflux, which increases the pressure in this venous system. The Trendelenburg test can be used to demonstrate reflux. Starting with the patient in supine position, the leg is elevated to empty the superficial veins and a rubber tourniquet is applied to the thigh. The patient stands up and the filling of the venous system below the tourniquet is observed. Normally, about 30 seconds are required for filling of the veins below the tourniquet. Faster filling indicates that reflux from the deep system is speeding the filling process. The examination is repeated with removal of the tourniquet as soon as the patient is standing. Immediate filling of the superficial veins indicates reflux down the great saphenous vein. Further information can be obtained by repeating the test with tourniquet placement at different levels to determine the site of the incompetent perforator contributing to reflux.

6.3 *Vascular laboratory*

The duplex scan is considered the primary diagnostic tool for deep-vein thrombosis. Both the imaging and the flow mapping show exactly where the thrombi are located, even when these do not occlude the lumen. In patients with chronic disease, the ultrasound study is used to document reflux in both the superficial and deep systems to develop an appropriate management plan.

7. Appendix — Noninvasive Vascular Laboratory

7.1 *CW Doppler*

The continuous-wave (CW) Doppler velocity detector is a simple, inexpensive, portable tool to evaluate vascular disease. A high-frequency signal (2–10 MHz) is emitted into tissues from a pencil probe. The ultrasound is reflected off tissues and off blood in vessels. Reflections from stationary tissues are received by the detector at the same frequency as transmitted, while those from moving interfaces, such as blood, have a shift in frequency proportional to the velocity of flow. When flow is toward the probe, the frequency is increased and when away, it is decreased (Doppler principle). In simple clinical devices, the Doppler-shifted signal is converted into an audio signal for interpretation by the examiner: the higher the pitch of the output, the higher the velocity through the vessel examined. Some of the CW Doppler detectors can provide a recording of the frequency shift, which is related to velocity in the blood vessel. In most cases, this is a simple tracing that represents the instantaneous mean shift (Usually there is no practical way to calibrate for actual velocity or flow determination.) (Fig. 1).

A portable Doppler detector can be used in patient examinations in many clinical situations, so it is important to acquire experience in using it. There are two important principles to apply. It is always necessary to have a liquid or gel interface between the surface of the probe and the skin in order to exclude air from the path of the ultrasound beam. High-frequency ultrasound is severely attenuated by air, leading to a loss of detectable signal. Instinctively, most people place the probe at a right angle to the course of the vessel. (Some publications even have illustrations showing this

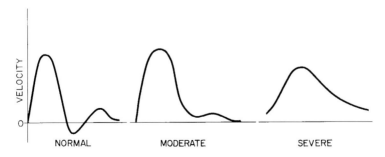

Fig. 1.   Doppler frequency shift tracings from CW Doppler detector, illustrating waveforms from normal, moderate, and severe disease. From Baker JD. In Moore WS (Ed.), *Vascular and Endovascular Surgery: A Comprehensive Review*, 7th Edition, 2006. Permission from Elsevier.

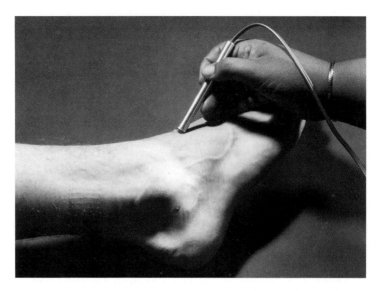

Fig. 2. Doppler probe should be held at a 45–60 degree angle to the course of the vessel. From Baker JD. In Ernst CB (Ed.), Current Therapy in Vascular Surgery, 3rd Edition, 1995. Permission from Elsevier.

erroneous technique.) A 90 degree angle of insonation produces the smallest possible frequency shift. The best practice in most clinical situations is to use a 45–60 degree angle (Fig. 2).

A decrease in pressure down an extremity reflects energy loss and the resulting decreased flow caused by an arterial stenosis. The most common application of the CW Doppler is the measurement of extremity pressures. In this situation, the device is placed distal to a sphygmomanometer cuff and replaces the stethoscope to determine when arterial flow returns after being arrested by cuff inflation. Since the velocity meter is only distinguishing between flow and no-flow, only the systolic endpoint can be determined. Extremity pressure measurements are primarily used for the evaluation of occlusive arterial disease in the legs. The pressure cuff is placed just above the malleoli and measurements are made using the dorsalis pedis and the posterior tibial arteries. Brachial artery pressures are taken in both arms so that the upper extremity pressure can serve as a reference value. The ratio of the higher of the ankle pressures to the higher brachial pressure provides a clinical parameter — ankle-arm index (AAI) or ankle-brachial index (ABI). This value gives an overall assessment of all occlusive disease from the aorta to the ankle level. When occlusive disease is present, additional information can be obtained by measuring segmental pressures with cuff placements at upper thigh, lower thigh, below knee, and ankle. With severe stenosis in the aorto-iliac segment high thigh pressure will be abnormal, while with superficial femoral artery lesions there will be normal pressure in the high thigh and a drop below this level. With significant multilevel disease, gradients can be found at more than one level.

7.2 *Doppler signal recording*

An important limitation of pressure measurements occurs with abnormal stiffening of the arterial wall. The assumption made when measuring pressure with a sphygmomanometer is that the only force opposing the pressure of the cuff to collapse the artery is the intra-arterial pressure. However, with arterial wall stiffening both the wall and the intra-arterial pressure oppose collapsing. This combination is often seen in patients with long-standing diabetes. The end result is that pressure taken with a sphygmomanometer technique can be artifactually elevated. In order to avoid errors, an additional test that is separate from pressure measurement should be used. Most commonly, this is done by a qualitative evaluation of the recording of the Doppler waveform. This parameter is not substantially affected by arterial stiffening. The normal peripheral tracing is triphasic — brisk systolic upstroke and downstroke, reversed flow in early diastole, and a low velocity forward flow in the later part of diastole. With development of stenotic disease, there is a loss of the reverse flow and blunting of the systolic upstroke and downstroke. (Figure 1 shows normal and progressively abnormal waveforms.) Any time that there is substantial disagreement between the results of pressure measurements and waveform findings, artifactual pressure elevations due to stiff arteries should be assumed.

7.3 *Pulse volume record*

The pulse volume recorder (PVR) is another technique for evaluating extremity occlusive disease that avoids the problem of arterial wall stiffening. The method uses a sensitive volume transducer to record changes in limb volume during the cardiac cycle. A pressure cuff is applied to the extremity and inflated to 60 mm Hg. During systole there is a measurable increase in the limb volume under the cuff with a decrease during diastole. This volume change phenomenon is not significantly altered by vessel stiffening. The interpretation of the test is based on qualitative analysis of the resulting volume waveform recorded. (Figure 3 shows normal and varying abnormal waveforms.) These waveforms have different configurations from the Doppler velocity waveforms — notably normal arteries do not have a negative component in early diastole.

7.4 *Lower extremity exercise test*

Most noninvasive tests are performed at rest, for the baseline studies are the most reproducible. However, when dealing with claudication patients it is sometimes useful to study the response to exercise. Patients with moderate stenosis may have adequate resting circulation and the stenosis only has a hemodynamic impact at the higher flow rates that occur with exercise. Many laboratories use a standardized

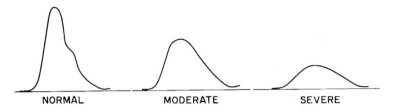

NORMAL   MODERATE   SEVERE

Fig. 3. Pulse volume recorder tracings, illustrating waveforms from normal, moderate, and severe disease. From Baker JD. In Moore WS (Ed.), *Vascular and Endovascular Surgery: A Comprehensive Review*, 7th Edition, 2006. Permission from Elsevier.

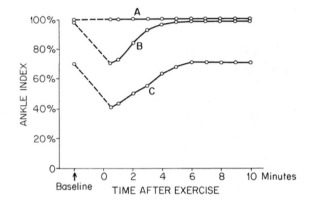

Fig. 4. Changes in AAI after exercise protocol (A, normal response; B, moderate disease; and C, severe disease).

treadmill test. The resting ankle and arm pressures are measured. Although different laboratories may use differing parameters, a typical protocol is for the patient to walk for five minutes at a two-mile-per-hour speed on a 12% incline. As soon as the exercise phase is completed, the patient lies down and the pressure measurements are repeated at 30 seconds after, then at 1 minute intervals from stopping out to five minutes after stopping. The level of exercise in the protocol is moderate: normal subjects will not have a drop in pressure ratios. In the presence of moderate occlusive disease, the resting pressures will be normal but there will be a drop following exercise, with return to baseline values within five minutes (Tracing B, Fig. 4). With severe occlusive disease the baseline values will be abnormal and there will be a substantial drop with stress (Tracing C, Fig. 4). In such patients, the recovery period may be 15 minutes; however, for practical reasons the test is limited to five minutes of recovery. The severity of pressure drop and the duration of recovery are parameters of severity of arterial insufficiency. Patients with very severe arterial disease cannot complete the five minute exercise protocol due to severity of claudication symptoms. Others stop early not because of leg symptoms but because of other symptoms, such as shortness of breath. Noting such a result is important because it documents that the patient's walking limitation is due to a factor other than arterial occlusive disease.

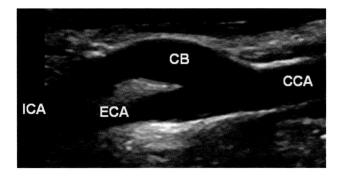

Fig. 5. Gray-scale ultrasound image of normal carotid bifurcation.

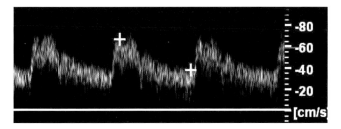

Fig. 6. Spectral waveform of normal internal carotid artery. The horizontal axis records time and the vertical axis records velocity. The white dots on the record represent the proportion of cell travelling at the given velocity. In this normal vessel there is uniform flow, with a narrow range of velocities at any point in time.

7.5 *Duplex ultrasound scan*

The duplex scanner is a complex diagnostic device that is used extensively for noninvasive diagnosis of arterial and venous disease. Two different modalities are available simultaneously: gray-scale image generation and Doppler detection of blood flow. The gray-scale imaging yields a real-time depiction of the anatomic structures and their pathology (Fig. 5). Resolution is fine enough so that arterial plaques and venous thrombi can be seen. In many situations, the image alone is insufficient to define severity of the disease process, but alterations of flow patterns are used diagnostically. The Doppler detector signal is processed by spectral analysis to provide detailed information on the flow characteristics at a given point in the vessel. The imaging system determines the angle between the ultrasound beam and the course of the vessel so that actual velocity calculations can be made (Fig. 6). This degree of quantification is very helpful both in the determination of severity of disease and in the comparison of repeat examinations. By using different ultrasound frequencies, studies can be made of a full range from superficial vessels to those deep in the abdomen or the skull.

Chapter 3
Surgical Anatomy of the Arterial and Venous Systems

Steven Farley

———————

Learning Objectives

- Learn the relevant arterial and venous anatomy most commonly involved in vascular surgical procedures and its relationship to surrounding structures.
- Become familiar with the various surgical procedures performed in the different anatomic regions described in this chapter.

1. Introduction

A vascular surgeon operates on the human body from head to toe, requiring broad knowledge of anatomy. Human anatomy is compact and efficiently designed. Major arterial and venous structures often course in a neurovascular bundle, requiring in-depth anatomic familiarity with the nervous system. Moreover, major vascular structures typically are well-protected by the musculoskeletal system. Therefore, vascular anatomy covers not only arteries and veins, but all of human anatomy. In the evolving vascular surgical field, less-invasive techniques are becoming more widely practiced, which has placed new emphasis on the anatomy of vascular access for percutaneous approaches and the interpretation of angiograms.

Entire text books covering vascular anatomy have been written. This chapter focuses on relevant vascular anatomy. First, the major vessels that circulate blood to and from the heart are described. Second, important relationships to nervous, musculoskeletal, and solid organs are included. Emphasis is placed on a more in-depth description of commonly encountered vascular anatomy, such as central venous access, angio-access for endovascular therapy, and surgical exposures of the great vessels.

2. Neck

2.1 *Arterial*

In the compact arrangement of the neck, vital structures pass between the head, arms, and chest. Oxygenated blood travels from the heart to the head by two paired ves-

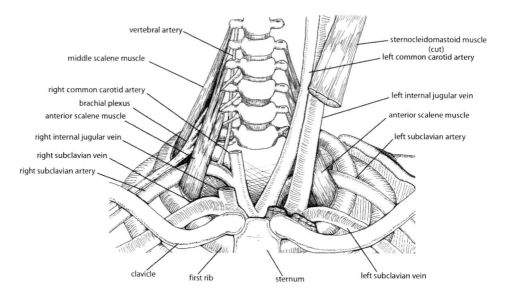

vertebral artery

middle scalene muscle

right common carotid artery

brachial plexus

anterior scalene muscle

right internal jugular vein

right subclavian vein

right subclavian artery

sternocleidomastoid muscle (cut)

left common carotid artery

left internal jugular vein

anterior scalene muscle

left subclavian artery

clavicle

first rib

sternum

left subclavian vein

Fig. 1.

sels — the carotid and vertebral arteries. The right common carotid artery typically originates from the brachiocephalic artery — the first artery arising from the aortic arch. The left common carotid artery is the second artery arising from the aortic arch. Originating in the thoracic cavity, both common carotid arteries travel through the thoracic outlet to reach the head. They course posterior to the sternocleidomastoid muscles and medial to the internal jugular veins (Fig. 1). The distal common carotid artery widens, forming the carotid bulb and gives off two branches — the internal and external carotid arteries (Fig. 2).

The external carotid artery provides branches to the oropharynx, face, and scalp. The vascular surgeon does not often operate on the branches of the external carotid, except for temporal artery biopsy. Branches of the external carotid are the superior thyroid, ascending pharyngeal, lingual, occipital, maxillary, posterior auricular, and temporal arteries.

Of particular interest to the vascular surgeon is the anatomy of the internal carotid artery. It supplies blood to the parietal and frontal lobes of the brain and does not give off its first branch, the ophthalmic artery, until it enters the skull. Associated with strokes and transient ischemia attacks (TIAs), atherosclerotic disease is common in the internal carotid artery and vascular surgeons operate on this artery for stroke prevention. Therefore, precise knowledge of the location of the carotid bifurcation and the surrounding structures is important. The common carotid artery bifurcation can vary, but landmarks to identify the level of the bifurcation include the hyoid bone and the facial vein as it enters the internal jugular vein. Surgical exposure involves

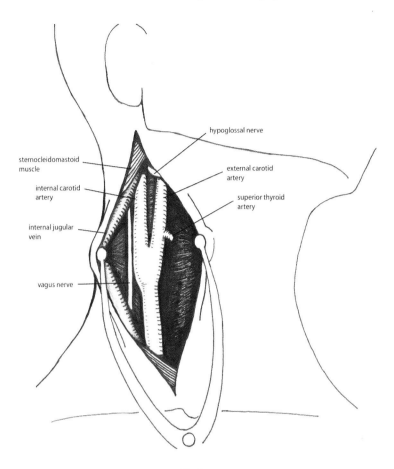

sternocleidomastoid muscle

internal carotid artery

internal jugular vein

vagus nerve

hypoglossal nerve

external carotid artery

superior thyroid artery

Fig. 2.

a vertical incision along the medial aspect of the SCM. After passing through the platysma muscle, the internal jugular vein and SCM are retracted laterally and the vagus nerve, lying in the carotid sheath, is protected. Superiorly, the hypoglossal nerve is commonly found coursing over the internal and external carotid arteries (Fig. 2).

The vertebral arteries are the second paired arteries which travel from the heart to the head. They originate as branches from the subclavian artery (Fig. 1) near the thoracic outlet, course posteriorly through fenestrations in the transverse processes of C6-C1, and enter the skull *via* the foramen magnum. The vertebral arteries coalesce in the skull, forming the basilar artery, and supply blood to the brain stem, cerebellum, and occipital lobe. Derangements in circulation present with dizziness, dysarthria, double vision, and balance disturbances. The vertebral arteries are exposed surgically only occasionally; however they are surgically relevant in the syndromes of subclavian steal, vertebral artery dissection, and coverage of the left subclavian artery for thoracic aortic endograft.

2.2 *Venous*

Whether performed using anatomic landmarks or ultrasound guidance, the venous drainage of the neck is a common source for central venous access. Needed acutely for critical care or electively for long-term access, the veins of the neck are large caliber and are in close vicinity to the heart. External landmarks and knowledge of the relationships of the external jugular vein, internal jugular vein, and carotid artery are, therefore, important.

The internal jugular vein lies within the carotid sheath, lateral to the carotid artery and behind the SCM (Fig. 1). External landmarks used for central venous access are the sternal and clavicular heads of the SCM. In conjunction with clavicle, the two heads of SCM form a triangle, the apex of which is used for percutaneous access of the internal jugular vein. The internal jugular veins join the subclavian veins, forming the brachiocephalic veins in the thoracic cavity.

The external jugular vein lies more superficially than the internal jugular vein and drains into the subclavian vein (Fig. 3). It lies deep to the platysma and courses in medial-to-lateral direction over the SCM. Cannulation of the external jugular vein can provide access to the superior vena cava through the subclavian vein for prolonged central venous access.

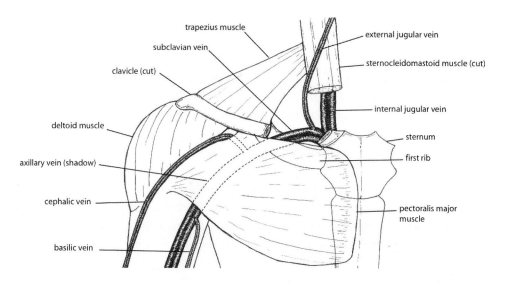

Fig. 3.

3. Arm

3.1 *Arterial*

The right subclavian artery arises from the brachiocephalic artery. The left subclavian artery originates directly from the aorta as the third branch of the aortic arch. Because the proximal extent of the subclavian artery arises in the bony thorax, surgical access can be challenging. The artery passes posterior the anterior scalene muscle and anterior to the brachial plexus and middle scalene muscle. The subclavian arteries are divided into three anatomic zones (Fig. 4). The first zone begins at the origin of the vessel and ends at the medial border of the anterior scalene muscle. The second zone of the artery lies behind the anterior scalene muscle. The third is defined by the section of the artery distal to the lateral border of the anterior scalene muscle up to the lateral edge of the first rib.

Branches of the subclavian artery are the internal mammary, vertebral, thyrocervical, and dorsal scapular arteries. Surgical exposure of the subclavian artery may be required emergently, as in trauma, or electively for carotid-subclavian bypass. In an elective setting, a supraclavicular incision is often employed (Fig. 5). The skin and platysma are opened and the omohyoid muscle is divided. The scalene fat pad is carefully retracted and the external jugular vein is often sacrificed as it enters the subclavian vein. Care must be taken to avoid injury to the phrenic nerve as it courses lateral-to-medial along the anterior surface of the anterior scalene muscle.

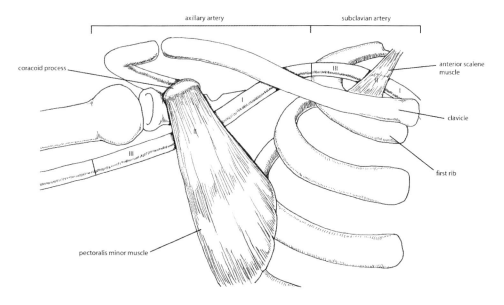

Fig. 4.

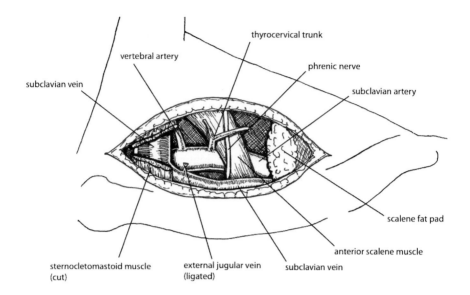

Fig. 5.

For traumatic injuries to the right subclavian artery, median sternotomy with cervical extension is recommended. The proximal left subclavian artery is more difficult to expose and an anterolateral left thoracotomy may be required.

After crossing over the lateral edge of the first rib, the subclavian artery becomes the axillary artery. Similar to the subclavian artery, the axillary artery is divided into three regions by anatomists (Fig. 4). The first zone begins at the lateral edge of the first rib and ends at the medial border of the pectoralis minor muscle. The second region of the axillary artery is defined by the segment of artery lying behind the pectoralis minor muscle, which originates from the rib cage and inserts on the coracoid process of the scapula. The third zone starts at the lateral border of the pectoralis minor muscle and ends at the lateral border of the teres major muscle.

Several named branches of the axillary artery exist including the thoracoacromial, lateral thoracic, thoracodorsal, and circumflex humeral arteries. Rich collaterals exist around the shoulder, made possible by the humeral circumflex arteries. Surgical exposure of the axillary artery is achieved by an infraclavicular incision and dissection through the pectoralis muscles. Exposure of the second zone often requires dividing the pectoralis minor muscle.

After crossing the lateral edge of the teres major muscle insertion to the proximal humerus, the axillary artery becomes the brachial artery (Fig. 6). It travels medially in the arm and it courses between the medial borders of the biceps and triceps muscles. The brachial artery can be used for vascular access in dialysis or in catheter-based therapy by percutaneous or open cut-down techniques. Also, the median nerve and brachial vein are contained in a fascial sheath with the artery. Bleeding inside the

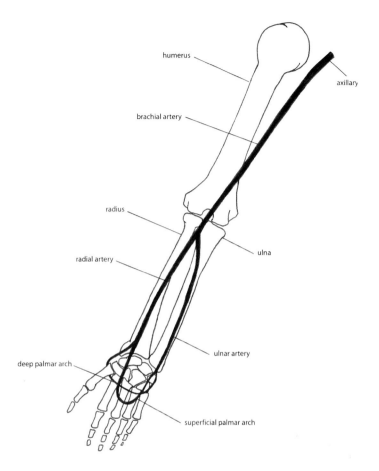

Fig. 6.

sheath can lead to nerve compression and permanent nerve damage. At the elbow, the brachial artery lies in the antecubital fossa, medial to the insertion of the biceps tendon. Due its proximity to the humerus, traumatic fractures of the humerus and elbow dislocations are associated with brachial artery injuries.

After crossing the elbow joint and reaching the level of the radial tuberosity, the brachial artery branches into the radial and ulnar arteries (Fig. 6). In the upper forearm, both the ulnar and radial artery lay deep to the muscles of the flexor compartment. Traveling distally at the wrist, both arteries assume more superficial positions. The radial artery can be found at the lateral border of the flexor digitorum superficialis muscle. The cephalic vein and superficial radial nerve are nearby and should be protected. The ulnar artery is found on the radial side of the flexor carpi ulnaris muscle. Importantly, the ulnar and radial arteries meet in the hand, forming deep and superficial palmar arches. The palmar arches allow for collateral flow to the hand when the radial artery is used for catheterization or arteriovenous fistula formation.

3.2 *Venous*

The venous system of the upper extremity is often utilized by the vascular surgeon. The superficial venous system includes the cephalic and basilic veins. The deep system, which communicates with the superficial system, is comprised of the brachial, axillary, and subclavian veins.

The superficial veins are used for surgical arteriovenous fistulas created for hemodialysis. The cephalic vein starts at the wrist along the radial aspect of the arm (Fig. 7). Its proximity to the radial artery makes it a common choice for arteriovenous fistula creation. The vein travels along the radial aspect of the forearm and moves to the antecubital fossa. From there, it courses along the lateral aspect of the biceps muscle, onto the chest wall in the deltopectoral groove before traveling deep to empty into the axillary vein (Fig. 3). At the wrist, the basilic vein lies along the ulnar side of the forearm and courses toward the medial aspect of the antecubital fossa (Fig. 7). In the upper arm, it travels medial and deep, emptying into the proximal axillary vein (Fig. 3).

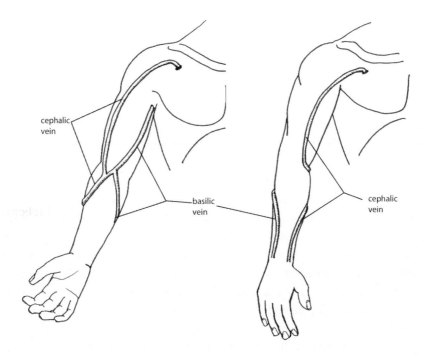

cephalic vein

basilic vein

cephalic vein

Fig. 7.

The deep venous system is accessed by the vascular surgeon for numerous procedures. Often the superficial venous system of a patient is inadequate for creation of an arteriovenous fistula. In this situation, a prosthetic graft is sewn to an artery in the arm and anastomozed to the deep venous system, creating a high-flow arteriovenous communication. Common veins accessed are the brachial and axillary veins. The brachial vein travels alongside the brachial artery in the brachial sheath of the upper arm. After crossing the lateral border of the teres major muscle, the vein is named the axillary vein (Fig. 3).

Once crossing the lateral edge of the first rib, the axillary vein becomes the subclavian vein as it courses anterior to the anterior scalene muscle (Fig. 2). Central venous access of the subclavian vein therefore requires passing a needle beneath the clavicle and superficial to the subclavian artery. Surrounding the vein are the subclavius muscle and clavicle anteriorly. The anterior scalene muscle, subclavian artery, and brachial plexus pass posteriorly and superiorly and the first rib lies inferiorly. This tightly arranged region is termed the thoracic outlet, which has been identified as an anatomically susceptible location of human anatomy. Repetitive use of the upper extremity can result in compression of the subclavian vein, subclavian artery, or brachial plexus in a disease process termed thoracic outlet compression syndrome.

4. Thorax

4.1 *Arterial*

The first artery of the body is the aorta as it arises from the left ventricle of the heart. The aorta arches in an anterior-to-posterior and slight right-to-left fashion to become the thoracic aorta (Fig. 8). In general, the aorta at the arch gives off three major branches — the brachiocephalic, left common carotid, and left subclavian artery. Embryonic formation of the aortic arch can vary so that other arch configurations are possible.

The thoracic aorta contributes intercostal branches and blood supply to the anterior spinal cord. Therefore, surgery on the thoracic aorta has the potential for spinal cord ischemia and paralysis. Considered a major component to spinal cord circulation, the artery of Adamkiewicz, also termed the anterior segmental medullary artery, can be found anywhere along the descending thoracic aorta, but most commonly along the T9–T11 segment of the thoracic aorta. The distal descending aorta passes caudally along the left side of the thoracic spine in the posterior mediastinum and pierces the diaphragm at T12.

A remnant of the fetal circulation, the ligamentum arteriosum is a fibrous connection between the aorta distal to the left subclavian artery and the pulmonary

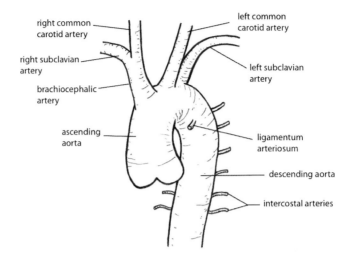

right common carotid artery

left common carotid artery

right subclavian artery

left subclavian artery

brachiocephalic artery

ascending aorta

ligamentum arteriosum

descending aorta

intercostal arteries

Fig. 8.

artery. The ligamentum arteriosum is a fixation point for thoracic aorta and common site for transaction of the aorta in blunt trauma. Also the ligamentum is the lead point for type B aortic dissection. During embryonic development, the ligamentum arteriosum prevents the left recurrent laryngeal nerve from migrating superiorly and traps the nerve in the chest.

4.2 *Venous*

The venous drainage of the upper thorax begins with the brachiocephalic veins, which are formed by the coalescence of the internal jugular and subclavian veins (Fig. 9). The left brachiocephalic vein crosses the midline anteriorly, underneath the sternum, and joins the right brachiocephalic vein, forming the superior vena cava. The SVC is positioned to the right of the ascending aorta and drains directly into the right atrium of the heart. The azygous vein provides venous drainage along the posterior mediastinum and enters the SVC near the right atrium. Also in the thorax, the venous return of the abdomen, pelvis, and lower extremities is provided by the inferior vena cava. The IVC pierces the diaphragm at T8, enters the pericardium, and drains into the right atrium.

5. Abdomen

5.1 *Arterial*

After traveling through the diaphragm, the aorta assumes a retroperitoneal position in the abdomen. The first major visceral branch is the celiac axis (Fig. 10). The

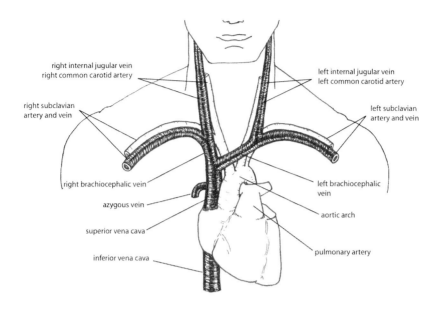

Fig. 9.

celiac trunk provides the blood supply to the embryonic foregut, which includes the hepatobiliary system, pancreas, stomach, spleen, and duodenum. The celiac axis quickly divides into the left gastric, common hepatic, and splenic arteries. The common hepatic artery passes over the inferior vena cava and branches into the gastroduodenal and proper hepatic braches. The proper hepatic artery gives off the right gastric artery on its way to the liver.

The second intestinal branch of the abdominal aorta is the superior mesenteric artery, which supplies blood to the embryonic midgut, which includes the distal duodenum, pancreas, jejunum, ileum, and colon up to the splenic flexure. The third intestinal branch of the aorta is the inferior mesenteric artery, which arises from the infrarenal aorta. The IMA supplies blood to the descending and sigmoid colon, as well as to the rectum. This artery is commonly ligated in open infrarenal aortic surgery, which can lead to ischemic colitis of the sigmoid colon.

Another set of important branches of the aorta are the renal arteries. The left renal artery commonly arises more cephalad than the right. Typically, the renal arteries originate at the L1–L2 interspace and lie posterior to the renal veins at the hilum of the kidney. The right renal artery passes posterior to the inferior vena cava to reach the right kidney.

Also relevant to the vascular surgeon, the lumbar arteries branch posteriorly from the aorta. During open aortic aneurysm surgery, these vessels must be over-sewn for hemostasis. In endovascular surgery, the lumbar arteries are a common cause of type II endoleaks, which can lead to aneurysm growth.

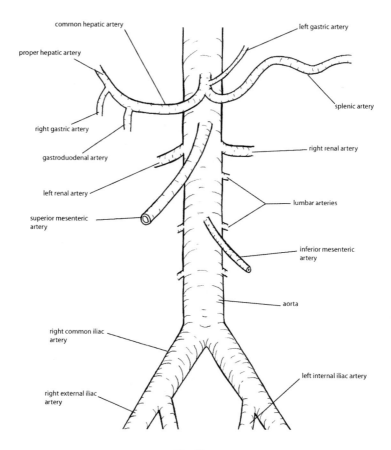

Fig. 10.

Due to the deep retroperitoneal position of the aorta, surgical access to the abdominal aorta can be complex. Both transperitoneal and retroperitoneal routes are used. Tranperitoneal supraceliac exposure involves a left medial visceral rotation by which the descending colon is freed from the retroperitoneum along the lateral attachments (Fig. 11). This dissection can be extended superior and lateral to the spleen. The spleen, tail of the pancreas, and left colon are carefully rotated to a midline position, and for greater proximal exposure the left crus of the diaphragm may be opened. The kidney can remain in the retroperitoneum or be mobilized medially along with the spleen. This results in lifting the left ureter from the retroperitoneum. Transperitoneal exposure of the infrarenal aorta can be achieved by retracting the transverse colon superiorly and the small bowel to the right upper quadrant. The parietal peritoneal covering of the aorta is incised and the aorta exposed. Mobilization of the ligament of treitz, duodenum, and pancreas can provide suprarenal access to the aorta (Fig. 12).

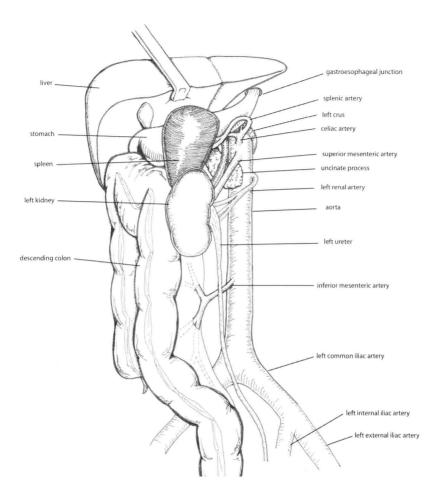

Fig. 11.

Because of its retroperitoneal position, the aorta can be readily accessed in this plane. Careful dissection of the three layers of the abdominal wall is required. The first layer of the abdominal wall, the external oblique, travels in an inferomedial direction and contributes its fibers to the anterior layer of the rectus sheath, passing over the rectus abdominus muscle (Fig. 13). The fibers of the internal oblique, the second layer, travel at a right angle to the external oblique and splits above the semilunar line to form layers of the anterior and posterior rectus sheath. The final abdominal wall layer, the transverse abdominus, runs in a horizontal plane and adds fibers to the posterior rectus sheath superior to the semilunar line. The peritoneum lies underneath the transverse abdominus layer, and gentle blunt dissection opens this potential space. Similar to transperitoneal exposure, the dissection can be carried behind or in front of the kidney to obtain exposure of the aorta.

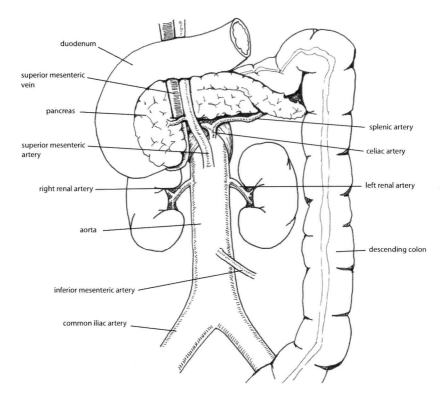

Fig. 12.

In the abdomen, the aorta divides at its distal extent into the right and left common iliac arteries near the lumbosacral junction of the spine. The common iliac arteries travel along the pelvic brim laterally and anteriorly. An important anatomic landmark is the ureter as it passes over the iliac artery and enters the pelvis (Fig. 14). The sympathetic fibers of the pelvis also course over the common iliac arteries. Operative exposure may require sacrificing these nerves and can lead to impotence.

The common iliac arteries divide into the internal and external iliac arteries (Fig. 10). The internal iliac artery carries blood to the pelvis, including organs such as the rectum, bladder, buttock muscles, and genitalia. The external iliac artery continues along the pelvic brim and passes underneath the inguinal ligament to supply blood to the lower extremity.

5.2 *Venous*

The venous circulation of the abdomen includes portal and systemic circulations. Portal circulation is defined as one capillary bed draining into a second capillary bed through veins without returning to the heart. The portal circulation of the liver is an example. Venous blood from the spleen, pancreas, and intestines drains *via* the

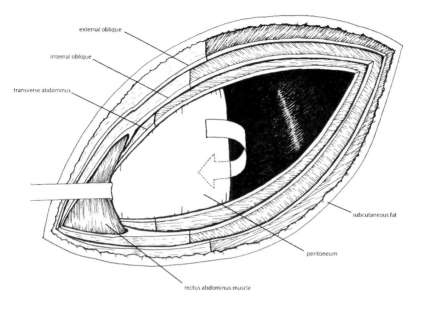

external oblique

internal oblique

transverse abdominus

subcutaneous fat

peritoneum

rectus abdominus muscle

Fig. 13.

superior mesenteric, inferior mesenteric, and splenic veins, eventually coalescing to form the portal vein. Venous blood in the portal vein is taken to the second capillary bed in the liver and eventually returns to the systemic venous system by way of the hepatic veins to the inferior vena cava (IVC).

Venous operations on the portal system of the abdomen have become less common. Previously surgical bypasses between the portal and systemic venous systems were employed to reduce portal venous pressures in patients, commonly suffering from cirrhosis, with portal hypertension.

The systemic venous system in the abdomen returns blood from the pelvis, retroperitoneum, and lower extremities to the heart by the iliac veins and inferior vena cava. Surgical exposure of the systemic venous system in the abdomen including the inferior vena cava and renal veins may be needed for trauma, tumors of the retroperitoneum, or lymphadenectomy. Exposure of the infrahepatic inferior vena cava requires a right medial visceral rotation (Fig. 14). The lateral attachments of the ascending colon are incised and the small bowel is freed from the retroperitoneum to the ligament of Treitz. An extensive Kocher maneuver (medialization of the duodenum) completes the exposure of the infrahepatic IVC. With this exposure the right and left renal veins can be isolated. Surgical access to the retrohepatic IVC involves mobilization of the right lobe of the liver, isolation of the right hepatic vein, and careful ligation of the communicating veins of the caudate lobe of the liver.

The common iliac veins travel in parallel to their arterial neighbors. The iliac veins at the aortic bifurcations lie deep to the iliac arteries, and surgical access to an

S. Farley

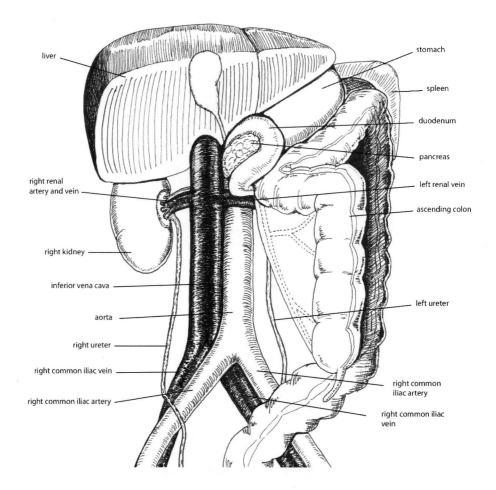

Fig. 14.

iliac vein injury can be difficult. The right common iliac artery crosses over the left internal iliac vein (Fig. 14) and can cause compression of the vein, leading to left leg swelling (May–Thurner syndrome) and deep-vein thrombosis.

The left renal vein usually crosses over the aorta to reach the vena cava (Fig. 14). Hence, the right renal vein is typically shorter than the left. Ligation of the left renal vein at the level of the IVC is possible because of adrenal and lumbar collaterals (Fig. 15). Exposure of the infrarenal aorta may require elevation of the left renal vein which is facilitated by division of the gonadal and lumbar branches. Occasionally, the left renal vein travels behind or circumferentially around the aorta.

In the percutaneous era of vascular surgery, inferior vena cava filters are commonly placed. Identification of the renal veins and the iliac vein bifurcation is important. Other vascular procedures involving the systemic venous drainage of

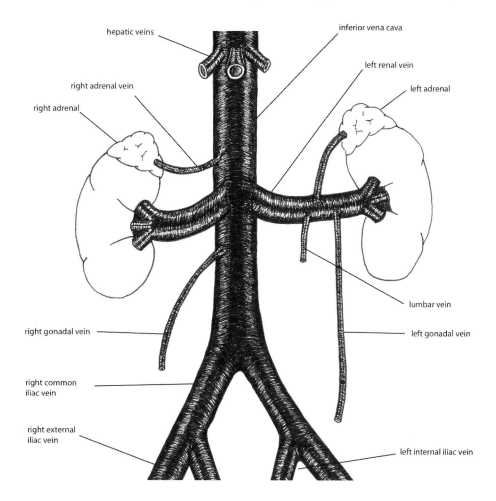

Fig. 15.

the abdomen included selective venous sampling of the adrenal veins for neuroendocrine tumors and embolization of gondal veins for pelvic varicose veins. Note, the left adrenal vein typically empties directly into the infrahepatic inferior vena cava and the right adrenal vein empties into the left renal vein. Also, the left gonadal vein drains into the left renal vein and the right gonadal vein typically drains directly into the inferior vena cava.

6. Lower Extremity

6.1 *Arterial*

The arterial supply of the lower extremity begins in the abdomen at the aortic bifurcation with the origin of the common iliac arteries. After passing underneath the inguinal ligament, the artery becomes the common femoral artery. Fibrous attachments connecting the inguinal ligament and the superior pubic ramus to the pubic tubercle are named the lacunar ligament. Along the superior surface of the superior pubic ramus runs the pectineal (Cooper's) ligament. The artery and vein are covered by the continuation of the transversalis fascia, named the femoral sheath. Proximal in the thigh, the common femoral artery divides into the superficial and profunda femoral arteries (Fig. 16).

The profunda femoral artery supplies major branches to the thigh and knee. It is the largest branch vessel of the common femoral artery and can supply adequate

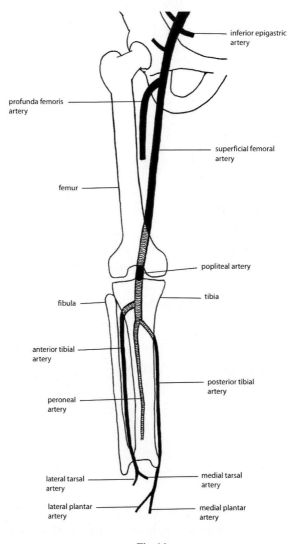

Fig. 16.

outflow for bypass surgery. The superficial femoral artery is a common site for peripheral vascular disease. Despite originating early in the thigh, the SFA does not branch in the upper leg and instead directs blood to below the knee. Traveling deep to the sartorius muscle, the SFA lies medial in the mid-thigh. Distally, it passes posterior through the adductor hiatus to reach the popliteal fossa. At this point, the artery name changes to the popliteal artery and is positioned posterior to the knee joint.

In the lower leg, the popliteal artery divides into three arteries — anterior tibial (AT), posterior tibial, and peroneal arteries. Typically the anterior tibial artery is the first branch. The AT originates in the popliteal space, courses through the interosseous membrane between the tibia and fibula, and into the anterior compartment of the lower leg. After the division of the AT from the popliteal artery, the remaining artery is termed the tibio-peroneal trunk, which soon divides into the posterior tibial and peroneal arteries. The posterior tibial artery courses medially in the deep posterior compartment. The peroneal artery also travels in the deep posterior compartment but branches before reaching the ankle.

At the foot, the dorsalis pedis artery is the continuation of the AT and travels along the dorsum of the foot. It gives off medial and lateral tarsal artery branches. At the ankle, the posterior tibial artery travels posterior to the medial mallelolus and divides into the lateral and medial plantar arteries.

As percutaneous interventions have increased in frequency, the anatomy of the femoral triangle is increasingly important. From lateral to medial, using the common pneumonic NAVEL, lie the femoral Nerve, common femoral Artery, common femoral Vein, Empty space (lymphatics), and the Lacunar ligament (Fig. 17). The common femoral artery, the target for percutaneous procedures, is found below the inguinal ligament. Using external landmarks, a line connecting the anterior superior iliac crest and the pubic tubercle delineates the inguinal ligament. In the obese or elderly patient, the inguinal ligament is located surprisingly cranial to the groin crease. Fluoroscopically, the middle of the femoral head is a reliable landmark for identifying the level of the common femoral artery. Percutaneous access achieved above the inguinal ligament can result in retroperitoneal bleeding which is difficult to recognize, difficult to control with manual pressure, and can result in exsanguination. Percutaneous access below the common femoral artery results in puncture of the superficial artery, which is smaller caliber and has poor collateral circulation.

6.2 *Venous*

Similar to the upper extremity, superficial and deep venous systems exist in the lower extremity. Important to venous disease of the lower extremity, perforating veins connect the deep and superficial systems.

S. Farley

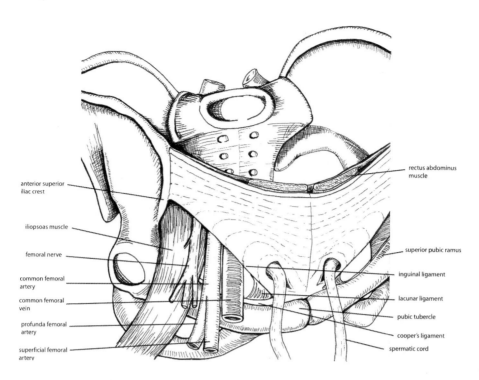

Fig. 17.

The main superficial veins of the leg are the greater and lesser saphenous veins (Fig. 18). The greater saphenous vein travels from the ankle to the upper thigh and is found consistently anterior to the medial mallelolus of the ankle. It travels along the medial aspect of the lower leg and knee and courses along the medial thigh in a slight posterior direction before meeting with the common femoral vein at the saphenofemoral junction. The lesser saphenous vein begins at the ankle posterior to the lateral mallelolus. It travels along the lateral lower leg and moves posteriorly behind the knee, where it empties into the popliteal vein. The superficial veins of the lower extremity are relatively long and of large caliber and commonly used by surgeons as conduits for bypass procedures. Of note, one-way valves which direct blood to the heart and prevent reflux of blood to the feet are found in the superficial veins. If used as vascular conduits, the valves must be oriented in the direction of flow or removed. Also, valvular incompetence is associated with venous reflux, venous hypertension, and varicose veins.

The deep venous system starts below the knee with the tibial veins. At the knee, the popliteal vein travels alongside the artery, often as paired veins. Popliteal artery aneurysms can compress the vein and lead to leg swelling. The popliteal vein continues cranially to become the femoral vein. The venous drainage of the thigh *via* the profunda vein connects with the femoral vein to become the common femoral

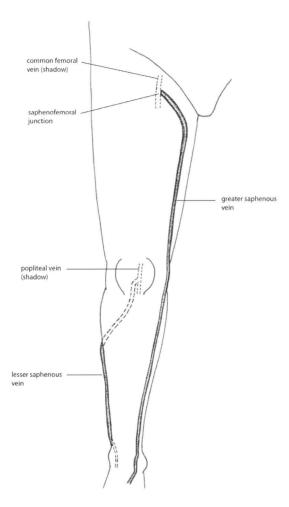

common femoral
vein (shadow)

saphenofemoral
junction

greater saphenous
vein

popliteal vein
(shadow)

lesser saphenous
vein

Fig. 18.

vein. The common femoral vein is often used for central venous access and is found medial to the common femoral artery. Similar to the superficial venous system, one-way valves present in the deep veins are oriented to prevent reflux in the standing position and are important in facilitating blood return to the heart.

Termed Cockett's perforators, perforating veins connect the superficial veins traveling in the subcutaneous tissue to the deep venous system traveling inside the fascial compartments of the leg. Perforators direct blood from the superficial to the deep system.

Venous hypertension of the lower extremity affects millions of patients in the United States. In severe presentations, large non-healing wounds of the lower extremity develop. Normal venous circulation of the lower leg involves the strong fascia covering of the lower leg (Fig. 19), the muscles of the lower leg, and the

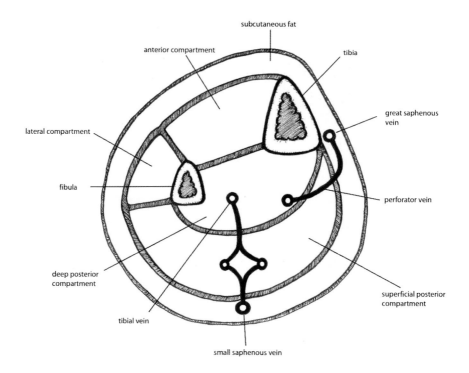

Fig. 19.

one-way valves of the venous system. Contraction of the muscles inside the fascia covering of the lower limb results in increased pressure, propelling venous blood back to the heart. During relaxation of the muscles, the pressure inside the compartments lowers, but the one-way valves of the venous system prevent blood from refluxing back to the foot. With valvular incompetence, the musculovenous pump fails and the result is increased venous pressure transmitted outside the fascial compartments and into the subcutaneous tissue. Over time, the increased venous pressure overcomes the subcutaneous tissues. Ischemia, tissue loss, and non-healing wounds, particularly at the sites of perforating veins, are the result.

The fibrous covering of the lower extremity important for the musculovenous pump is implicated in a disease process termed lower extremity compartment syndrome. After acute ischemic events, the muscles of the lower extremity swell. The four compartments of the lower limb — anterior, lateral, deep posterior, and superficial posterior — are rigid and cannot accommodate the swelling muscles and compartment pressures rise, causing ischemia and possible tissue death. Longitudinal incisions of the fascial compartments (fasciotomy) are employed to release the pressure.

All figures with this chapter are original works of Steven Farley MD.

Chapter 4
Diagnostic Imaging of the Vascular System

Juan Carlos Jimenez

Learning Objectives

- Understand the basic principles of computed tomography angiography, its advantages, and limitations for imaging of the vascular system.
- Understand the basic principles of magnetic resonance angiography, its advantages, and limitations for imaging of the vascular system.
- Understand the basic principles of conventional angiography, its advantages, and limitations for imaging of the vascular system.
- Be familiar with the clinical applicability of the described imaging modalities to the different anatomic regions presented.

1. Computed Tomography Angiography: Basic Principles

Computed tomography angiography (CTA) is a noninvasive imaging modality that has emerged as a powerful tool to image rapidly and accurately the vascular structures. Third-generation CT scanners contain a rotating gantry with a tube and a detector opposing each other, which obtain images by passing a rotating beam of x-rays through the patient, and calculate the transmission at several different points. Images are then obtained as a series of transverse (axial) slices. The emergence of multidetector CT (MD-CT) scanners and dual source detectors has allowed increased speed, resolution, and flexibility in the diagnosis of both arterial and venous disorders. MD-CT decreases breath holding times and reduces the overall amount of contrast administered compared with earlier CT technology. CTA produces volume data sets, which can be reformatted and viewed in several distinct projections to obtain detailed three-dimensional (3D) reconstructions. In order to obtain images of superior quality, CTA requires administration of iodinated contrast during a precise timed bolus for optimal intraluminal enhancement. Factors that influence arterial enhancement include: the volume of contrast administered, the rate of injection, and the concentration of iodine in the contrast.

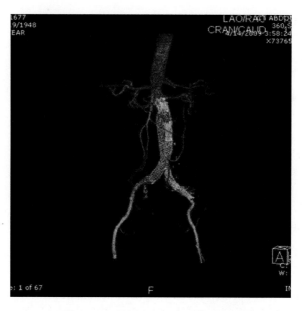

Fig. 1. 3D computed tomography reconstruction of abdominal aorta and iliac arteries following endovascular abdominal aortic aneurysm repair.

Compared with digital subtraction angiography, CTA is less invasive, faster, and less expensive. Accurate 3D renderings can be obtained to visualize vessels from any angle from a single set of acquired data (Fig. 1). This technique is also able to delineate the vessel wall in detail and evaluate the abnormalities such as mural thrombus, aneurysm, intraluminal plaque, penetrating ulcers, and dissection. The relationship of the vessel with nearby organs and structures can also be visualized, whereas conventional angiography is largely limited to the imaging of intraluminal pathology.

1.1 *Limitations of CT angiography*

Limitations of CTA include the required intravenous administration of iodinated contrast, which is associated with allergic (and sometimes anaphylactic) reactions and nephrotoxicity. This technique also requires patient exposure to ionizing radiation and its cumulative effects. The radiation dose of CTA, however, is generally lower than that of conventional angiography. Severely calcified arteries can cause corresponding artifact, which may decrease the accuracy of vessel wall evaluation. Intraluminal stents may also impede luminal visualization. Rapid infusion of contrast requires large-bore intravenous access, which may be difficult to obtain in patients with advanced peripheral vascular or end-stage renal disease.

2. Magnetic Resonance Angiography: Basic Principles

Advancements in magnetic resonance angiography (MRA) have allowed it to become a reasonable and noninvasive alternative to conventional angiography for imaging of the vascular system. This technique utilizes radiofrequency waves and magnetic field gradients to produce images. A variety of pulse sequences can be administered to permit the enhancement or reduction of signal from different tissues based on their hydrogen density and their response to differing magnetic field gradients. These sequences include time of flight (TOF) angiography, phase-contrast angiography, and 3D contrast-enhanced MRA. A detailed description of the principles and physics of MRI is beyond the scope of this book.

2.1 *Time of flight and phase contrast magnetic resonance angiography*

Time of flight magnetic resonance angiography (TOF-MRA) is an older technique, which is performed by saturating stationary tissues in the volume or slice of interest with repeated radiofrequency pulses (Fig. 2). Inflowing blood (unsaturated) not subjected to these radiofrequency pulses retains its signal intensity and creates a contrast when compared to the stationary background tissues. The limitations of this technique include longer acquisition times, turbulence-induced signal loss distal to stenoses, and in-plane saturation.

Phase-contrast angiography (PC-MRA) utilizes velocity-induced phase shifts of moving protons by bipolar flow-encoding gradients to create images of both moving and nonmoving systems. Both 2D and 3D acquisition techniques can be applied. PC-MRA minimizes distal signal loss associated with TOF-MRA, however, turbulent flow can still cause artifact at sites of vessel stenosis. Although newer MRA techniques are now available to better evaluate the vascular system, TOF-MRA and PC-MRA are most useful when patients have a contraindication to gadolinium infusion.

2.2 *Contrast-enhanced magnetic resonance angiography*

3D contrast enhanced MRA(CE-MRA) has emerged as an accurate and efficient method for imaging vascular structures without the limitations of the previously described techniques (Fig. 3). It combines the enhanced tissue contrast obtained with conventional MRI with superior vessel visualization, and it can provide a 3D image that can be rotated 360° for improved evaluation following postprocessing. CE-MRA utilizes the intravascular infusion of the paramagnetic contrast agent, gadolinium chelate, to shorten the T1 relaxation time of blood compared with surrounding tissues. This technique is less flow sensitive because, unlike TOF and PC-MRA,

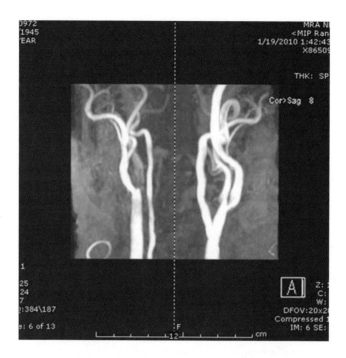

Fig. 2. Time of flight magnetic resonance angiography of the extracranial carotid arteries.

the signal of the blood is based on its intrinsic T_1 signal and less on flow effects. More rapid scan times can be achieved with increasing spatial resolution. Maximum intensity projection (MIP) images can then be obtained through postprocessing. Because the intravascular signal is dependent on T1 relaxation as opposed to inflow or phase accumulation required with TOF-MRA and PC-MRA, in-plane saturation and turbulence-induced signal loss are reduced. Careful timing of the contrast bolus is required to ensure a high concentration of gadolinium at the desired station during image acquisition. More detailed descriptions of these techniques are beyond the scope of this book.

2.3 *Limitations of magnetic resonance angiography*

Because patient cooperation is necessary to obtain high-quality images, motion artifact and inadequate breath holding may result in nondiagnostic or suboptimal studies. Claustrophobic patients who exhibit anxiety should be administered intravenous sedatives (*i.e.* diazepam or fentanyl) prior to testing. Sometimes, conscious sedation and/or general anesthesia may be required. Morbidly obese patients may not be able to undergo MRA due to size and weight limitations of most scanners.

Although gadolinium-based contrast is rapidly excreted in most patients and considered less nephrotoxic than iodinated contrast agents, their relationship with

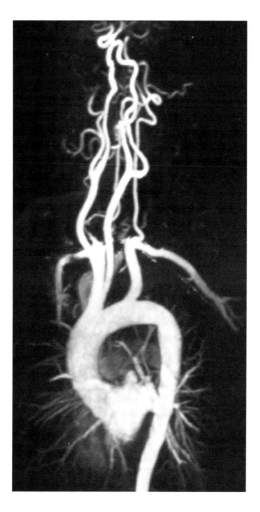

Fig. 3. Magnetic resonance angiography of the aortic arch and its branches.

a systemic fibrotic syndrome has been recently observed. Nephrogenic systemic fibrosis has been linked to gadolinium-based contrast and is a potentially fatal condition, which is most common in patients with Stages IV and V kidney disease. Patients typically present with progressive fibrosis and hyperpigmentation of their skin, which can lead to generalized visceral involvement. Because little is known about this disorder, patients with compromised renal function should not undergo CE-MRA with gadolinium-based contrast agents.

Metallic stents imaged with MRA exhibit signal dropout due to magnetic susceptibility and radiofrequency shielding. Thus, vessels with previously placed metallic stents may not be imaged accurately. Subsequently, patients with magnetic, electrically conductive, or RF-reactive implants (*i.e.* pacemakers, defibrillator, *etc.*) cannot undergo MRA due to potential interaction between magnetic and radiofrequency fields elicited during these examinations. Titanium implants are generally considered safe.

3. Digital Subtraction Angiography: Basic Principles

Digital subtraction angiography (DSA) has long been considered the gold standard for obtaining high-resolution images of the vascular system (Fig. 4). This technique involves recording and computer processing of a fluoroscopic image in order to "subtract" or mask the surrounding radiodensities (bones, soft tissues, air densities, and calcifications) of the vessel wall and surrounding tissues. Once this subtraction has been performed, the image is comprised exclusively from the subsequent local injection of intraluminal contrast (Figs. 5(a) and 5(b)). Angiographic wires, sheaths, and catheters are advanced to the desired intravascular location for contrast injection. Any movement after the initial subtraction image has been obtained results in motion artifact and image deterioration and a new mask image must be obtained

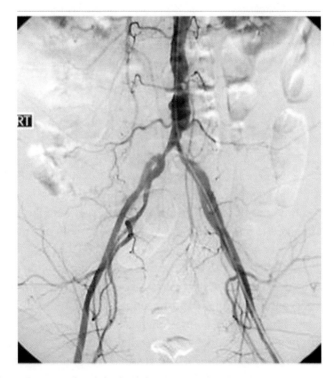

Fig. 4. Digital subtraction angiography of the abdominal aorta demonstrating critical stenoses of the bilateral common iliac arteries.

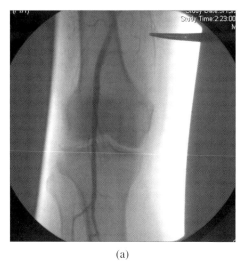 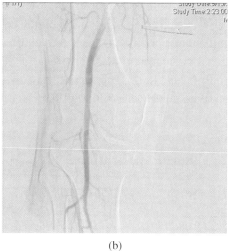

(a)   (b)

Fig. 5.   (a) Conventional angiogram demonstrating the popliteal artery and tibial vessels prior to subtraction. (b) "Subtracted" image of the popliteal artery and tibial vessels demonstrated in Fig. 5(a).

prior to further injection of contrast. Although iodinated contrast materials are most common, alternative agents such as gadolinium and carbon dioxide can also be used.

DSA maintains several advantages over less invasive imaging modalities such as CTA and MRA. Techniques such as "road mapping" allow a previously recorded image of a contrast-filled vessel to be viewed on the monitor while real-time movement of angiographic wires and catheters are passed through the "road mapped" image. This technique is used to facilitate cannulation through tortuous or calcified arteries.

With conventional angiography, superior opacification of small and low flow vessels can be achieved using subtraction and digital magnification techniques with minimal contrast administration. Dynamic information regarding collateral pathways, the number, extent, and severity of arterial stenoses can be obtained with superior image resolution and clarity. Furthermore, interventions (*i.e.* angioplasty, stenting, atherectomy, thrombolysis, *etc.*) can be performed using catheter-based techniques at the time of diagnostic angiography.

3.1 *Limitations of conventional angiography*

The main limitation of conventional angiography is its invasiveness. It requires percutaneous vessel cannulation with the introduction of intravascular wires, catheters, sheaths, and devices. Potential complications include vessel thrombosis, rupture, dissection, pseudoaneurysm, and arteriovenous fistula formation. Most studies require the use of iodinated contrast agents, which can be nephrotoxic and cause allergic

69

reactions. With conventional angiography, the amount and concentration of contrast can be determined and limited by the angiographer as opposed to CTA where large and defined contrast boluses are required for optimal vessel opacification. Conventional angiography also requires a dedicated imaging suite with trained technical and medical staff. The overall cost of this modality is generally greater than the other noninvasive techniques described.

4. Clinical Applications

4.1 *Aorta, visceral, and iliac arteries*

4.1.1 *Computed tomography angiography*

CTA is the diagnostic modality of choice to evaluate both acute and nonacute pathology within the thoracic and abdominal aortas and iliac arteries. With 64-slice MDCT, it is possible to scan the entire aorta with less than one-millimeter collimation within a single breath-hold. The rapid speed of image acquisition makes it especially useful in patients with acute aortic syndromes (*i.e.* aortic dissection, penetrating aortic ulcer, unstable aortic aneurysms, *etc.*). In patients with aortic dissection, CTA can accurately provide information regarding the site of the entry tear, branch artery involvement, distinction between the true and false lumen, and the presence of aortic rupture. This technique can also reliably assess the diameter of both the true and false lumens and measure the diameter of the iliac and femoral arteries for the planning of endovascular repair. Compared with transesophageal echocardiography for evaluating thoracic aortic pathology, CTA is less invasive, provides the ability to visualize the aorta beyond the root, limits the reliability of operator dependence, and visualizes the entire aortic arch and great vessels.

In the abdominal aorta, this technique can be reliably used for the diagnosis and surveillance of abdominal aortic aneurysms and aortoiliac occlusive disease and to determine accurately the extent of visceral and renal artery involvement. 3D reconstructions of the infrarenal abdominal aorta and iliac arteries are especially useful in the preoperative planning of endovascular repair where the precise measurement of aortic diameters, neck length, and size of access arteries are required (Fig. 6). CTA is also useful for postoperative surveillance following endovascular AAA repair to monitor the presence or development of endoleaks, graft positioning, and aneurysm sac enlargement (Figs. 7(a) and 7(b)).

The visceral and renal arteries can be visualized reliably using CTA, especially with the recent advancements of MD-CT. Renal artery stenosis originates from either atherosclerotic lesions or fibromuscular dysplasia and CTA can provide high-resolution and thin-section images of the renal arteries for evaluation. Detection of

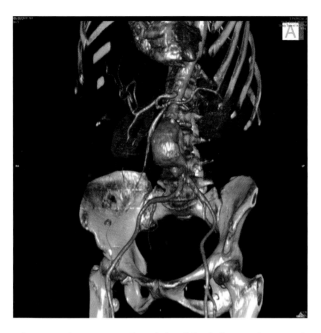

Fig. 6. 3D computed tomography reconstruction of the abdominal aorta demonstrating a large infrarenal abdominal aortic aneurysm.

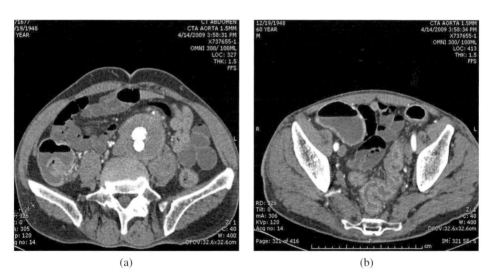

(a)   (b)

Fig. 7. (a) CT angiogram in a patient who presented two weeks after endovascular AAA repair with severe abdominal pain. No evidence of endoleak was present. (b) The abdominal CT scan revealed the source of the abdominal pain to be a diffusely thickened colon consistent with *Clostridium difficile* colitis. The ability to visualize contiguous structures with CT, as well as the vascular structures makes it the imaging modality of choice for suspected aortic pathology.

thrombosis or embolism within the mesenteric arteries can be achieved with a high degree of sensitivity and specificity. In patients with acute mesenteric ischemia, CTA is the initial procedure of choice for rapid diagnosis. When acute embolization to the superior mesenteric artery occurs, the occlusion is most commonly encountered distal to the middle colic artery origin with minimal collateralization present. In patients with chronic mesenteric ischemia, the celiac trunk, superior mesenteric artery, and inferior mesenteric artery can be accurately visualized for either stenosis or occlusion. In these patients, more abundant collaterals are present and the region of stenosis and/or occlusion is at the level of the vessel origin at the aorta. Calcification in the visceral and renal arteries may sometimes cause artifact, which may obscure the vessel lumen. In these cases, conventional angiography may provide additional information regarding the true degree of arterial occlusive disease. Associated findings such as bowel wall thickening, dilatation, and perforation can also be visualized accurately with CTA.

4.1.2 *Magnetic resonance angiography*

MRA also provides excellent visualization of the thoracic and abdominal aortas, and iliac arteries for all the indications mentioned above (Fig. 8). MRA has lower spatial resolution and image acquisition times can be longer compared with CTA. Recent multicenter controlled trials, however, have found equivalent sensitivity and specificity when compared to digital subtraction angiography for evaluation of renal

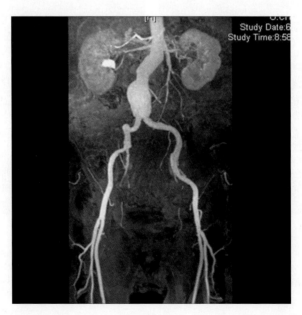

Fig. 8. Magnetic resonance angiography of the abdomen demonstrating the presence of an infrarenal abdominal aortic aneurysm.

artery stenosis. Because patients with RAS frequently present with moderate to severe renal dysfunctions, the avoidance of the large boluses of iodinated contrast associated favors MRA. However, in patients with Stages IV and V chronic kidney disease, MRA should be avoided over the concerns of associated nephrogenic systemic fibrosis. Conventional angiography is likely the best imaging modality in these cases.

Because arterial calcification is not visualized, reliably assessing areas of stenosis within the visceral and renal arteries may be easier with MRA compared with CTA. However, preoperative knowledge of the extent of aortic calcification may be useful for planning both endovascular and open interventions of the thoracic and abdominal aortas. Longer scan times compared with CTA make MRA less favorable for acute aortic pathology.

4.1.3 *Conventional angiography*

Conventional angiography provides superior resolution images of the flow lumen within the thoracic and abdominal aortas, their branches, and the iliac arteries (Figs. 9(a) and 9(b)). However, for the evaluation of aortoiliac pathology, CTA and MRA are initially preferred because the aortic wall and contiguous structures are visualized. For example, in patients with AAA, conventional angiography provides information regarding the size and integrity of the aortic lumen but excludes any visualization of mural thrombus or aortic wall pathology. Angiography is especially unreliable for patients with aortic dissection, because distinct imaging of both the true and false lumens cannot be achieved as accurately as either CTA or MRA. This

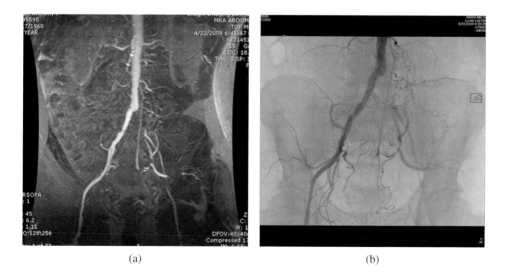

(a)   (b)

Fig. 9. A comparison of MRA (9a) and DSA (9b) in the same patient with a left common iliac occlusion.

technique does, however, provide the opportunity to intervene simultaneously (*i.e.* placement of a proximal balloon for vascular control during ruptured AAA, *etc.*) and cannot be performed during other noninvasive studies.

DSA is the gold standard and provides the best resolution for accurately imaging stenoses of the visceral and renal arteries. The ability to perform balloon angioplasty and stenting is another advantage. In patients with mesenteric ischemia, it is preferable to perform either CTA or MRA prior to invasive imaging, because the extent of visceral organ involvement can be imaged simultaneously. Findings such as bowel thickening and dilatation, mesenteric edema, and free peritoneal fluid cannot be visualized with conventional angiography.

4.2 *Lower limb peripheral arterial disease*

4.2.1 *Computed tomography angiography*

In most cases, DSA remains the gold standard for evaluating infrainguinal PAD; however, CTA and MRA provide excellent and noninvasive alternatives. The advent of multidetector CTA has enhanced its use dramatically in the diagnosis of lower extremity peripheral arterial disease. In a recent meta-analysis of 909 studies comparing CTA with DSA, the sensitivity of CTA for detecting more than 50% stenosis or occlusion was 95% and the specificity was 96%. The ability to visualize the extent of arterial calcifications and the ability to perform multiplanar reconstructions are additional advantages over conventional angiography. Patients with previously placed peripheral stents are better evaluated with CTA compared with MRA because of the associated signal dropout seen with the latter. In our experience, this technique is especially useful in patients with suspected vascular trauma because of rapid scan times and the ability to evaluate simultaneously the intracranial, intrathoracic, or intraabdominal injuries.

4.2.2 *Magnetic resonance angiography*

MRA provides several advantages over CTA for evaluating infrainguinal arterial occlusive disease. (Figs. 10(a) and 10(b)). As mentioned prior, no radiation exposure or iodinated contrast is required. Newer advancements such as time-resolved imaging of contrast kinetics (TRICKS) has been shown to enhance visualization of the popliteal and infrapopliteal arteries when compared to DSA. TRICKS-MRA is a newly available method of data acquisition that eliminates the need for bolus-chase techniques and permits high spatial and temporal resolution with the elimination of venous-phase contamination. In a recent study, this technique correctly identified significant disease of the popliteal artery with a sensitivity of 94% and a specificity of 92%. Disease of the tibial arteries was imaged with a sensitivity and specificity of

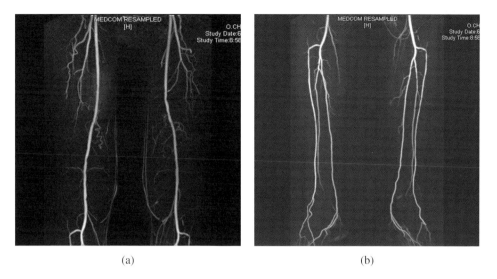

(a)   (b)

Fig. 10. MRA demonstrating the femoropopliteal and tibial arteries. There is no evidence of peripheral arterial occlusive disease in this patient.

100% and 84%, respectively. Patients with peripheral stents, advanced renal disease, and implanted pacemakers and defibrillators should avoid MRA for reasons already mentioned.

4.3 *Extracranial carotid and vertebral arteries*

4.3.1 *Computed tomography angiography*

CTA is an excellent study for evaluation of the extracranial carotid arteries. Sixty-four-section CTA can be performed from the aortic arch through the intracranial vessels at submillimeter collimation in 3–4 seconds. Postprocessing techniques can produce 3D reconstructions using a variety of algorithms. With 64-section MDCT, the timing of bolus administration becomes critical since acquisition times can be faster than the flow of contrast-opacified blood. Visualization of both the plaque and vessel lumen is readily achieved. Potential sources of artifact include stents in the great vessels, dental hardware, and venous contamination. Severe calcification can obscure evaluation of the vessel lumen in high-grade stenoses.

4.3.2 *Magnetic resonance angiography*

MRA also provides an excellent and noninvasive imaging modality for imaging the extracranial carotid arteries. This technique can achieve excellent sensitivity and specificity for evaluating carotid artery pathology and for planning both carotid stent and open carotid reconstructions. Advantages include an increased number of

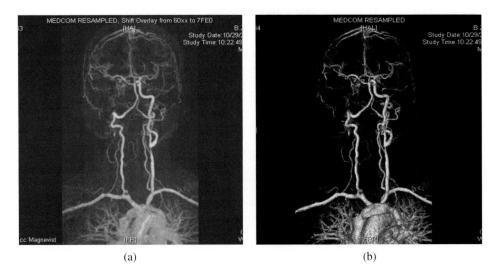

(a)   (b)

Fig. 11. MRA of the extracranial carotid arteries (11a) with the corresponding 3D reconstruction (11b).

projections and high spatial resolution, which allow the visualization of the aortic arch to the circle of Willis. Increasingly shortened acquisition times and enhanced postprocessing techniques proved detailed pictures of the cerebrovascular circulation. (Figs. 11(a) and 11(b)). Aortic arch and branch calcifications are not visualized with MRA, which may be a limitation in patients being preoperatively evaluated for carotid stenting. In these patients, as well as patients with pacemakers, metallic implants, and prior stents, CTA is the preferred imaging test.

4.3.3 *Conventional angiography*

DSA remains the gold standard for imaging the extracranial carotid and vertebral arteries; however, a small but substantial stroke risk exists compared with noninvasive imaging. (Fig. 12). This technique provides the highest spatial and temporal resolution for determining accurately the degree of vessel stenosis. Noninvasive studies of the carotid arteries (duplex, MRA, and CTA) are usually performed for planning both endovascular and open carotid interventions in most patients prior to conventional angiography. Arch and carotid angiography is performed routinely in conjunction with carotid angioplasty stenting procedures.

4.4 *Venous system*

4.4.1 *Computed tomography venography*

The contrast bolus administered during MD-CT can be timed for delayed opacification to visualize accurately the entire venous system. Timing parameters can also be

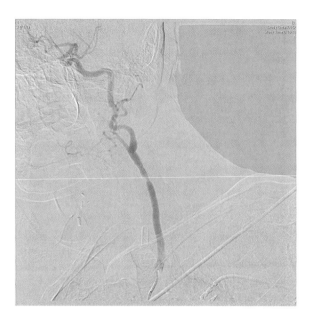

Fig. 12. Digital subtraction angiogram of the carotid arteries demonstrates a critical stenosis in the left common carotid artery. This was later treated with angioplasty and stenting.

set for scanning of both the arterial and venous phases during the same examination. Although duplex scanning is generally the initial test of choice for assessment of the peripheral veins of the upper and lower extremities, CT venography (CTV) can be used to image the deep veins of the thorax, abdomen, and pelvis, which are not readily amenable to ultrasound scanning. This technique can be used for accurate diagnosis of portal and mesenteric vein thromboses. As with mesenteric ischemia from arterial insufficiency, abnormalities in the abdominal viscera and solid organs can also be assessed. Other features such as engorgement of mesenteric veins and mesenteric edema can be clearly visualized. Imaging of both the superior and inferior venae cavae and their major branches can also be performed with excellent spatial and temporal resolutions in multiple planes allowing for high-quality image reconstructions.

4.4.2 *Magnetic resonance venography*

3D contrast-enhanced MR venography provides similarly sensitive and specific imaging of both the central and peripheral venous systems compared with CTV. Some advantages of MRV include the more favorable safety profile of gadolinium compared with iodinated agents, the lack of exposure to ionizing radiation, and the increased ease of 3D reconstruction. CTV is favored in patients with advanced renal disease due to concerns over NSF. Spatial resolution of MRV is generally lower compared with that of computed tomography and overestimation of vessel stenosis

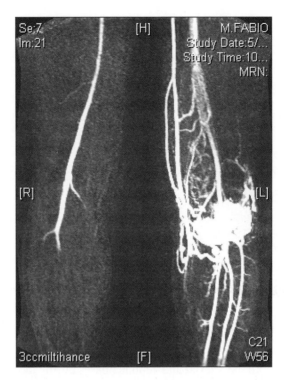

Fig. 13.   MRA is useful for delineating the anatomy of peripheral arteriovenous malformations as shown in this image.

severity may occur due to turbulence-related signal degradation. Scan times are also generally longer than CTV.

MRV of the peripheral veins can be used as an adjunct to duplex scanning for more comprehensive evaluation of both the deep and superficial venous systems of the upper and lower extremities. It is useful for detailed noninvasive evaluation of arteriovenous malformations, fistulas, and venous aneurysms and in the preoperative planning for both open and endovascular procedures. MRV (as well as CTV) can also be used to evaluate malformations associated with a variety of peripheral venous disorders including Klippel–Trenaunay and Sturge–Weber syndromes (Fig. 13).

4.4.3 *Conventional angiography*

Due to the superior applicability of the aforementioned noninvasive imaging modalities, conventional venography is generally reserved for use with planned endovascular treatment of venous pathology. Common interventions include placement of vena cava filters, recanalization of acute and chronic venous occlusions, angioplasty and stenting, thrombolysis, and coil embolization.

References

Barth A, Arnold M, Mattle HP, *et al.* Contrast-enhanced 3-D MRA in decision making for carotid endarterectomy: A 6-year experience, *Cerebrovasc Dis* 2006; **21**:393–400.

Borisch I, Horn M, Butz B, *et al.* Preoperative evaluation of carotid artery stenosis: Comparison of contrast-enhanced MR angiography and duplex xonography with digital subtraction angiography, *Am J Neuroradiol* 2003; **24**:1117–1122.

Bradbury MS, Kavanagh PV, Bechtold RE, *et al.* Mesenteric venous thrombosis: Diagnosis and non-invasive imaging, *Radiographics* 2002; **22**:527–541.

Chan D, Anderson ME, Dolmatch BL. Imaging evaluation of lower extremity infrainguinal disease: Role of the noninvasive vascular laboratory, computed tomography angiography, and magnetic resonance angiography, *Tech Vasc Intervent Radiol* 2009; **13**:11–22.

Heijenbrok-Kal MH, Kock MCJM, Hunink MGM. Lower extremity arterial disease: Multidetector CT angiography-meta-analysis, 2007; **245**:433–439.

Horton KM, Fishman EK. Multidetector CT angiography in the diagnosis of mesenteric ischemia, 2007; **45**:275–288.

Kalva SP, Mueller PR. Vascular imaging in the elderly, *Radiol Clin N Am* 2008; **46**:663–683.

Lakshminarayan R, Simpson JO, Ettles DF. Magnetic resonance angiography: Current status in the planning and follow up of endovascular treatment in lower-limb arterial disease, *Cardiovasc Intervent Radiol* 2009; **32**:397–405.

Met R, Bipat S, Legemate DA, Reekers JA, Koelemay MJW. Diagnostic performance of computed tomography angiography in peripheral arterial disease: A systematic review and meta-analysis, *JAMA* 2009; **301**:415–424.

Muhlenbruch G, Das M, Mommertz G, *et al.* Comparison of dual-source CT angiography and MR angiography in preoperative evaluation of intra- and extracranial vessels: A pilot study, *Eur Radiol* 2010; **20**:469–476.

Rogalla P, Kloeters C, Hein PA. CT technology overview: 64-slice and beyond, *Radiol Clin N Am* 2009; **47**:1–11.

Shah DJ, Brown B, Kim RJ, *et al.* Magnetic resonance evaluation of peripheral arterial disease, *Cardiol Clin* 2007; **25**:185–212.

Shareghi S, Gopal A, Gul K, *et al.* Diagnostic accuracy of 64 multidetector computed tomographic angiography in peripheral vascular disease, *Catheter Cardiovasc Interv* 2010; **75**:23–31.

Shih MCP, Hagspiel KD. CTA and MRA in mesenteric ischemia: Part I, Role in diagnosis and differential diagnosis, *AJR Am J Roentgenol* 2007; **188**:452–461.

Yoo SM, Lee HY, White CS. MDCT evaluation of acute aortic syndrome, *Radiol Clin N Am* 2010; **48**:67–83.

Yu T, Zhu X, Tang L, *et al.* Review of CT angiography of aorta, *Radiol Clin N Am* 2007; **45**:461–483.

Chapter 5

Management of Extracranial Cerebrovascular Disease

Wesley S. Moore

Learning Objectives

- Provide background information regarding thrombo-embolic cerebral infarction (stroke).
- Discuss related pathology and pathogenetic mechanisms of stroke and associate it with extracranial cerebrovascular disease.
- Review risk factors and their options for modification.
- Outline essentials of patient workup.
- Outline treatment options for primary stroke prevention and results.

1. Stroke Facts

Stroke is the third leading cause of death in the United States and is the number one leading cause of adult disability. There are approximately 700,000 new strokes recorded in the United States each year. Approximately 70% of strokes are ischemic and are related to thrombo-embolic phenomena. The remainder are hemorrhagic. In the past, anywhere from 40 to 60% of ischemic strokes could be traced to disease in the extra-cranial carotid and vertebral arteries. This number has now dropped to about 10% due to a variety of factors, which may include better medical management of risk factors and the steady removal of patients from the pool of those with extracranial cerebrovascular disease by their identification and surgical correction of appropriate lesions. At the present time, approximately 150,000 patients undergo carotid endarterectomy or other interventional procedures each year. This number has been steadily increasing since the 1960s, when carotid endarterectomy began to become performed more frequently.

2. Pathology of Extracranial Cerebrovascular Disease

Atherosclerosis accounts for more than 90% of the pathology seen in the extracranial vessels of patients studied in the United States and Europe. Less common lesions include fibromuscular dysplasia of the internal carotid arteries, and arteritis, of which Takayasu's arteritis is its most common manifestation.

Atherosclerotic lesions are most typically located in the bulb of the internal carotid artery. It is thought that this anatomic location has a propensity for the formation of an atherosclerotic plaque due to turbulence and increased boundary layer separation, which is related to its normal anatomic dilatation. Plaques in this location can contain a mixture of calcific, lipid, and thrombotic components. Other anatomic locations for atherosclerotic plaques include the origin of the supra-aortic trunks, including the innominate, innominate bifurcation, left common carotid, and left subclavian arteries. The origin of the vertebral arteries can also be involved in the atherosclerotic process. These lesions are typically within the subclavian arteries and encroach upon the ostia of the vertebral arteries.

Fibromuscular dysplasia involves the cervical internal carotid artery anywhere from its origin to the base of the skull. Four variations have been described, which include intimal fibroplasia, medial hyperplasia, medial fibroplasia, and paramedial dysplasia. Of these, the medial fibroplasia is the most common type. Angiographically, it appears as a "chain of lakes" created by a series of septae along the course of the lesion.

Takayasu's arteritis typically involves the supra-aortic trunks and usually stops short of the carotid bifurcation. The lesion is firm and rubbery, and during the acute phase will have a giant cell and lymphocyte infiltration into the media of these large vessels. During the chronic phase, the inflammatory infiltrate is gone, leaving behind a chronic stenotic or occluded major trunk.

Other abnormalities that can involve the extracranial vasculature include redundancy of the carotid arteries producing coiling or kinking. Coils are usually asymptomatic unless associated with an atherosclerotic plaque in a critical location. Kinking may become symptomatic with head turning, resulting in temporary reduction of flow through the internal carotid artery.

Rarely, aneurysms of the cervical internal carotid artery can be found. Most often these are associated with fibromuscular dysplasia.

Patients who have undergone radiation therapy for cervical malignancies are at increased risk of developing radiation-associated atherosclerosis of the carotid arteries.

3. Pathogenetic Mechanisms of Cerebral Ischemic Events

The most common mechanism for a cerebral ischemic event, either transient or permanent, is related to thrombo-embolism. A less common mechanism for ischemic symptoms is the presence of a hemodynamically significant stenosis in an extracranial artery that slowly and progressively reduces flow through that vessel. The reason that this is less common is the fact that the cerebral circulation has abundant collateral primarily through the interrelationships involved in the Circle of Willis.

An atherosclerotic plaque in the bulb of the internal carotid artery has a strategic relationship relative to thromboembolic phenomenon as it affects the ipsilateral hemisphere. If the plaque in the internal carotid artery goes on to sudden occlusion of that vessel, there can be thrombotic propagation of the internal carotid artery to occlude the middle cerebral artery. Since the internal carotid artery is essentially an unbranched vessel, with the exception of the ophthalmic artery, thrombotic propagation from a sudden occlusion of the internal carotid artery can result in either a transient ischemic event or cerebral infarction. If flow reversal takes place in the ophthalmic artery and/or if other flow is contributed to the middle cerebral artery through the Circle of Willis, then the thrombotic propagation may not pass the ophthalmic artery, and occlusion of the internal carotid artery can be a silent event.

If the intimal covering of a plaque in the internal carotid artery ruptures, then the contents from the atherosclerotic plaque can be released into the circulation of the internal carotid artery and be carried to smaller arteries, usually in the distribution of the middle cerebral artery. If the embolic material that is released is thrombotic in nature, it can undergo breakup and thrombolysis resulting in temporary rather than permanent damage. On the other hand, if the embolic fragment is made up of cholesterol or calcific atherosclerotic material, it is unlikely that this will break up, and certainly will not undergo lysis. Therefore, the size of the embolic fragment as well as its composition will depend upon the extent of the ischemic damage.

Once there has been discharge of atheromatous debris from the plaque, a defect is left within the plaque. This defect, on angiography, will appear to be a punched-out area reminiscent of an ulcer. An ulcerated plaque can be a source of continued embolization from the plaque itself, or it can be a location for platelet aggregate or thrombotic material to reside. If the platelet aggregate or thrombotic material, resting within an ulcer crater, is dislodged, then this can be a source of secondary embolization with further ischemic damage.

Atherosclerotic plaques can remain stable over many years, or they can slowly develop an increase in atherosclerotic burden compromising the flow lumen. On occasion, hemorrhage can occur within the substance of the atherosclerotic plaque, which will cause the plaque to suddenly expand. The expansion can be the cause of intimal rupture with embolization, or can be the cause of a sudden occlusion of the internal carotid artery.

4. Risk Factors Associated with Ischemic Stroke

The risk factors associated with symptomatic extracranial arterial occlusive disease are primarily those associated with atherosclerosis in general. These include (1) cigarette smoking, (2) advancing age, (3) hypertension, (4) diabetes mellitus, (5) hyperlipidemia, or (6) the identification of atherosclerosis in another anatomic region.

The presence of multiple risk factors has an exponential effect on the development of extracranial cerebrovascular atherosclerotic disease.

5. Symptomatic Manifestations of Extracranial Cerebrovascular Disease

The two principal manifestations of extracranial cerebrovascular disease are transient ischemic attacks (TIA) and infarction (stroke). Infarction can take place in either the retina or the brain.

Transient ischemic attacks can occur in the retina or the brain. When it occurs in the retina, there is a characteristic shade that partially covers the visual field of one eye. The shade can come from above down, from below up, or from one side to the other, depending upon which branch of the retinal artery is the recipient of an embolic fragment. If the embolic material breaks up and is carried through the microcirculation, then the episode of visual disturbance will last for only seconds or minutes. If the embolic fragment is large and occludes a principal branch of the retinal artery, this will result in retinal infarction in the distribution of that vessel. Similar phenomenon can occur in the brain. For example, if emboli are released from plaque of the internal carotid artery, those emboli can be carried up to the distribution of the internal carotid artery, usually the middle cerebral artery or the anterior cerebral artery. If the emboli pass out through the middle cerebral artery, then the neurologic manifestations can be either sensory or motor or a combination of the two. Depending upon when part of the cortex is affected, this can result in a monoplegia or hemiplegia. Likewise, if this occurs in the dominant hemisphere and the embolus goes to the part of the cortex that controls speech, the result can be an expressive dysphasia. On occasion it can also cause a receptive aphasia or difficulty with expression with writing, dysgraphia. Once again, if the emboli are relatively small and break up, the neurologic events can last a matter of minutes to a few hours. By definition, if the event lasts more than 24 hours, it is deemed to have caused permanent damage or infarction. Recent studies with better imaging techniques suggest that a TIA is actually a small infarct with a good functional recovery. Larger infarcts can also be associated with a good functional recovery depending upon collateral circulation and the age of the patient. Younger patients have greater recovery potential due to increased plasticity of the brain as opposed to older patients, in whom recovery is less likely.

Transient ischemic attacks can also be the result of a temporary drop in bloodflow to an affected area. This can occur in the presence of a high-grade stenosis and a transient drop in systemic pressure resulting in malperfusion of the retina or a portion of the hemisphere.

Malperfusion and embolization can also take place in the posterior circulation as a result of disease in the subclavian-vertebral system. These events can involve sensory, motor, or cranial nerve dysfunction. Occasionally, the symptoms can be nonfocal with symptoms such as dizziness or vertigo. These symptoms, however, are relatively common and are most likely caused by something other than vertebrobasilar flow dysfunction.

6. Evaluation of the Patient with Cerebrovascular Disease

6.1 *History*

Perhaps the most important part of the evaluation of patients with cerebrovascular disease is a careful history. The history should be obtained not only from the patient, but also from a close relative such as a spouse. One of the manifestations of chronic cerebrovascular disease is memory impairment, which will limit the accuracy of history taken from the patient. Having the spouse in the room at the same time that history is obtained is extremely helpful. The history should include directed questions as to whether or not the patient has experienced manifestations of symptomatic cerebrovascular disease and, if so, to what degree has the patient been physically limited by one or more events. The history should also include careful documentation of associated risk factors. A smoking history is of importance. A simple question of "Do you smoke?" is often answered by saying no. The next question should be "When did you quit?" and the occasional answer to that question is "Yesterday". Besides a smoking history, documentation of hypertension under treatment, diabetes mellitus, or other manifestations of atherosclerosis such as symptomatic coronary artery disease and peripheral vascular disease should be noted. Finally, it should be kept in mind that advancing age is also a risk factor.

6.2 *Physical examination*

In addition to a general physical examination, blood pressure should always be obtained in both arms. This may be the first clue that there is associated subclavian arterial occlusive disease if there is an important difference in blood pressure between the two arms. The presence of documented subclavian disease can also suggest that other arch vessels such as the left common carotid or innominate arteries may be involved as well. A careful pulse examination beginning with the presence and quality of the carotid pulses should be documented. If there is a difference in pulse amplitude between the two sides, this can also suggest proximal arch vessel occlusive disease. The carotid artery should be checked for the presence of a bruit. Patients with aortic valve disease can often radiate a valve murmur into the carotid arteries and be confused with the presence of a bruit. In order to differentiate between a radiated murmur from an intrinsic plaque-producing bruit in the carotid artery, auscultation should begin at the base of the neck and extend up to the angle of the jaw. Isolated carotid bruits will be best heard over the carotid bifurcation, but the location of that anatomically can vary. Not every bruit means that there is significant disease in the carotid artery, and patients can have significant carotid artery disease without a bruit. Some of the loudest bruits are caused by stenoses of the external carotid artery, which are usually of no clinical consequence. Occasionally this can be picked up by palpating the temporal pulses to see if there is an amplitude difference between the two sides. Once examination of the carotid arteries is complete, palpation of the subclavian arteries as well as auscultation in the supraclavicular fossi is helpful in detecting the presence of occlusive disease in that distribution. The brachial, radial, and ulnar pulses should also be checked. Finally, lower extremity pulsation including femoral, popliteal, dorsalis pedis, and posterior tibial pulses should be examined as abnormalities in that area would indicate the associated finding of peripheral arterial occlusive disease, which is clearly a risk factor for cerebrovascular disease.

In patients who have symptomatic cerebrovascular disease, a basic neurologic examination should be carried out. Even though the history may suggest a transient ischemic event, if there is residual abnormality on neurologic examination this will indicate that, in fact, a cerebral infarction has taken place. Motor examinations of the upper and lower extremities are particularly helpful, as well as checking for a pronator drift. This is done by having the patient extend their hands and supinate both hands while asking the patient to keep that position. Patients who have had an infarction will tend to rotate from supination to pronation involuntarily. This pronator drift is perhaps one of the more subtle findings of prior infarction.

6.3 *Noninvasive testing*

The principal noninvasive test utilized in the diagnosis of extracranial cerebrovascular disease is the duplex scan. A duplex scan combines B-mode imaging of the artery of interest and allows the sonographer to place a Doppler beam in the center of the artery in order to assess velocity. Areas of stenoses are identified by a velocity acceleration through the stenotic region, and the ratio of the peak systolic velocity through the stenotic lesion when compared with the velocity proximal to the lesion allows the sonographer to identify a percent stenosis. The problem with duplex scanning is that it is both machine- and technician-dependent. Therefore, it is very important that one have confidence in the laboratory in which the duplex scan is performed. If there is a high level of confidence, the duplex scan can be a stand-alone study and may be sufficient for preoperative planning. If there is any question regarding the accuracy of the duplex scan, then a second study should be employed. Studies can include MR angiography with gadolinium enhancement and CT angiography. MR angiography notoriously overestimates the percent of stenosis in the extracranial vessels. However, imaging of the intracranial vessels is quite accurate using this modality. CT angiography is also quite accurate, but has the disadvantage of requiring a large intravenous contrast infusion, which may be detrimental to the patient, particularly those with compromised renal function or diabetes. In the past, intra-arterial contrast angiography was required for diagnosis and was considered the gold standard. With improvements in noninvasive technology, catheter-based intra-arterial contrast angiography is rarely required.

Imaging of the brain is usually not required in the asymptomatic patient. However, patients who have had transient ischemic attacks or a completed stroke should undergo either CT or MRI to investigate the brain, the extent of any damage, and alternative diagnoses. Occasionally, intracranial masses such as brain tumors can present as transient ischemic episodes. While the coexistence of extracranial carotid artery disease and a brain tumor is rare, it does happen, and serious clinical errors in management can occur if both are not identified.

7. Treatment

The objective of treatment of patients with extracranial cerebrovascular disease is either the primary prevention of stroke or the secondary prevention of recurrent stroke. To this end, a combination of medical and interventional management has been well documented to achieve significant reduction of stroke risk.

7.1 *Medical management*

The medical management of patients with documented extracranial cerebrovascular disease involves, first of all, risk factor reduction. This includes cessation of tobacco exposure, careful control of blood pressure, and tight control of diabetes mellitus. Patients with documented atherosclerosis of the extracranial cerebral vessels by definition have generalized atherosclerosis. Therefore, they should be on statin drugs irrespective of their cholesterol levels. Statins, in addition to lowering serum cholesterol levels, also have an anti-inflammatory effect, which may be more important for plaque stabilization. Patients who have experienced one or more transient ischemic attacks who were found to have only modest stenoses in the appropriate extracranial vessel, should be tried initially on antiplatelet drugs. The simplest and cheapest antiplatelet drug is low-dose aspirin. There is a category of patients who are aspirin resistant, and this is most often seen among women. In cases of aspirin resistance, the use of clopidogrel (Plavix) is advisable. Aggrenox is a drug that combines aspirin and Persantine, and in recent trials has been found to be quite effective. It can be reasonably argued that patients with documented extracranial arterial occlusive disease, in the absence of symptoms, should also be placed on aspirin. The use of Warfarin (Coumadin) in patients with symptomatic carotid artery disease has been extensively studied and found to be of no benefit. The only absolute indication for the use of Warfarin is in patients with atrial fibrillation in order to prevent thromboembolic complications of cardiac origin.

7.2 Surgical management of the carotid artery

7.2.1 Indications for carotid endarterectomy

Carotid endarterectomy can be indicated for patients who are asymptomatic as well as for those who are symptomatic. The objective for operating on the asymptomatic patient is to prevent a high-grade stenosis of the bulb of the internal carotid artery from going on to total occlusion or intimal rupture with dislodgement of atherosclerotic content resulting in ischemic stroke. A high-grade stenosis can be defined as a diameter-reducing lesion of 60% or greater when using contrast angiography or the highest grade stenosis using duplex ultrasound criteria. Patients who are experiencing symptoms in the territory of the internal carotid artery in question, such as a stroke over the last six months with good functional recovery, hemispheric transient ischemic attacks, or ipsilateral transient monocular blindness, particularly if these symptoms occurred or persist while on optimal medical management, are also candidates for carotid endarterectomy. This is particularly true if the lesion of the internal carotid artery has a diameter-reducing stenosis of 70% or greater by contrast angiography or 50% or greater when the symptoms are not controlled on antiplatelet therapy.

7.2.2 Preoperative preparation

Patients who are considered for carotid endarterectomy should have their hypertension well controlled, be on a statin medication, be receiving either an ACE inhibitor or a beta blocker, and be taking an antiplatelet agent. Patients with carotid bifurcation disease also have a high likelihood of concurrent coronary artery disease, and therefore their heart should be carefully evaluated for the presence of a critical lesion that may require treatment prior to carotid endarterectomy.

7.2.3 *Anesthesia and perioperative monitoring*

Carotid endarterectomy can be performed using either cervical block (local) anesthesia or general endotracheal anesthesia. At the present time, most surgeons favor general anesthesia because of considerations of patient comfort, a stable operative field, good airway management, and oxygenation during operation. It had been assumed that there would be fewer cardiac events under local anesthesia. However, clinical trials have failed to demonstrate a difference between local and general anesthesia with respect to cardiac complications. An arterial line should be inserted in the radial artery for continuous blood pressure monitoring as well as for intermittent blood gas measurement. Careful management of blood pressure during operation is of great importance in that hypotension should be avoided, particularly during clamping of the carotid artery, as well as uncontrolled hypertension.

7.2.4 *Surgical technique*

The patient is positioned supine on the operating table with a pad placed under the shoulders to produce a slight neck extension and the head turned away from the side of operation. The potential line of incision is defined as a line extending from the mastoid process to the suprasternal notch along the anterior border of the sternomastoid muscle. The incision is positioned along this line and centered over a point that the surgeon anticipates to be the location of the carotid bifurcation. This can often be marked in advance with the use of carotid ultrasound to designate the location. Alternatively, an oblique incision gently curved toward the mastoid process can also be used and is often thought to result in a more cosmetic scar, but at the expense of potentially compromising proximal exposure.

The incision is carried down through the platysmal layer, and sternomastoid muscle is mobilized off the carotid sheath and held in place with a self-retaining retractor. The jugular vein is identified, and the carotid sheath is entered along the anterior border of the internal jugular vein. The common facial vein as it drains into the internal jugular vein represents an important landmark for the carotid bifurcation. The common facial vein is the venous analog of the external carotid artery, and therefore the carotid bifurcation, most of the time, will lie immediately beneath the common facial vein. The vein is divided between ligatures, and the internal jugular vein is retracted laterally. Care should be taken to identify the vagus nerve as its location can be variable within the carotid sheath. Trauma to the vagus nerve can result in temporary or permanent vocal cord paralysis. The common carotid artery is then identified and circumferentially mobilized within the perivascular plane. Dissection is then carried distally to expose the internal and external carotid arteries. The vessels should be handled gently in this location in order to prevent any loose atheromatous plaque material within the bulb from being dislocated with the result of embolization and intraoperative cerebral infarction. The internal carotid artery, distal to the plaque, is circumferentially mobilized at a point where the vessel is free of atheromatous disease. The external carotid artery is mobilized in a similar manner. In the case of a high carotid bifurcation, it may be necessary to divide the nerve to the carotid sinus in order to allow the carotid bifurcation to be drawn downward and provide additional exposure to the internal carotid artery distally. Once the carotid bifurcation is fully mobilized, intravenous heparin should be administered. The exact heparin dose has not been established and is subject to individual surgeon preference. On the average, 5000 units of heparin intravenously is a reasonable dose. If the patient is on both aspirin and clopidogrel, the dose of heparin should be revised downward in order to minimize bleeding following completion of endarterectomy. At this point, the surgeon has a choice regarding intraoperative circulatory support. The choice includes the routine use of an intraoperative shunt versus selective shunting. If routine shunting is to be employed, no specific neurologic monitoring is required. If selective shunting is the surgeon's choice, and if the patient is under general anesthesia, then some method must be employed to determine which patient will require a shunt for cerebral circulatory support by determining whether or not collateral circulation is adequate during temporary clamping. The most common method for making this determination is the use of intraoperative EEG monitoring. Other techniques include the measurement of internal carotid artery backpressure as a measure of collateral circulation. Other techniques have included measure of transcranial Doppler flow or somatosensory evoked potential measurement. Patients who have had a prior infarction on the side of operation, or those with EEG change during a trial of clamping, are best managed by the placement of a shunt. After the patient has received heparin anticoagulation, the internal, external, and common carotid arteries are clamped. An arteriotomy is begun on the common carotid artery and extended distally, opening the atherosclerotic plaque and extending the arteriotomy onto normal internal carotid artery distally. A dissection plane between the plaque and the adventitia is established circumferentially, and the atherosclerotic plaque is removed optimally with a tapering and feathered endpoint in the internal carotid artery at the distal point of the plaque, and usually with a sharp division of the thickened intima proximally. The plaque is also delivered from the external carotid artery by circumferentially removing this and allowing the clamp on the external carotid artery to define the endpoint. Once the plaque is removed, the luminal surface of the artery is gently irrigated with heparinized saline, and small bits of medial debris are carefully removed. The arteriotomy should then be closed with a patch angioplasty as it has now been well documented that the use of patch angioplasty can reduce the incidence of perioperative neurologic complication as well as reduce the incidence of postoperative recurrent stenosis. Once the arteriotomy has been repaired with a patch angioplasty, flow is restored first to the external, then to the internal carotid artery. It is strongly recommended that the technical result of the operation be documented before completion of the operation. The most direct way to do this is with intraoperative angiography. This will allow the surgeon to look at the technical result of the endarterectomy as well as to examine the intracranial circulation to rule out any intracranial occlusive or aneurysmal disease. Alternative techniques include intraoperative duplex scanning to evaluate the proximal and distal endpoints. Once the surgeon is satisfied that there is a good technical result, the platysmal layer and skin are then closed.

7.2.5 *Postoperative care*

Once the patient awakens from general anesthesia, a neurologic assessment of both hemisphere and cranial nerve function should be carried out. The patient should be observed initially in a post-anesthesia recovery room for neurologic function and blood pressure control. Once it is determined that the patient has returned to baseline, further follow-up can be carried out in a regular hospital room. Intensive care monitoring is no longer routinely required. Antiplatelet drugs should be continued postoperatively, and careful monitoring of blood pressure to avoid either hyper- or hypotension is critical. The patient is usually observed overnight, and if vital signs are stable the following morning, the patient can be discharged. The first visit postoperatively is usually approximately three weeks after operation. At this time the incision can be checked, and a postoperative duplex scan can be obtained to provide the new baseline for subsequent follow-up. The next visit should be in six months, when a second duplex scan is obtained. This is done because, if the patient is going to develop intimal hyperplasia, this usually occurs within a period of six months to a year and should be identified. The next duplex scan can be done at the 12-month visit, and yearly thereafter.

7.3 *Surgical management of the vertebral artery*

Operations directed toward the vertebral artery are relatively rare. Lesions in the vertebral artery can occur at its origin or anywhere along the course of the vertebral artery up to the point where the vessel enters the base of the skull. Lesions at the origin of the vertebral artery are actually within the subclavian artery and encroach upon its origin. The simplest way to remove a lesion of the origin of the vertebral artery is through a subclavian approach. The subclavian artery is mobilized through a supraclavicular incision. The vessel is clamped proximal and distal to the vertebral artery, and a longitudinal arteriotomy is made opposite the vertebral artery orifice. An endarterectomy plane is developed, and the orifice of the vertebral artery can be cleared. The arteriotomy in the subclavian artery can then be closed primarily. Alternatively, the vertebral artery can be transected and reimplanted into the side of the common carotid artery through the same incision. Many surgeons prefer this approach, although it is a more complicated operation. Lesions in the distal vertebral artery cannot be approached directly because of the intravertebral course of the vertebral artery. The alternative is to carry out a bypass to the vertebral artery as it emerges from the intravertebral canal at the level of C2. This is a very specialized procedure and is only done by a few surgeons.

7.4 Surgical management of the aortic arch trunks

The innominate artery, the left common carotid artery, and the left subclavian artery are also subject to the development of hemodynamically significant atherosclerotic plaques. Of all the locations for atherosclerosis in the extracranial circulation, arch vessel occlusive disease accounts for about 6.0% of the lesions. Of these, a lesion of the left subclavian artery is the most common. Most of the time these lesions are asymptomatic. On occasion, a high-grade stenosis at the origin of the left subclavian artery will result in flow reversal of the vertebral artery as the vertebral artery then becomes a collateral to the subclavian circulation. On occasion, this can result in either symptoms of arm ischemia or, with the exercise of the arm, symptoms of inadequate flow in the distribution of the vertebrobasilar system. The so-called symptomatic subclavian steal syndrome can be treated by restoration of flow to the subclavian artery. This is best accomplished by either providing a bypass from the left common carotid artery to the subclavian artery or transposing the subclavian, proximal to the vertebral artery, to the side of the common carotid artery. Symptomatic lesions of the innominate artery are best approached through a median sternotomy, with a graft being placed on the ascending aorta and bypass to the innominate bifurcation. Lesions at the origin of the left common carotid artery can be treated with an extrathoracic approach by placing a graft from the right common carotid artery, passing the graft retropharyngeal, and anastomozing it to the left common carotid artery in an end-to-side fashion. Alternatively, if there is no disease in the left subclavian artery, then the left common carotid artery can be transected and reimplanted onto the side of the subclavian artery.

7.5 *Endovascular surgical management of carotid bifurcation and the aortic arch trunks*

The use of balloon angioplasty with stent placement has recently emerged as an alternative to direct surgical repair of lesions of the extracranial cerebral circulation. These techniques can be applied to the lesions of the bulb of the internal carotid artery, the origin of the innominate artery, the left common carotid artery, and the left subclavian artery. Most commonly, arterial access is achieved through a femoral puncture with passage of guidewire into the aortic arch and placement of a sheath at this location. Selective catheterization of the aortic arch trunks can be carried out, and balloon angioplasty and stent placement of appropriate lesions of the origin of the arch vessels can be performed. In the case of carotid bifurcation disease, selective catheterization of the individual carotid artery is carried out. An antiembolism device is then passed distal to the lesion toward the base of the skull in order to trap any large atherosclerotic fragments that are dislodged at the time of balloon angioplasty. A stent is then deployed across the stenotic lesion, and a balloon expanded to dilate the stenotic area to the size appropriate to the stent is carried out. The embolic protection device is then retrieved. Patients undergoing stent angioplasty of the carotid arteries are managed pre- and postoperatively in the same manner as patients undergoing open operation with the exception that double antiplatelet therapy consisting of aspirin and clopidogrel is routinely used. Postprocedure management and follow-up are identical with carotid endarterectomy.

8. Results of Treatment

While there have been multiple publications from individual centers describing the 30-day morbidity, mortality, and long-term follow-up of patients undergoing carotid endarterectomy and carotid angioplasty, the most important data come from prospective randomized trials, which compare carotid endarterectomy to best medical management as well as carotid endarterectomy to carotid angioplasty and stenting.

8.1 *Randomized trials of asymptomatic carotid stenosis*

The first randomized trial comparing carotid endarterectomy with best medical management for asymptomatic carotid stenosis was carried out in the Veterans Administration and reported in 1986. About 444 men with carotid stenosis in excess of 50% occlusive as documented by contrast angiography were randomized to carotid endarterectomy plus medical management versus best medical management alone. The five-year event rate, including composite of TIA, stroke, and death, was 8.0% for carotid endarterectomy versus 20.6% for medical management. This difference was significant at p < 0.001. This benefit in favor of carotid endarterectomy occurred in spite of a relatively high 30-day stroke morbidity and mortality for the operation of 4.3%. The next major trial comparing prophylactic carotid endarterectomy plus best medical management versus best medical management alone was entitled Asymptomatic Carotid Atherosclerosis Study (ACAS) and was sponsored by the National Institutes of Health. The study took place in 34 centers in the United States and Canada. This study is of importance in that it included women, and the endpoints were limited to death and stroke. The study was concluded in 1994. The Data, Safety, and Monitoring Committee called a halt to the study at that point stating that an endpoint had been reached in favor of carotid endarterectomy. About 1662 patients with diameter-reducing stenosis of 60% or greater as measured by contrast angiography were randomly allocated to carotid endarterectomy plus best medical management versus best medical management alone. The aggregate risk of death and stroke over five years was 5.1% for the surgical patients and 11% for those treated medically. This resulted in an absolute risk reduction of 5.9% and a relative risk reduction of 53% in favor of carotid endarterectomy. Furthermore, the perioperative stroke and death rate for carotid endarterectomy was 2.3%. However, this included the risk of preoperative angiography. The risk of a preoperative angiogram was 1.2%. Those patients actually receiving carotid endarterectomy had a 30-day stroke morbidity and mortality of 1.52%. The last asymptomatic randomized trial was entitled the Asymptomatic Carotid Surgery Trial (ACST) and took place primarily in the United Kingdom. The results were reported in 2004. A total of 3128 asymptomatic patients with carotid stenoses >70% as measured by duplex ultrasound were randomized to carotid endarterectomy versus best medical management. The 30-day stroke and death rate for the surgical group was 3.1%. The five-year event rate, including perioperative events, was 6.4% in the surgical group versus 11.8% in the medical group. This difference was statistically significant with p < 0.0001. The results were quite similar to the results reported in ACAS.

8.2 *Randomized trials of symptomatic carotid stenosis*

The first large prospective randomized trial comparing carotid endarterectomy with best medical management was entitled the North American Symptomatic Carotid Endarterectomy Trial (NASCET). This trial entered patients who had carotid stenoses ranging from 30% to 99% occlusive and was stratified to the 30–69% group and the 70–99% group. In February of 1991, a clinical alert was issued by the Data, Safety, and Monitoring Committee, which reported a clear difference in endpoint in the high-grade (70–99%) category. This group was stopped after 295 patients received medical management and 300 patients received surgical management. The 30-day stroke morbidity and mortality for the surgically managed group was 5.0%.

At the end of 18 months of follow-up, the incidence of fatal and nonfatal strokes in the surgical group was 7.0% compared with 24% in the group treated with medical management alone. This represented a 17% absolute risk reduction and a 71% relative risk reduction in favor of patients undergoing carotid endarterectomy. At that time, no clear endpoint had occurred in patients with lesser stenoses. That part of the trial went on to conclusion and was reported in 1998. The trial demonstrated a beneficial effect in favor of surgery. The 30-day mortality and stroke rate was 6.7% in the surgically treated group. The five-year event rate for the surgically treated patients was 15.7% compared with 22% for those treated medically. At the same time that the study was being carried out in North America, a large European trial was being done and sponsored by the Medical Research Council of Great Britain. They stratified their patients into mild stenosis (10–29%), moderate stenosis (30–69%), and severe stenosis (70–99%). This showed no benefit of carotid endarterectomy in the mild stenosis category. Carotid endarterectomy done for patients in the severe category had a clear benefit in favor of endarterectomy. In spite of a higher perioperative stroke morbidity and mortality of 7.5%, there was a sixfold reduction in subsequent strokes over a three-year interval with the difference being statistically significant (p < 0.0001). The final prospective randomized trial among symptomatic patients was started relatively late in the Veterans Administration and stopped early once the NASCET and ECST trial results were reported. With a mean follow-up of 11.9 months, 7.7% of patients randomized to surgical care experienced either a stroke or crescendo TIA. In contrast, patients randomized to medical management alone experienced a 19.4% incidence of stroke or crescendo TIA. The difference was statistically significant (p = 0.01%).

8.3 *Carotid endarterectomy versus carotid angioplasty and stenting*

While there have been several reports of industry-sponsored registry data documenting that carotid angioplasty and stenting was competitive with reports of carotid endarterectomy in randomized trials. However, it must be kept in mind that carotid endarterectomy data from the randomized trials are now approximately 15 years old. Therefore, the important comparative data must come from the current randomized trials, of which there are several. The first prospective randomized trial comparing carotid endarterectomy with carotid angioplasty and stenting was carried out in what was described as a "high-risk" group. High risk can be defined as having major medical comorbidity or high risk due to technical factors such as prior endarterectomy with recurrent stenosis, radiated neck, prior radical neck surgery with tracheostomy, or a high carotid bifurcation. The Stenting and Angioplasty with Protection in Patients at a High Risk for Carotid Endarterectomy (SAPPHIRE) reported their initial results in 2002. About 307 patients were randomly allocated to stenting (156) or carotid endarterectomy (151). This study used as their end-points the conventional death and stroke parameters, but also added, for the first time, myocardial infarction as a primary endpoint. There was no significant difference in the endpoints of death and stroke when one compared stent angioplasty to carotid endarterectomy in this high-risk group. However, when the endpoint of myocardial infarction was added, a statistically significant difference occurred in favor of carotid angioplasty and stenting, with 5.8% of patients undergoing stent angioplasty incurring the combined endpoint and 12.6% of patients undergoing carotid endarterectomy incurring the combined endpoint (p = 0.047). This study has been criticized in that the majority of myocardial infarctions were non-Q wave or chemical in nature, and therefore the impact of that endpoint could not really be compared in severity with such endpoints as stroke and death. The study also compared symptomatic and asymptomatic subgroups, but the study was underpowered to look at any difference, and in fact no difference between the two treatment modalities could be identified in these subcategories. When the two groups were followed out to four years, the event-free survival was equivalent. The next major prospective randomized trial, entitled Endarterectomy Versus Stenting in Patients with Symptomatic Severe Carotid Stenosis (EVA-3S), was reported in 2006. The 30-day event rate of death and stroke following carotid endarterectomy was 3.9% versus 9.6% in patients undergoing angioplasty and stenting. These patients were then followed out to four years, with the difference being maintained at the end of four years in favor of carotid endarterectomy. The event-free survival at the end of four years in patients undergoing carotid endarterectomy was 6.2% compared with 11.1% for those undergoing angioplasty and stenting. The next major trial, carried out in German-speaking countries, was entitled SPACE. The hypothesis that was being tested was that carotid angioplasty and stenting was not inferior to carotid endarterectomy. About 1200 symptomatic patients were randomized. The study was ultimately stopped because of futility analysis, which indicated that the primary hypothesis would be unlikely to be proven. At that time, the 30-day death and stroke rate for carotid angioplasty and stenting was 7.7% versus 6.5% for carotid endarterectomy. The SPACE trial also demonstrated that the incidence of recurrent carotid stenosis was less in carotid endarterectomy, at 4.6% versus 10.7% for carotid angioplasty and stenting. The next trial to report was entitled Carotid Artery Stenting Compared with Endarterectomy in Patients with Symptomatic Carotid Stenosis (ICSS). About 1713 patients drawn from Europe, the UK, Canada, Australia, and New Zealand were randomly allocated to carotid artery stenting (855) or carotid endarterectomy (858). The primary endpoints included stroke, death, or periprocedural myocardial infarction. The results favored carotid endarterectomy. The combined event rates in the endarterectomy group was 5.2% versus 8.5% in the stenting group (p = 0.006). This study also carried out a pre- and post-MR study in a subgroup of patients in order to look at the incidence of both overt and silent brain infarction. The incidence of new infarction in the carotid stenting group was 50% versus 17% in the carotid endarterectomy group. The most recent trial to report, the Carotid Revascularization Endarterectomy versus Stent Trial (CREST), was the largest prospective randomized trial to date. This included both symptomatic and asymptomatic patients and drew upon centers in the United States and Canada. This trial was unique in that they had a rigidly controlled method of selecting highly skilled interventionists to participate in the carotid angioplasty portion of the trial. Individuals who wished to participate had to document abundant experience in angioplasty, and in particular carotid angioplasty, before being considered. Those selected from the initial screening then had to prospectively submit the results of up to 20 carotid angioplasty and stent patients. Once those results were reviewed, and if the Interventional Management Committee found the results to be satisfactory, then and only then could they be permitted to participate in the randomized portion of the study. As a result, only interventionists who had the best technical expertise were allowed to randomize patients and be compared with surgeons performing carotid endarterectomy. About 2502 patients were randomized to either carotid endarterectomy (1240) or carotid angioplasty and stenting with protection (1262). The primary endpoints were death, stroke, and myocardial infarction. The 30-day event rate for carotid endarterectomy was 4.9% versus 5.9% in the angioplasty and stent group. However, this difference was not statistically significant. When the important events of death and stroke were looked at, independent of myocardial infarction, the event rate was 2.6% for carotid endarterectomy versus 4.8% for carotid angioplasty and stenting. This difference was highly statistically significant in favor of carotid endarterectomy, with p = 0.005. It was also found that older patients did better with carotid endarterectomy than stenting. Patients over the age of 70 had better long-term results with carotid endarterectomy, and patients who were younger had better results with angioplasty. Quality of life assessment was also carried out among patients who have had complications. It was determined that stroke had both a physical and a mental component that patients reported as being significant as compared with myocardial infarction, which after a recovery was deemed to be insignificant.

While there have been a number of registries reporting results of angioplasty, the Society for Vascular Surgery responding to the Center for Medicare and Medicaid Services Mandate established a registry not only for carotid angioplasty and stenting but also for carotid endarterectomy from institutions doing both procedures. This registry provided a unique opportunity to compare the results of both techniques. The registry recorded the results of 645 symptomatic patients undergoing carotid angioplasty and stenting and compared them with 506 symptomatic patients undergoing carotid endarterectomy. The combined event rates of death, stroke, and myocardial infarction were 7.13% for carotid angioplasty and stenting versus 3.75%

for carotid endarterectomy. The difference was significant, with p = 0.014. About 805 asymptomatic patients underwent carotid angioplasty and stenting and were compared with 606 asymptomatic patients undergoing carotid endarterectomy. The combined event rates of death, stroke, and myocardial infarction were reported to be 4.6% in patients undergoing angioplasty and stenting versus 1.97% in patients undergoing carotid endarterectomy. The difference was statistically significant, with p = 0.003. Similar comparisons were also available from the National Hospital Discharge Database for the target year 2005. The morbidity and mortality for patients undergoing carotid endarterectomy who were asymptomatic was 1.2% versus patients undergoing carotid angioplasty and stenting at 1.9%. For symptomatic patients, the event rate was 3.1% for carotid endarterectomy versus 7.7% for those undergoing carotid angioplasty and stenting. It was also noteworthy that the cost of carotid angioplasty and stenting was more expensive than carotid endarterectomy. The average charge for asymptomatic patients undergoing carotid endarterectomy was $21,700 versus $32,400 for angioplasty and stenting. In symptomatic patients, the cost of carotid endarterectomy was $37,000 versus $63,000 for angioplasty and stenting.

Therefore, at this particular point in time, carotid endarterectomy continues to hold an edge over angioplasty and stenting with respect to both stroke morbidity and mortality and cost.

References

Berguer R. Surgical reconstruction of the supra-aortic trunks and vertebral arteries. Chapter 36 In: Wesley S. Moore MD (Ed.), *Vascular and Endovascular Surgery: A Comprehensive Review*, 7th Edition, WB Saunders, Elsevier, 2006.

Barnett HJ, Taylor DW, Eliasziw M, *et al.* Benefit of carotid endarterectomy in patients with symptomatic moderate or severe stenosis. North American Symptomatic Carotid Endarterectomy Trial Collaborators, *N Engl J Med* 1998; **339**:1415–1425.

Brott TG, Hobson II RW, Howard G, *et al.* Stenting compared to endarterectomy for treatment of carotid artery stenosis, *N Engl J Med* (in press).

Executive Committee for the Asymptomatic Carotid Atherosclerosis Study. Endarterectomy for asymptomatic carotid stenosis, *JAMA* 1995; **273**:1421–1428.

Mas JL, Chatellier G, Beyssen V, *et al.* Endarterectomy versus stenting in patients with symptomatic severe carotid stenosis, *N Engl J Med* 2006; **355**:1660–1671.

Moore WS. Extracranial cerebrovascular disease: The carotid artery. Chapter 35 In: Wesley S. Moore MD (Ed.), *Vascular and Endovascular Surgery: A Comprehensive Review*, 7th Edition, WB Saunders, Elsevier, 2006.

Chapter 6
Management of Chronic Aortoiliac and Infrainguinal Arterial Occlusive Disease

Brian G. DeRubertis and Gavin Davis

1. Incidence, Etiology, and Risk Factors

Chronic lower extremity ischemia is a common manifestation of atherosclerosis and causes significant morbidity and mortality worldwide. In the United States, between 5% and 7% of individuals over the age of 50 years will report symptoms consistent with claudication (pain in the legs or calves with ambulation due to insufficient oxygen delivery) and aortoiliac and infrainguinal occlusive diseases have been demonstrated to cause disabling claudication in six of every 1000 persons. Additionally, chronic lower extremity occlusive disease results in over 400,000 hospital admissions yearly in the United States and contributes to most of the 75,000 amputations per year.

Aortoiliac and infrainguinal occlusive disease is caused by atherosclerosis in the same manner as disease of other arterial beds. Plaque deposition is often more prominent at arterial bifurcations, likely due to changes in arterial wall sheer stress resulting in endothelial injury.

Risk factors for aortoiliac and infrainguinal occlusive disease are similar to those for atherosclerotic disease of the coronary and cerebral circulations. While genetic predisposition of the development of vascular pathology is likely an important determinant of the disease, there are a number of modifiable risk factors that can significantly affect the progression of disease. Tobacco abuse is among the most important of these, as ex-smokers have a seven-fold increased risk of chronic lower extremity ischemia and current smokers have a 16-fold increased risk. In most series, 75–90% of patients evaluated and treated for claudication have a history of prior or current tobacco abuse. Diabetes is another important risk factor, as the Framingham Study demonstrated a 3.5-fold increased risk of claudication in men with diabetes and an 8.5-fold increased risk in women with diabetes. Other risk factors include hyperlipidemia, obesity, and increased age. Evidence suggests that medical therapy of patients with aortoiliac and infrainguinal occlusive disease with statins, aspirin, b-blockers, and ACE-inhibitors can reduce the incidence of cardiovascular events in this population. Screening for asymptomatic aortoiliac and infrainguinal occlusive disease should be performed in patients over the age of 50 years for the primary purpose of directing risk-factor modification rather than identification of patients requiring intervention, as these procedures (either percutaneous or open surgical reconstruction) are reserved for patients with disabling claudication or limb-threatening ischemia.

2. Natural History of Aortoiliac and Infrainguinal Occlusive Disease

While atherosclerosis is generally a progressive disease, the natural history of patients with chronic lower extremity ischemia from aortoiliac or infrainguinal occlusive disease depends largely on the patient's initial presentation and the patient's symptoms can generally be assigned to one of two categories: (1) claudication or (2) limb-threatening ischemia. These categories have important implications for the natural history of the disease process and the goals of therapy.

2.1 *Claudication*

Claudication is defined as burning or cramping pain that develops in the buttock, thighs, or calves with ambulation. It is caused by lack of blood flow to the muscles involved with ambulation due to occlusive disease that prevents the increased amount of blood flow required by these muscles when they are in use. This pain generally is reproducible each time the patient walks the specific distance that elicits the pain, and resolves with several minutes of rest. Patients with claudication that is sufficiently severe to warrant intervention have a significant risk of death due to coronary atherosclerosis or cerebrovascular disease, with a five-year mortality rate of up to 30% in many series. Although as many as 20–30% of claudicants may ultimately progress to limb-threatening ischemia, the risk of major lower extremity amputation is relatively low in these patients, and less than 5% require major amputation within five years of presentation. The goal of therapy in these patients should be directed at improving or maintaining quality of life with treatment designed to reduce or eliminate the patient's symptoms. While percutaneous intervention and open surgical revascularization are appropriate treatment options in selected patients, initial management should consist of risk-factor modification, exercise programs, and consideration of pharmacotherapy.

2.2 *Limb-threatening ischemia*

Limb-threatening ischemia is defined as lower extremity rest pain, nonhealing ulceration, or gangrene in the presence of aortoiliac and/or infrainguinal occlusive disease. The occlusive disease in these patients is often complex multi-level disease. Rest pain is caused by insufficient blood flow and oxygen delivery required to carry out the basic metabolic processes required by the extremity, and the pain results from nerve ischemia. Rest pain is generally experienced as exquisitely severe burning pain in the forefoot, tends to be most pronounced at night, and often wakes patients from sleep. The pain is often relieved by placing the affected foot in a dependent position. Patients with limb-threatening ischemia often have a very limited life expectancy due to their comorbid coronary and cerebrovascular disease and have five-year mortality rates as high as 75% in many series. Unlike claudicants, these patients are at high risk of limb loss without intervention, as over 50% will eventually require amputation if revascularization is not performed. Thus, all patients with limb-threatening ischemia should be considered for revascularization if feasible. Because of the numerous and severe comorbidities in these patients, percutaneous intervention is often favored over open surgical reconstruction, as it is a less invasive modality that can often achieve limb salvage with nearly equivalent rates as surgical bypass.

3. Evaluation

3.1 *History and physical examination*

Obtaining a thorough history is the first step in evaluating the patient with symptoms or signs of lower extremity occlusive disease, and when this history is combined with the physical examination and simple noninvasive vascular lab studies, one can pinpoint the severity and location of disease with a high degree of accuracy. For patients with claudication, the duration, progression, location, and severity of symptoms are important factors to determine. Claudication can be caused by single level disease, with aortoiliac disease resulting in thigh and buttock claudication, impotence, and, occasionally, thigh muscle atrophy (Leriche's Syndrome), and femoropopliteal disease resulting in calf claudication. Nerve root impingement due to lumbar stenosis may mimic intermittent claudication symptoms of vascular etiology, though patients with lumbar stenosis generally must sit, lean over a walker or chair, or do a similar activity that results in increased curvature of the spine and widening of the spinal foramina, while patients with vascular claudication can get symptom relief by simply standing still. The history should also elicit other comorbidities and behavioral habits that put the patient at risk for arterial occlusive disease.

Physical examination should be focused on pulses and the appearance of the lower extremities. A thorough pulse examination is performed, evaluating for bruits over the carotid, iliac, and femoral locations and palpable pulses at the carotid, radial, femoral, popliteal, and pedal locations. While several methods of describing the quality of a palpable pulse have been utilized, many prefer a 4-point scale in which 0 indicates no pulse, 1+ indicates diminished but present pulse, 2+ is a normal pulse, and 3+ indicates an abnormally strong or aneurismal pulse. A diminished or absent pulse indicates occlusive disease at the level immediately above the abnormal pulse examination (*i.e.* absent femoral pulse indicates aortoiliac disease and absent popliteal pulse indicates femoral disease). The patient's legs should be examined for any sign of muscle atrophy, hair loss, ulceration, swelling, or discoloration. Chronic lower extremity occlusive disease can give rise to nonhealing ulcers as well as gangrene of the distal extremity. The patient's feet should be examined carefully, especially the heel and between the toes, for evidence of ischemic ulcers or tissue infection.

3.2 *Non-invasive vascular lab/hemodynamic assessment*

The vascular lab has become an integral part of the initial assessment of patients with lower extremity occlusive disease as well as an important method for surveillance following revascularization. The modalities described below should be readily available to the vascular surgeon and should be considered an extension of the physical examination. These tests have the benefit of being relatively inexpensive, simple to perform, noninvasive, and they can be used effectively to provide risk stratification and to guide interventional or operative management.

3.2.1 *Ankle: brachial index and doppler waveforms*

The Ankle: Brachial Index (ABI) is a simple screening method that can be performed at the bedside to assess of the severity of occlusive disease for the affected extremity. An ABI is measured as the ankle pressure divided by the higher of the two brachial pressures. Normal ABI values are greater than 1.0 and any value under 0.95 is considered abnormal. Generally, ABI values between 0.4 and 0.95 are indicative of sufficient occlusive disease to result in claudication and ABI values below 0.3 are generally found in patients with rest pain, ischemic ulceration, or gangrene.

ABI values, although helpful, do not give you a definitive assessment of disease. Some patients may have higher ABIs than symptoms indicate due to arterial wall calcification causing ankle pressure measures to be elevated. When the ABI is greater than 1.3 or is not congruent with the symptoms describes stiff vessels should be considered. In addition, in patients with aortoiliac disease, collateral reconstitution may provide normal ankle pressures.

Diabetic patients or others with heavily calcified arteries may have noncompressible tibial vessels and, therefore, have "suprasystolic" ABIs of >1.2. In these patients, the ABI is not helpful and a more reliable assessment of disease can be obtained with a Toe: Brachial Index (TBI) or by observing the quality of the Doppler waveform at the ankle level.

3.2.2 *Segmental pressures and pulse-volume waveforms*

Segmental pressure evaluation can be done to further localize the occlusive lesion. This is done by taking pressure measurements at the thigh, the upper calf, and above the ankle. These measurements are then compared to the brachial pressure, and a pressure difference of 20 mm Hg or more is indicative of disease above the cuff site. While segmental pressures cannot reliably distinguish between aortoiliac disease and common femoral disease, they can be used to clearly identify between inflow disease (aortoiliac and common femoral) and infrainguinal disease, and can pinpoint the level of occlusive disease throughout the infrainguinal circulation.

Pulse volume waveforms can be performed at the same time as segmental pressures. To collect waveforms, the cuff is inflated to 65 mm Hg and a transducer is attached to measure the pressure change in the cuff caused by the artery during systole. The resulting waveforms are then analyzed and categorized as normal, mildly, moderately, or severely abnormal. A normal waveform has a steep up-slope to a sharp systolic peak and often has a prominent dicrotic notch. As the waveform becomes abnormal, the first characteristic to vanish is the dicrotic notch followed by the steep up-slope. Eventually, in severe disease, the entire waveform becomes flattened and wide. Bilateral testing may be advantageous to detect amplitude differences between the legs for unilateral disease. When a patient has bilateral disease standardization against an arm, waveform may allow better comparison. Waveform analysis may also be used as a monitoring technique where diminishing amplitude indicates disease progression. Pulse volume waveforms can be helpful especially in patients with noncompressible vessels.

3.2.3 *Arterial duplex*

Arterial duplex scanning allows for an accurate assessment of the entire lower extremity arterial system. With this technique, stenotic or occlusive areas can be identified with accuracy. Increased velocity is an indication of stenosis in a given vessel. To gauge the degree of stenosis in a vessel, the peak systolic velocity at a point of narrowing is compared to the velocity at a normal point in the same artery. When this ratio is greater than 2.0, there is a greater than 50% reduction in diameter of the vessel. Some groups consider there to be a 75% stenosis when the ratio passes 4.0 and the peak systolic velocity at the stenotic site is greater than 400 cm/second.

3.3 *Axial imaging and angiography/anatomic assessment*

Many patients can be adequately assessed by the combination of symptom history, physical examination, and noninvasive vascular lab studies without the need for more expensive imaging modalities before proceeding to intervention. This is especially true for patients in whom the treatment of choice is percutaneous intervention, as these procedures begin with the use of angiography to delineate the target lesions requiring treatment. In patients who have aortoiliac disease or patients who are being treated with open surgical revascularization, additional axial imaging or diagnostic contrast angiography is generally utilized for operative planning.

3.3.1 *CT angiography*

CT angiography (CTA) is a common imaging technique used to visualize the arterial system. It requires the use of iodinated contrast material, similar to conventional angiography, and carries the same risks of nephrotoxicity and idiosyncratic allergic reaction. Modern CT scanners that expose patients to less radiation than conventional angiography are extremely fast, provide exceptional resolution, and can offer three-dimensional (3D) reconstructions of the arterial tree. Unlike MRA, implants such as pacemakers are not a contraindication to imaging with CTA. Limitations of CTA include patients with chronic renal insufficiency in whom contrast nephropathy could result in further deterioration of renal function and patients who have heavily calcified arteries, as this prevents adequate luminal visualization.

3.3.2 *MR angiography*

MR angiography (MRA) is an alternate technology used to visualize the arterial system. MRA is often used in patients with contraindications to the use of iodinated contrast and those who should not be exposed to ionizing radiation. While the image quality of MRA varies by institution, high-quality studies can offer tremendous resolution that can even match or exceed images obtained by contrast angiography.

3.3.3 *Conventional angiography*

Although the above-mentioned methods have gained popularity in visualizing the arterial system, there are still benefits to conventional angiography including high resolution, the ability to repeat studies at the time of viewing, the ability to visualize small vessels, and the ability to therapeutically intervene immediately. For screening, many physicians lean away from angiography due to its invasive nature, need for sedation, and length of study.

4. Classification of Disease Severity

Prior to intervention on patients with aortoiliac or infrainguinal occlusive disease, it is important to classify the disease severity both clinically and anatomically. The clinical categorization of the severity of ischemia is determined by the history and physical examination and has important implications regarding the need for intervention and the goals for therapy, as outlined above in the discussion regarding the difference between claudicants and limb-threat patients. The anatomic classification of the disease pattern is determined by the patient's imaging studies, and this classification can help direct the most appropriate form of intervention.

4.1 *Rutherford clinical categories of lower extremity ischemia*

The Rutherford classification system is used to objectively describe patients' clinical status (Table 1). Patients who fall into Categories 1–3 are considered claudicants and patients in Category 4 or higher are those with limb-threatening ischemia. It is important to classify patients by such a system not only to help determine the need for therapy and goals of intervention, but also to quantify the degree of clinical improvement following intervention in order to follow outcomes after percutaneous or open surgical intervention.

4.2 *Transatlantic consensus classification*

The Transatlantic Consensus Classification document serves as a guideline for describing the degree of aortoiliac and femoropopliteal occlusive diseases in a particular patient and provides recommendations regarding the appropriateness of different types of treatment modalities (Table 2). A premise leading to the establishment of this document included the fact that while percutaneous endovascular interventions offered less invasive means of treating patients with aortoiliac or femoropopliteal occlusive disease, there are some disease patterns that respond less well and demonstrate poorer patency rates when treated with endovascular therapy as opposed to open surgical reconstruction. This document, therefore, acts as an evidence-based guideline to assist in making appropriate decisions regarding treatment selection. An equally important contribution it makes is the ability to use this system to stratify patients in terms of anatomic disease severity, which then allows for comparative outcome analysis among groups of patients with similar levels of disease severity.

Table 1. Rutherford clinical categories of chronic lower extremity ischemia.

Grade	Category	Clinical description	Objective criteria
0	0	Asymptomatic — no hemodynamically significant occlusive disease	Normal treadmill or reactive hyperemia test
	1	Mild claudication	Completes treadmill exercise; ankle pressure after exercise >50 mm Hg but at least 20 mm Hg lower than resting value
I	2	Moderate claudication	Between categories 1 and 3
	3	Severe claudication	Cannot complete standard treadmill exercise and ankle pressure after exercise <50 mm HG
II	4	Ischemic rest pain	Resting AP <40 mm Hg, flat or barely pulsatile ankle of metatarsal pulse volume recording; toe pressure <30 mm Hg
III	5	Minor tissue loss — nonhealing ulcer and focal gangrene with diffuse pedal ischemia	Resting AP <60 mm Hg, flat or barely pulsatile ankle of metatarsal pulse volume recording; toe pressure <40 mm Hg
	6	Major tissue loss — extending above the transmetatarsal level and functional foot no longer salvageable	Same as category 5

5. Medical Management of Aortoiliac and Infrainguinal Occlusive Diseases

The first steps in the management of any patient with symptomatic or asymptomatic aortoiliac or infrainguinal occlusive disease should include (a) medical optimization and (b) risk factor modification.

Patients with peripheral arterial occlusive disease have been shown to have reduced rates of stroke, myocardial infarction, and vascular-related death with the

Table 2.   TASC classification for aortoiliac and femoropopliteal occlusive disease.

Type	Criteria (aortoiliac)	Criteria (femoropopliteal)	Treatment
A	• Single stenosis < 3 cm of the CIA or EIA (unilateral/bilateral)	• Single stenosis < 3 cm in length, not at the origin of the superficial femoral artery (SFA) or the distal • popliteal artery	Endovascular therapy is the treatment of choice
B	• Single stenosis 3–10 cm in length and not extending into the CFA • Total of two stenoses < 5 cm long in the CIA and/or EIA and not extending into the CFA • Unilateral CIA occlusion	• Single stenoses or occlusions 3 cm to 5 cm long not involving the distal popliteal artery • Heavily calcified stenoses up to 3 cm in length • Multiple stenoses or occlusions, each < 3 cm • Single or multiple lesions in the absence of continuous tibial runoff to improve inflow for distal surgical bypass	Endovascular therapy is more often used, but there is insufficient evidence to make a firm recommendation
C	• Bilateral 5–10 cm-long stenoses of the CIA and/or EIA and not extending into the CFA • Unilateral EIA occlusion not extending into the CFA • Unilateral EIA stenosis extending into the CFA • Bilateral CIA occlusions	• Single stenoses or occlusions longer than 5 cm • Multiple stenoses or occlusions, each 3 cm to 5 cm, with or without heavy calcification	Surgical treatment is more often used, but there is insufficient evidence to make a firm recommendation

(Continued)

Table 2. (*Continued*)

Type	Criteria (aortoiliac)	Criteria (femoropopliteal)	Treatment
D	• Diffuse multiple unilateral stenoses involving the CIA, EIA, and CFA (usually >10 cm) • Unilateral occlusion involving both the CIA and EIA • Bilateral EIA occlusions • Diffuse disease involving the aorta and both iliac arteries • Iliac stenoses in a patient with an abdominal aortic aneurysm or other lesion requiring aortic or iliac surgery	• Complete common femoral artery or SFA occlusions, or complete popliteal artery and proximal trifurcation vessels occlusion	Surgery is the treatment of choice

use of antiplatelet therapy. Additionally, there is growing evidence from nonrandomized trials that antiplatelet therapy may slow the progression of atherosclerotic disease. Statin therapy has likewise been shown to slow symptom progression in patients with lower extremity occlusive disease and has demonstrated reduced rates of overall mortality, cardiovascular-related mortality, and stroke in patients with coronary atherosclerosis. The benefit of statin therapy has been demonstrated even in patients with normal total cholesterol levels. Treatment with peri-operative β-blockers has been shown to reduce mortality in patients undergoing major vascular surgery, and may have long-term benefit for patients with lower extremity occlusive disease. Finally, evidence suggests that the renin-angiotensin system plays an important role in the development and progression of atherosclerosis, and angiotensin-converting enzyme (ACE) inhibitors have been shown to reduce overall mortality, cardiovascular mortality, and the likelihood of cardiac/peripheral revascularization procedures in patients with known coronary atherosclerosis regardless of the presence of hypertension. For these reasons, medical optimization for all patients with peripheral arterial occlusive disease should include consideration of the use of antiplatelet therapy (with aspirin or clopidogrel), statin therapy, β-blockade, and an ACE inhibitor. Additionally, strict glucose control should be instituted in all patients with diabetes, as uncontrolled diabetes has a considerable impact on progression of atherosclerosis.

Risk factor modification is also imperative and consists of smoking cessation, preventative foot care, and weight reduction in obese patients. The single most important controllable risk factor for the development and progression of atherosclerotic disease is tobacco abuse, and aggressive efforts toward smoking cessation, including pharmacotherapy to prevent recidivism, are warranted in these patients.

For claudicants, it is imperative to weigh the risk: benefit ratio for any invasive intervention designed to reduce symptoms, as all of these procedures are associated with some degree of risk of major morbidity or mortality. All claudicants should undergo a trial of an exercise program prior to invasive interventions, as most patients will derive substantial improvement in walking distance with a well-structured program. Standard programs involve walking until symptoms are experienced, resting until they abate, then repeating this cycle for 30–40 minutes daily. Additionally, pharmacotherapy with cilostazol or pentoxifylline has been demonstrated to be effective at increasing walking distances in up to 50% in responders (roughly one half of patients) and can be used in conjunction with an exercise program to alleviate symptoms. For those patients who fail to respond sufficiently to these therapies and continue to suffer from lifestyle-limiting claudication, revascularization should be considered.

For patients with limb-threatening ischemia, medical optimization and risk factor modification remain imperative, but these patients generally require revascularization in order to assure limb-salvage. Significant delays in revascularization can increase the likelihood of amputation and should be avoided.

6. Revascularization for Aortoiliac Disease

6.1 *Open surgical treatment*

6.1.1 *Aortobifemoral bypass*

Open surgical revascularization of the aortoiliac circulation by aortobifemoral bypass has been performed for over 40 years and has evolved considerably with the advances in surgical technique and perioperative care. Currently, this procedure can be performed with low morbidity and mortality rates, has exceptional long-term durability, and serves as the "gold-standard" by which other methods are evaluated.

Careful preoperative evaluation and thorough cardiovascular risk stratification are essential to select patients who are fit enough to undergo a procedure of this magnitude. Preoperative imaging (*i.e.* computed tomography and angiography) is performed to ensure a proximal infrarenal aortic neck suitable for aortic cross-clamping and suturing to the graft, as well as to identify concomitant infrainguinal disease.

The operation is carried out under general anesthesia in the supine position with the arms extended to allow access for IV catheters and hemodynamic monitoring devices. While the abdominal aorta can be exposed through a retroperitoneal approach, many prefer utilizing a vertical midline incision to expose the abdominal aorta for this operation. After the incision is made, the transverse colon is elevated and retracted cephalad and the small bowel is eviscerated and retracted to the patient's right. The posterior parietal peritoneum is then incised to the left of the duodenum, the ligament of Trietz is divided to mobilize the duodenum off the anterior surface of the aorta, and the aorta is dissected out. Next, longitudinal incisions are made over each groin to expose the common femoral, superficial femoral, and profunda femoris arteries. Next, retroperitoneal tunnels are created from the proximal infrarenal aorta to the groin incisions, using caution to stay directly anterior to the common and external iliac arteries and posterior to the ureters. Once these are completed, the patient is systemically anticoagulated, the aorta is clamped and transected, and an end-to-end anastomosis with 3–0 prolene suture is performed between the proximal infrarenal aorta and the proximal end of a bifurcated Dacron or PTFE graft. For patients with large accessory renal arteries or external iliac occlusions, an end-to-side anastomosis is performed without transecting the aorta, thus preserving accessory renal, inferior mesenteric, and hypogastric blood flow. Following the proximal aortic anastomosis, the graft limbs are tunneled to the level of the femoral arteries and the distal anastomoses are performed in an end-to-side fashion after a longitudinal incision in the common femoral artery is made and extended distally toward the profunda femoris artery. After completing the anastomoses and reestablishing flow to the lower extremities, the groin incisions are closed in multiple layers and the peritoneum is closed over the graft in the abdomen to prevent graft-enteric fistulae.

6.1.2 *Extra-anatomic bypass*

While aortobifemoral bypass provides a durable operation with exceptional long-term patency rates, it can be associated with significant morbidity and mortality and may not be well tolerated in patients with significant comorbidities. Open surgical alternatives to this operation include axillobifemoral bypass and femorofemoral bypass.

Axillobifemoral bypass is generally reserved for patients with limb-threatening ischemia, significant aortic and/or bilateral iliac disease, and contraindications to general anesthesia or aortic cross-clamping. The surgical exposure in this operation includes dissection of the axillary artery through an infraclavicular incision as well as exposure of both common femoral arteries in the groins. Following exposure of these vessels, the patient is systemically anticoagulated, clamps are applied to the axillary artery, and a subcutaneously tunneled PTFE or Dacron bypass is performed between the axillary artery and the ipsilateral common femoral artery. This second graft is tunneled subcutaneously anterior to the pubic symphysis. Following these anastomoses, a second bypass is performed between the femoral hood of the graft and the contralateral common femoral artery. For patients with unilateral iliac occlusive disease, a femorofemoral bypass from the common femoral artery on the donor side to the common femoral artery ipsilateral to the occlusive disease can be performed. End-to-side anastomoses are created at each common femoral artery, generally through obliquely oriented arteriotomies designed to allow the graft toe to extend toward the profunda femoris artery as a profundoplasty. Each of these extra-anatomic bypasses can be performed under local anesthesia in patients who are unfit for a general anesthetic because of other comorbid conditions.

6.2 *Endovascular treatment*

6.2.1 *Angioplasty and stenting*

Endovascular treatment of aortoiliac occlusive disease has emerged as an attractive alternative to aortobifemoral bypass or extra-anatomic bypass in selected patients. While the patency rates of aortofemoral bypass are exceptional, extra-anatomic bypass procedures carry much less encouraging results. Additionally, there is considerable morbidity associated with these procedures in terms of cardiovascular events, pulmonary complications, wound or graft infections, and overall recovery.

Alternatively, percutaneous endovascular therapy for aortoiliac atherosclerotic stenoses or occlusions can be performed with minimal morbidity and mortality, often with a single-day hospital stay. The long-term durability of these interventions in properly selected patients approaches that of aortobifemoral bypass, and for this reason, endovascular therapy has supplanted aortobifemoral bypass in many centers as first-line therapy for this disease process.

Endovascular treatment of occlusive disease begins with obtaining arterial access and performing diagnostic angiography to identify target lesions for revascularization. For aortoiliac disease, noninvasive axial imaging (CTA or MRA) can be helpful for planning the endovascular approach and ruling out patterns of disease that are unlikely to be amenable to endovascular treatment. Arterial access is aided by the use of ultrasonography, as duplex-guided puncture of the artery can help to assure that the puncture occurs in the common femoral artery rather than the profunda femoris or the superficial femoral artery. Access is generally obtained in a retrograde fashion ipsilateral to the lesion of interest, and then a guidewire is advanced into the iliac artery. The puncture needle is exchanged over the wire for a 5Fr sheath through which retrograde angiography is performed. For patients without total occlusions, it is helpful to advance a side-hole catheter through this ipsilateral sheath up to the aorta in order to perform antegrade aortography to identify all target lesions throughout the aortoiliac circulation. In patients with total iliac occlusions, puncture of the contralateral femoral artery followed by sheath and catheter placement through this side can assist in imaging during the recanalization procedure. Additionally, bilateral access can be helpful or even required in the event of proximal bilateral iliac disease.

Focal stenoses can often be easily traversed utilizing a relatively floppy guidewire and angled catheter. For total occlusions, a more rigid hydrophilic guidewire can be used to cross the occlusion, using caution to keep the wire centered in the occluded vessel to prevent vessel perforation. Once the lesions are crossed, the patient is anticoagulated and an appropriately sized angioplasty balloon can be used to dilate the lesion. Primary stenting of the lesion without pre-dilation is often done with complete occlusions in order to reduce the risk of embolization and because stenting has been demonstrated to have superior patency rates to balloon angioplasty alone in the iliac circulation.

Bilateral proximal common iliac stenoses or occlusions generally require bilateral access that enables simultaneous balloon inflation and/or stent implantation in each iliac artery to prevent shifting of plaque to the contralateral lumen. Angioplasty and stenting can be used in the aorta and both the common and external iliac arteries, though caution should be used to avoid extending iliac stents past the inguinal ligament into the common femoral arteries, as stents in these locations are likely to fracture and occlude due to the flexion at this region. Care should also be used to avoid unnecessary coverage of the hypogastric arteries, as this may result in occlusion of these vessels.

6.3 *Results of aortoiliac revascularization*

As demonstrated in Table 3, aortobifemoral bypass results in superior long-term patency relative to both extra-anatomic bypass and endovascular treatment of aortoiliac occlusive disease. However, the results of angioplasty and stenting for TASC A–C lesions in many series approaches direct in-line surgical revascularization with aortobifemoral bypass, and it does so at a considerably reduced cost in terms of morbidity and mortality for the patient. Though three-year primary patency rates of these lesions with endovascular treatment range from 73% to 85%, secondary

Table 3.   Patency and complication rates with aortoiliac revascularization.

	Five-Year patency	Complication rate
Aortobifemoral bypass	85–90%	5–8%
Axillo-bifemoral bypass	50–80%	5–15%
Femorofemoral bypass	−80%	5%
	Three-Year patency primary (secondary)	
Iliac angioplasty and stenting	76%	1–5%
TASC A	>80% (>90%)	—
TASC B	78% (95%)	—
TASC C	73% (93%)	—
TASC D	80% (83%)	—

patency rate in most series are >90%, which compares favorably to the 85–90% five-year patency rates seen with aortobifemoral bypass. For this reason, endovascular therapy is now considered an appropriate first-line treatment for most patients with aortoiliac occlusive disease.

7. Revascularization for Infrainguinal Disease

7.1 *Open surgical reconstruction*

As with aortobifemoral bypass for aortoiliac occlusive disease, open surgical bypass with autogenous conduit remains the "gold standard" for infrainguinal reconstruction for occlusive disease. There are several important principles that must be observed when performing lower extremity bypass for patients with either claudication or limb-threatening ischemia. First, adequate arterial inflow must be established (*i.e.* absence of untreated aortoiliac occlusive disease) prior to performing an infrainguinal bypass. Second, an appropriate bypass target with adequate distal runoff is required. Third, bypass patency rate is strongly correlated with choice of conduit for infrageniculate bypass, with autogenous greater saphenous vein being the conduit of choice for femoral to below-knee popliteal or tibial/pedal bypass. Finally, all levels of disease should be bypassed in operations for patients with limb-threatening ischemia, as a palpable pulse in the foot is the goal of revascularization procedures done for tissue loss or gangrene. The exception to this rule includes patients with rest pain, whose symptoms can often be ameliorated by improving a single level of disease (*e.g.* endarterectomy and profundoplasty for patient with rest pain and significant common femoral disease).

Lower extremity bypass with reversed or *in-situ* saphenous vein is the mainstay of open surgical treatment of infrainguinal occlusive disease. Preoperative workup includes appropriate imaging studies including a contrast angiogram or a high-quality MRA to identify the bypass target and rule out inflow disease or atherosclerotic disease of the distal runoff vessels. Preoperative cardiac risk stratification is important, as this procedure requires either regional or general anesthesia. A longitudinal incision is made in the groin and the common femoral, superficial femoral, and profunda femoris arteries are circumferentially dissected. Next, an incision is made over the target vessel at the popliteal, tibial, or pedal level and this vessel is circumferentially dissected and controlled with vessel loops. Once the target vessel has been evaluated and is determined to be adequate for the distal anastomosis, the vein is harvested. In the reversed saphenous technique, the favored approach at our institution, the vein can be harvested through a series of longitudinal skip incisions or through an endoscopic vein harvest technique to reduce the morbidity of the vein harvest incision. Once the vein is harvested, it is prepared by flushing with heparinized saline and ligating any side branches with silk ties. With *in-situ* bypass, the saphenous vein remains in its anatomic location; however, valve lysis with a valvulotome and thorough ligation of venous side branches are required to ensure maximal bypass patency. When using reversed vein, the subcutaneous tunnel between the femoral artery and the target vessel is created with a tunneling device, with counter incisions placed where necessary to facilitate the tunneling. The tunnel may be made either anatomically (along the course of the vessels) or subcutaneously based on surgeon preference. The patient is then anticoagulated, the femoral artery is clamped, and an arteriotomy is made. An end-to-side anastomosis between the femoral artery and the reversed saphenous vein is then performed with running 5-0 or 6-0 prolene suture; then after completing the anastomosis, the artery is unclamped and the bypass is pressurized. This step facilitates passing the vein through the tunneling device without twisting or kinking the graft. Next, the distal anastomosis is performed after assessing the correct length of the graft with the leg fully extended. Finally, the wounds are closed in layers and the skin is re-approximated with subcuticular sutures or staples.

For patients with isolated infrageniculate disease of the popliteal or tibial circulation, popliteal to tibial or popliteal-to-pedal artery bypass can be performed. In these cases, the distal superficial femoral artery or the popliteal artery is used as the inflow vessel rather than the femoral artery, thus substantially reducing the length of the bypass and required conduit.

While saphenous vein is favored by most as the conduit of choice in all bypass procedures, evidence suggests that femoropopliteal artery bypass grafts with PTFE have similar patency as saphenous vein provided the bypass target is located in the above-knee popliteal artery. Even in these cases, however, saphenous vein has the advantage of decreased propensity for infection. PTFE or other disadvantaged conduit (lesser saphenous vein, spliced arm vein, and cryopreserved cadaveric saphenous vein) can be used for infrapopliteal bypass if adequate greater saphenous vein is not available, but these grafts would be expected to have inferior patency rates.

7.2 *Endovascular treatment*

As with aortoiliac occlusive disease, infrainguinal occlusive disease can be treated effectively with open surgical reconstruction with excellent results. However, the morbidity associated with infrainguinal bypass is not inconsequential, with some series reporting perioperative mortality and complication rates as high as 10% and 50%, respectively. Even in the absence of complications, recovery can be prolonged, with one series reporting that only 50% of patients returned to their baseline level of function by six months postoperatively. Therefore, endovascular treatment has been increasingly adopted to treat claudication and limb-threatening ischemia while minimizing the physiologic insult to the patient.

For infrainguinal intervention, percutaneous access is generally obtained through retrograde puncture of the contralateral common femoral artery, and after sheath placement, a side-hole catheter is introduced into the aorta for aortography and iliac and femoral runoff angiograms. Next, a curved-tip catheter (*i.e.* Omniflush or VCF catheter) is used in conjunction with a guidewire to cross the aortic bifurcation. The wire is then used to exchange the curved-tip catheter for an end-hole catheter to perform selective femoropopliteal and tibial angiography. Upon identification of lesions appropriate for endovascular treatment, the initial femoral sheath is exchanged over a stiff wire for a 45-cm sheath that is brought to the contralateral common femoral artery. The patient is systemically anticoagulated at this time.

The primary requirement for successful endovascular treatment of a target lesion is successful traversal of the lesion followed by luminal re-entry of the distal target vessel. When treating stenoses, care should be taken to maintain the intraluminal position at all times during wire advancement, avoiding the creation of subintimal dissection planes. This can be performed using a hydrophilic guidewire and angled catheter. The wire tip should be kept in constant motion using a torque device affixed to the wire, and creating a J-loop with the wire tip should be avoided.

Total occlusions can be crossed using a similar technique, but often require stiffer guidewires. For these lesions, creation of a J-loop in the wire and dissection along the subintimal plane is generally necessary until reaching the reconstituted vessel distally. Once the catheter is advanced to the region of the reconstituted vessel, the wire is removed to confirm back-bleeding. Angiography through the catheter will then confirm re-entry into the true lumen of the vessel, and the wire can be reinserted to guide delivery of the treatment device.

The most commonly utilized method for percutaneous lower extremity revascularization involves balloon angioplasty with or without stent placement (Fig. 1). The noncompliant angioplasty balloons and self-expanding nitinol stents currently utilized today are available in a wide range of diameters and lengths, though most commonly utilized nitinol stents are approved only for use in the biliary system and are placed in the infrainguinal location as "off-label" devices. For selective (rather than primary) stenting, the balloon is used to dilate the target lesion, then repeat angiography is performed, with stenting reserved by residual stenosis after angioplasty of >30% of the lumen or for flow-limiting dissections.

There are several alternatives to the use of angioplasty and bare-metal nitinol stents. These include cryoplasty (angioplasty with a thermal-controlled $-10°C$ balloon), excisional and laser atherectomies, and implantation of PTFE-covered stents. While each of these devices has specific advantages that can be exploited in different disease patterns or anatomic locations by the skilled interventionalist, no single device or technique has shown clear superiority over the others.

7.3 Results of treatment of infrainguinal occlusive disease

Surgical bypass for infrainguinal occlusive disease has been demonstrated to be an effective treatment for claudication and results in excellent limb-salvage rates in patients with limb-threatening ischemia. Outcomes following revascularization depend on a number of factors but overall primary patency rates for infrainguinal bypass with autogenous greater saphenous vein ranges from 60% to 70% at five years, while secondary patency and limb-salvage rates approach 75% and 85%, respectively at most centers. Five-year outcome for infrainguinal bypass with disadvantaged vein or PTFE is significantly worse, with primary patency of less than 20% in some series. The poor outcome with sub-optimal conduits, combined with the fact that overall five-year survival in patients undergoing lower extremity bypass ranges from 40% to 70%, justifies consideration of less invasive modalities in some patients. For this reason, endovascular therapy has become an important tool in the armamentarium of the vascular surgeon.

Unfortunately, there is no available data from randomized trials between lower extremity bypass and percutaneous endovascular therapy, and most data available

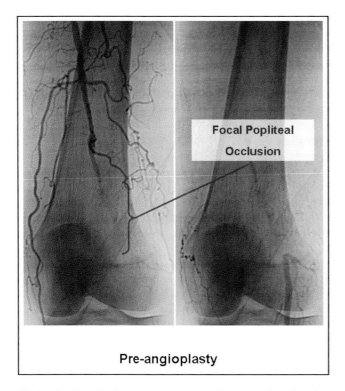
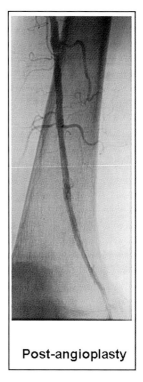

Fig. 1. Focal popliteal occlusion treated by balloon angioplasty. Stenting is avoided near flexion points such as the inguinal region or in the popliteal artery near the knee.

to date results from prospective device registries or reports from single institutions. Nevertheless, this data does suggest that endovascular therapy is a safe and effective treatment for both claudication and limb-threatening ischemia and is increasingly being utilized as a first-line treatment for these problems with surgical bypass reserved for failures of endovascular therapy. Technical success rates over 90% have commonly been reported, and while primary patency rates at two years in contemporary series is commonly quoted at roughly 50%, repeat intervention can result in secondary patency rates in claudicants of greater than 75% and limb-salvage rates in patients with limb-threatening ischemia of over 80%.

References

Brewster DC. Clinical and anatomical considerations for surgery in aortoiliac disease and results of surgical treatment. *Circulation* 1991; **83**(2 Suppl):I42–I52.

Conte MS, Bandyk DF, Clowes AW, *et al.* Results of PREVENT III: a multicenter, randomized trial of edifoligide for the prevention of vein graft failure in lower extremity bypass surgery. *J Vasc Surg* 2006; **43**(4):742–751; discussion 751.

DeRubertis BG, Faries PL, McKinsey JF, *et al.* Shifting paradigms in the treatment of lower extremity vascular disease: a report of 1000 percutaneous interventions. *Ann Surg* 2007; **246**(3):415–422.

Kudo T, Chandra FA, Ahn SS. The effectiveness of percutaneous transluminal angioplasty for the treatment of critical limb ischemia: a 10-year experience. *J Vasc Surg* 2005; **41**(3):423–435.

Szilagyi DE, Elliott JP Jr, Smith RF, *et al.* A thirty-year survey of the reconstructive surgical treatment of aortoiliac occlusive disease. *J Vasc Surg* 1986; **3**(3):421–436.

Timaran CH, Prault TL, Stevens SL, *et al.* Iliac artery stenting versus surgical reconstruction for TASC (TransAtlantic Inter-Society Consensus) type B and type C iliac lesions. *J Vasc Surg* 2003; **38**(2):272–278.

Chapter 7
Management of Aortic Aneurysms, Iliac Aneurysms, and Aortic Dissection

William J. Quinones-Baldrich

Learning Objectives

- Understand the incidence, risk factors, and natural history in patients with abdominal aortic aneurysm, descending thoracic aneurysms, and thoracoabdominal aneurysms.
- Learn the clinical presentation, the physical and radiologic diagnoses, and indications for treatment of patients with nonruptured and ruptured abdominal aortic, iliac, descending thoracic, and thoracoabdominal aneurysms.
- Learn the endovascular and open options for treatment of abdominal aortic, iliac, descending thoracic, thoracoabdominal aneurysms.
- Understand the natural history and pathogenesis of aortic dissection.
- Learn the appropriate medical and surgical managements of aortic dissection.

1. Aortic and Iliac Aneurysms

An aneurysm is defined by reporting standards as a localized dilation of an artery of at least 50% increase in diameter compared to the expected normal diameter. In practical terms, the reference diameter is the adjacent normal portion of the same artery. When several arterial segments have an increase in diameter of greater than 50% of normal, in the absence of a normal segment, the condition is termed arteriomegaly. When several dilated segments are involved with intervening normal diameter artery, the condition is termed aneurysmosis.

Aneurysms can be classified by location, size, shape, and etiology. In addition, the layers of the artery involved in the aneurysm define whether the aneurysm is true or the aneurysm is false. True aneurysms are those in which all layers of the artery are involved. False aneurysms represent a contained hematoma, which has been localized by the inflammatory reaction of the surrounding tissue. Thus, no layer of the artery is involved. When there is aneurysm formation after dissection, part of the aneurysm is formed by portions of the media and adventitia with the septum of the dissection formed by the intima and the inner part of the dissected media.

The shape of the aneurysm can be saccular or fusiform. Saccular aneurysms describe an eccentric dilation with a normal appearing segment of the artery forming the opposite wall of the aneurysm. Fusiform aneurysms represent a diffuse circumferential enlargement of the affected artery.

Most aortic and iliac aneurysms were formerly thought to be secondary to atherosclerosis. In reality, although they are associated frequently with atherosclerotic disease, these aneurysms are degenerative in nature. Histologically, the affected arterial wall shows elastin fragmentation and degeneration. Elastin has a half-life of 40–70 years and is not synthesized in the adult aorta. This explains the predilection for aortic aneurysms to develop in the older population. In addition, decreased nutrition, by the relative paucity of vasa vasorum in the infrarenal aorta and increased resistance to circulation below the renal arteries, may explain the increased incidence of aneurysm formation in this location. More recently, increased activity of matrix metalloproteinases (proteolytic enzymes) has been described in the wall of aortic aneurysms leading to degradation of the aortic media.

Other etiologies of aortic and iliac aneurysms include congenital, infectious, inflammatory arteritis, poststenotic dilation, and arterial rupture or an anastomotic disruption leading to pseudoaneurysm formation (false aneurysm). Infectious aneurysms (mycotic aneurysms) may occur secondarily due to sepsis or an adjacent infection, which can erode the arterial wall usually presenting as a saccular aneurysm. These are contained ruptures of the arterial segment and thus false aneurysms.

Degenerative abdominal aortic aneurysms (AAA) are most commonly seen in the infrarenal aorta. In an autopsy study of aortoiliac aneurysms, the abdominal aorta was involved in 65% of cases, the thoracic aorta in 19%, the abdominal aorta and iliac arteries in 13%, the thoracoabdominal aorta in 2%, and an isolated iliac aneurysm in 1%. It is estimated that AAAs occur in 21 per 100,000 person years compared to 6% per 100,000 person years for thoracic aortic aneurysms. Peripheral aneurysms, particularly popliteal and femoral aneurysms, are seen in approximately 3% of patients with abdominal aortic aneurysm. In contrast, approximately 30% of patients with popliteal aneurysms, and a higher percentage in patients with femoral aneurysms, will have an associated AAA.

2. Abdominal Aortic Aneurysms

AAAs are two to six times more common in men than in women and are most common in elderly white men. Approximately 20% of first-degree relatives with an abdominal aortic aneurysm have a first-degree relative with a history of an aortic aneurysm. Up to 7% of siblings older than 55 years old, of patients with AAA, will have an aneurysm 3 cm or larger. A twin of a monozygotic twin with an AAA has 71 times the likelihood of having an AAA compared with a heterozygotic twin of an individual without aneurysms.

Almost all AAAs involve the infrarenal aorta. Only 5% of AAA undergoing repair involve the suprarenal aorta. By definition, a juxtarenal AAA starts at the renal arteries but does not involve them. A pararenal aneurysm extends above one or both renal arteries but below the superior mesenteric artery and repair involves reimplantation and/or revascularization of at least one renal artery. A suprarenal aneurysm also involves the superior mesenteric artery. A total abdominal aortic aneurysm involves the entire visceral segment and the infrarenal aorta but does not involve the descending thoracic aorta. Approximately 25% of patients with infrarenal abdominal aortic aneurysm have involvement of the iliac arteries.

Inflammatory AAA is a rare form of aneurysm characterized by marked thickening of the aortic wall. The inflammatory process often causes significant adhesion to the surrounding organs, particularly the duodenum. Patients with an inflammatory AAA frequently present with abdominal or back pain. Retroperitoneal fibrosis may cause ureteral obstruction. The inflammatory process is seen as a halo around the aneurysm on a CT scan. This inflammatory process does not seem to decrease the risk of rupture and indications for repair are the same as for a degenerative aneurysm.

2.1 *Clinical presentation*

Most AAAs are asymptomatic. They are usually discovered on routine physical examination and most commonly, on imaging studies done for other pathology. Symptoms may include abdominal or back pain, early satiety secondary to duodenal compression, urinary symptoms secondary to hydronephrosis, organ or extremity ischemia secondary to distal embolization, or acute rupture. Symptoms of acute rupture include abrupt onset of abdominal pain that may radiate to the flank or groin. Most patients experience transient hypotension, which may develop into shock. Most ruptures, however, occur posteriorly and the retroperitoneum may contain the hematoma, thus limiting the degree of hypotension. These patients may present with a chronic contained rupture, which often makes the diagnosis difficult. A high index of suspicion is necessary. Rarely, the aneurysm may rupture into the iliac vein or inferior vena cava. In these cases, patients may present with high output congestive heart failure. A continuous bruit in the abdomen may help the clinician suspect this diagnosis.

Smoking is the risk factor mostly associated with abdominal aortic aneurysms. Other risk factors include hypertension, coronary artery disease, atherosclerosis, and high cholesterol. Hypertension has been found to be an independent risk factor in the incidence of abdominal aortic aneurysm and the risk of rupture. Other important factors increasing the risk of rupture include chronic obstructive pulmonary disease and large aneurysm size.

Routine physical examination alone will detect an abdominal aortic aneurysm smaller than 5 cm in less than 50% of patients. Abdominal ultrasound can confirm the diagnosis and with current technology is fairly accurate in determining size. It is also the study of choice for screening and follow-up when conservative treatment is elected. CT scan with contrast is the study of choice to accurately determine location, size, and plan treatment. Although MRI can also establish the diagnosis, it is more expensive and less useful to plan management. In addition, patients with abdominal aortic aneurysm frequently have pacemakers or other implants that contraindicate MRI. It is most useful in patients with iodine contrast allergy and or renal insufficiency. Arteriography, which used to be routine in the evaluation of patients with abdominal aortic aneurysm, is reserved for patients with occlusive disease or other specific indication.

A significant number of patients with AAA will have atherosclerotic occlusive disease. This includes peripheral and visceral involvement. Most importantly, the presence of renal and mesenteric occlusive disease must be evaluated, as it will influence management. Patients with symptoms of chronic mesenteric ischemia secondary to superior mesenteric artery and celiac artery disease present particularly high risk for intervention, as the circulation to the intestines may depend on the inferior mesenteric artery and thus may be significantly affected during aneurysm repair.

2.2 *Management of abdominal aortic aneurysms*

Management of patients with AAA must incorporate control of risk factors. This includes smoking cessation, control of hypertension, and evaluation for coronary artery disease. Control of their lipid profile with statins is highly recommended. Use of beta-blockers has been suggested to decrease the rate of abdominal aortic aneurysm expansion.

The decision between conservative management and intervention must take into account the risk of rupture of the aneurysm, the overall risk of repair, life expectancy, and patient preference. The risk of rupture of an abdominal aortic aneurysm increases progressively with aneurysm size where beyond 5–6 cm the risk appears to be high.

The estimated annual rupture risk for aneurysms 3–4.4 cm is approximately 2.1% per year whereas for aneurysms 4.5–5.9 cm, it is 10% per year. A higher rupture risk is estimated for aneurysms greater than 6 cm. Patients with a family history of aneurysms are at an even higher risk of rupture.

An important factor in patients under observation is the expansion rate. There is general consensus that aneurysms expand more rapidly, as they increase in size. Expansion rates for aneurysms 3–3.9 cm is estimated at 0.33 cm per year whereas those greater than 5 cm average 0.51 cm per year. Continued cigarette smoking is associated with more rapid expansion. In our current practice, we recommend consideration for intervention for aneurysms that grow more than 0.5 cm per year in patients with a reasonable life expectancy and acceptable risk for repair.

The risk of repair of AAA varies depending on location of the aneurysm and patient risk factors. The most important risk factors that increase mortality are renal dysfunction (creatinine greater than 1.8 mg/dL), history or presence of congestive heart failure, ischemic changes on electrocardiogram, and chronic obstructive pulmonary disease. Older age and female gender also increase operative risk. Aneurysms that involve the renal or other visceral arteries present a higher risk and, therefore, must take into account operator experience, life expectancy of the patient, and associated risk factors. In this regard, higher volume surgeons and or centers have been found to have a lower mortality.

2.3 *Options for repair*

2.3.1 *Surgical repair*

In modern practice, surgical repair is recommended for patients that are not candidates for an endovascular approach. Younger patients may also elect surgical repair to avoid the need for repeated imaging studies required after an endovascular procedure. Surgical repair of infrarenal AAA involves prosthetic graft replacement of the infrarenal aorta with either a tube or bifurcated graft depending on whether or not there is involvement of the iliac arteries (Fig. 1). A transperitoneal or retroperitoneal approach is utilized. This procedure is termed aneurysmorrhaphy. The technical aspect of this intervention is beyond the scope of this chapter.

For aneurysms involving the renal or other visceral arteries, surgical repair using a retroperitoneal approach is preferred with reimplantation and/or bypass to the affected visceral vessels. The location of the aortic clamp above the aneurysm will depend which visceral vessels are involved. Clearly, the risk of organ dysfunction, particularly renal failure, is increased. As endovascular technology evolves, the use

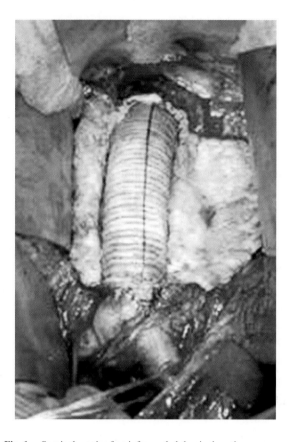

Fig. 1. Surgical repair of an infrarenal abdominal aortic aneurysm.

of branched or fenestrated grafts for aneurysms with visceral involvement may be an option.

The treatment of an infected or mycotic aneurysm will depend on the location of the process. When it occurs in the infrarenal aorta, aortic exclusion with extra-anatomic revascularization (axillofemoral graft) is recommended. When visceral involvement is present, *in situ* reconstruction with a prosthetic graft after thorough debridement of the infectious process has yielded excellent results. Alternatively, *in situ* revascularization with a homograft avoids the use of prosthetic material within an infected field.

Preoperative preparation and planning is essential in obtaining acceptable results. A CT scan with contrast is preferred to determine the exact location of the aneurysm and plan the reconstruction. Evaluation prior to intervention should include an assessment of coronary risk with selective use of cardiac stress testing. This will allow addressing significant coronary pathology prior to surgery. The patient should be adequately hydrated and mechanical bowel preparation is highly recommended.

Prophylactic antibiotics are routinely administered. Patients are routinely type and crossed for a minimum of two units of blood. Autologous donation is encouraged.

During anesthesia, maintenance of normal temperature decreases the risk of cardiac arrhythmias and coagulopathy. Use of arterial lines to monitor blood pressure and selective use of pulmonary artery catheters to monitor central pressures is recommended. In our practice, the use of intraoperative auto transfusion is reserved for suprarenal aneurysms and those that involve the visceral segment of the abdominal aorta.

Mortality after surgical repair of an AAA varies depending on whether or not the visceral arteries are involved. For purely infrarenal abdominal aortic aneurysms, the overall mortality in high-volume centers averages about 4%. This risk doubles when there is involvement of the visceral vessels mostly due to the need for suprarenal aortic cross-clamping. Furthermore, the risk of complications in these aneurysms increases with longer aortic cross-clamp times.

Bleeding after surgical repair of an abdominal aortic aneurysm may be secondary to a technical error or coagulopathy secondary to intraoperative bleeding, inadequate coagulation factor replacement, and/or hypothermia. Serial hematocrit measurements should be routine in the early postoperative period. Hypotension in the absence of cardiac dysfunction is most likely due to postoperative bleeding. Correction of hypothermia and coagulopathy, if present, is essential. Patients who do not respond to these initial measures should undergo early reoperation.

Myocardial infarction is the most common complication associated with mortality. Most events occur within the first 48 hours after surgery and thus patients with documented coronary artery disease should be monitored during the early postoperative period. In the absence of suprarenal clamping, renal failure is rare but highly morbid. We recommend the use of mannitol intraoperatively to induce diuresis particularly in the cases where suprarenal clamping is needed. It is wise to delay surgery after a CT scan with contrast to avoid the complication of renal toxicity from the iodinated contrast during the early postoperative period. Other causes postoperative renal insufficiency includes hypotension, decreased cardiac output, and intraoperative cholesterol embolization secondary to juxtarenal aortic clamping.

Respiratory failure after surgery is most often seen in patients with pre-existing pulmonary disease. Other important causes include aspiration, fluid overload, and sepsis. Aggressive pulmonary toilet, chest physical therapy, and incentive spirometry should be routinely utilized following surgical repair of AAA. Although controversial, the retroperitoneal approach seems to decrease the risk of pulmonary complications following surgery.

Gastrointestinal complications may be secondary to intraoperative injury or ischemia due to interruption of collateral circulation to the left colon in the presence of significant superior mesenteric and celiac artery occlusive disease. Table held retractors might further compromise blood flow to the colon by compression of the superior mesenteric artery superiorly and the inferior mesenteric collaterals inferiorly as necessary in a transperitoneal approach. This may explain why colon ischemia is extremely rare after a retroperitoneal approach. Ischemia to the left colon may also be secondary to exclusion of the internal iliac arteries by the reconstruction. Patients who have a bowel movement during or immediately after surgery, particularly if bloody, should be suspected of having ischemia of the left colon until proven otherwise.

Lower extremity ischemia after aneurysm repair may be secondary to graft thrombosis and or distal embolization. The former is usually secondary to a technical error or in some instances to an unrecognized hypercoagulable state. Micro-embolization can lead to toe ischemia also known as the blue toe syndrome. We routinely compress the femoral arteries manually during removal of the aortic clamp. This shunts the blood into the internal iliac system and may decrease the risk of distal extremity embolization.

Paraplegia is a rare complication after abdominal aortic aneurysm repair. It is most commonly seen when there is interruption of both internal iliac arteries leading to lumbar plexus ischemia. This usually presents as a mixed sensory and motor deficit. In suprarenal and total abdominal aortic aneurysm repairs, paraplegia may be secondary to spinal cord ischemia due to interruption of the anterior spinal artery. This usually presents mostly as a motor neurologic deficit.

Sexual dysfunction can occur after surgical repair of an abdominal aortic aneurysm in the form of retrograde ejaculation from sympathetic plexus injury and or impotence secondary to interruption of internal iliac blood flow. Maintaining the incision of the sac of the aneurysm to the right of the midline and avoiding longitudinal division of the left common iliac artery helps avoid sympathetic plexus injury. We routinely will tunnel an aortoiliac graft through the left common iliac artery to decrease the risk of sympathetic plexus injury.

Late complications associated with surgical repair of AAA include anastomotic disruption with pseudoaneurysm formation, graft infection, graft thrombosis and aorto enteric fistula. It is recommended that patients have a follow-up CT scan a minimum of five years after aneurysm repair.

2.3.2 *Endovascular repair*

Endovascular repair of infrarenal abdominal aortic aneurysms has emerged as the preferred approach in patients who have suitable anatomy. There is now sufficient follow-up of patients repaired with an endovascular graft more than 10 years ago to consider this approach as an effective intervention to reduce the risk of rupture.

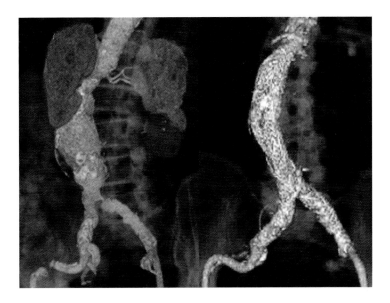

Fig. 2. Endovascular repair of an infrarenal abdominal aortic aneurysm.

This less invasive approach has reduced mortality and morbidity. A mean 30-day mortality of 2.4% with an overall morbidity of 9% represents a significant decrease compared to open surgical repair.

Endovascular repair of an abdominal aortic aneurysm involves the deployment of a prosthetic graft delivered through an access artery (usually the femoral arteries), which excludes the aneurysm sac from the circulation (Fig. 2). The intent is to thrombose the aneurysm sac around the graft to eliminate the risk of rupture. Currently available devices are mostly modular in design but vary in the method of deployment. Planning for the procedure is best done using a CT scan with intravenous contrast and thin (3-mm) cuts. Three-dimensional (3D) reconstructions are helpful but not essential. The technical aspects of endovascular repair are beyond the scope of this chapter.

The ideal anatomy for an endovascular repair include an appropriate proximal seal zone of 1.5 cm of normal diameter aorta and distal seal zone of at least 1 cm of normal iliac artery. With improved endovascular technology, these limitations have been reduced and vary according to the particular manufacturer. Use of adjunctive techniques such as internal iliac coil embolization and extension of the repair to the external iliac artery allows endovascular repair in the presence of iliac aneurysms. The tortuosity and shape of the proximal neck will also influence the suitability for endovascular repair.

Access for delivery of the endovascular components is an important aspect in planning repair. Deployment systems vary in size but most, at present, require an artery of at least 7 mm with minimal calcification. In most instances, these devices can be delivered through the femoral arteries either with a cutdown or percutaneously. If the size of the external iliac artery is inadequate, creation of a conduit by surgical placement of a graft to the common iliac artery using a retroperitoneal approach can provide adequate access for endograft delivery.

Most systemic complications following endovascular abdominal aortic aneurysm repair are similar to open surgical repair. Their incidence, however, is decreased by this less invasive approach. There are complications that are specific to the endovascular approach. Arterial bleeding can occur secondary to rupture of the access artery usually at the level of the external iliac artery. It is important during removal of the access sheath that the surgeon communicates with anesthesia so that changes in vital signs are immediately reported. A sudden change in heart rate and or blood pressure is indicative of retroperitoneal bleeding secondary to arterial rupture until proven otherwise. Rapid angiographic assessment of the access route with balloon tamponade can be life saving. Retroperitoneal bleeding can also be secondary to infrarenal aortic rupture at the level of the neck where aggressive ballooning can lead to tears of the aorta. Rapid resolution may be accomplished with placement of an aortic cuff but most often requires operative intervention.

An endoleak is a persistent flow of blood within the excluded aneurysm sac. It may be seen on completion angiography after implantation of the endograft or on follow-up CT scans. Endoleaks can be seen in up to 40% of cases with 70% of them resolving spontaneously within the first month. The cause of the endoleak has led to its classification in five different types.

Type I endoleak is secondary to an incomplete seal either at the proximal aortic neck or in the distal iliac landing zone.
Type II endoleak is due to persistent blood flow between branches of the aneurysm sac, most frequently between the inferior mesenteric artery and a lumbar artery.
Type III endoleak is due to separation or incomplete seal between endograft components.
Type IV endoleak is secondary to loss of integrity of the graft material.
Type V endoleak is secondary to ultrafiltration of serum through the graft material, also referred to as endotension and will not be evident on completion angiography.

Type I endoleaks represent continued pressurization of the aneurysm sac and, therefore, require additional intervention for their correction. Similarly, Type III and IV endoleaks should be treated as the risk of aneurysm rupture persists until their resolution. Type II endoleaks, seen on completion of the procedure, may be observed as they frequently resolve spontaneously and do not require treatment unless there is continued aneurysm growth during follow-up. A Type V endoleak was seen during follow-up in a specific graft manufactured before 2004. It is characterized by continued aneurysm growth in the absence of a detectable endoleak. Relining with a second endograft has been affective in its resolution. Most endoleaks that required treatment can be resolved with additional endovascular intervention. The specific endovascular treatment will depend on the type of endoleak. Surgical conversion is reserved for patients who have continued aneurysm growth with an unresolved endoleak. Acute surgical conversion during the initial endovascular graft deployment is associated with increased mortality and should be limited to those patients who have a life- or limb-threatening complications during implantation. Chronic surgical conversion can be performed with low morbidity and mortality.

Other complications specific to endovascular repair include graft limb thrombosis secondary to kinks that may occur due to morphology changes in the aneurysm during follow-up. As the aneurysm shrinks in diameter, it may also shorten in length. Options for treatment include surgical thrombectomy or thrombolysis with stenting of the affected limb. Graft migration can occur and its treatment will depend on the integrity of the repair. Observation is indicated in the presence of graft migration provided that no endoleak is present. In most instances, however, graft migration can result in sudden endoleak development and aneurysm rupture and thus should be addressed.

Aneurysm rupture following endovascular AAA repair occurs at an annual rate of 0.2% to 1%. It is most often due to a persistent endoleak and or graft migration. Not infrequently, it occurs in patients with inadequate surveillance or those lost to followup. Patients undergoing endovascular repair of abdominal aortic aneurysm must be followed on a yearly basis with imaging of the repair to avoid this complication. We recommend that patients have a CT scan with IV contrast within a month of the repair, at six months, and yearly thereafter. The sensitivity of the CT scan is increased when a delayed phase scan is done. In patients who have a shrinking aneurysm without evidence of endoleak or a stable aneurysm without evidence of endoleak, follow-up may consist of duplex scan of the abdomen (provided that the vascular laboratory is familiar with this type of evaluation) with assessment of the aneurysm size. When using this protocol, a CT scan should be done every few years. In patients with contraindication for iodinated contrast, MRI imaging is an excellent alternative. If an endoleak is detected, treatment will depend on the type of leak. If aneurysm growth is evident, treatment is indicated regardless of whether or not an endoleak is detected. The cumulative overall rate of reintervention after endovascular repair of abdominal aortic aneurysms can be as high as 10% per year. This underscores the importance of postoperative surveillance.

2.4 *Ruptured abdominal aortic aneurysm*

Rupture of an abdominal aortic aneurysm is associated with mortality of 90% when patients who do not reach the hospital are included. Patients who reach the hospital alive have a mortality that ranges between 40% and 70%. The classic presentation of a ruptured abdominal aortic aneurysm is a patient with severe abdominal or back pain, hypotension, and a pulsatile mass. Rapid evaluation is of critical importance. A plain film of the abdomen will frequently show calcification in of the aortic wall, with or without the loss of the psoas shadow, indicating the diagnosis. Abdominal ultrasound may be rapidly performed to establish the presence of an aortic aneurysm. With the use of rapid multislice CT scanner, computed tomography is the study of choice if the patient's conditions allows. This is particularly important when an endovascular approach is an option. A CT scan will help plan the appropriate procedure.

Perhaps most important in the management of a patient with a ruptured AAA is to avoid aggressive resuscitation until aortic control is accomplished. Thus, patients should be given enough intravenous fluids and blood to maintain consciousness and or a systolic blood pressure no higher than 100 mm Hg. Transfer to an operating room with endovascular capabilities should proceed without delay. The technical aspects of management of a ruptured abdominal aortic aneurysm are beyond the scope of this chapter. Suffice to say that an endovascular approach is an encouraging alternative to decrease the risk of death and morbidity. Unfortunately, not all patients are candidates for an endovascular repair and not all centers are prepared to proceed in that fashion on an emergency basis. When specific protocols for endovascular repair of ruptured abdominal aortic aneurysms are established, a significant decrease in mortality has been documented.

3. Iliac Aneurysms

Isolated iliac artery aneurysms are rare. They occur in less than 1% of all aortoiliac aneurysms. Isolated iliac aneurysms are more common in men (male to female ratio 5–16 to 1) older than 65 years old. The common iliac artery is involved in more than 70% of cases, the internal iliac in approximately 20–30% of cases and approximately 50% of the patients will present with bilateral involvement. External iliac artery aneurysms are extremely rare. Iliac aneurysms are most often asymptomatic. Symptoms of compression of adjacent structures have been reported including ureteral or rectal obstruction. The risk of rupture increases with size but the natural history of isolated iliac artery aneurysms is not well defined. Mortality from rupture ranges from 25% to 75% and, therefore, elective repair is recommended. In our practice, we recommend elective repair in acceptable risk patients for iliac aneurysms greater than 3 cm.

Options for repair include surgical graft replacement or endovascular treatment. The former is usually performed for unilateral aneurysms using a retroperitoneal approach with aneurysmorrhaphy. Endovascular repair may be accomplished using a bifurcated aortoiliac graft or an endovascular tube graft if an appropriate proximal landing zone is present. Frequently, endovascular repair involves coil embolization of the internal iliac artery with extension of the repair to the external iliac artery.

Treatment of internal iliac artery aneurysms is accomplished by proximal surgical ligation, with or without endoaneurysmal occlusion of the outflow tract. Surgical ligation alone, without distal occlusion of the outflow track, can be associated with continued aneurysm growth from back perfusion. We prefer an endovascular approach with distal outflow occlusion, accomplished with either coil embolization or deployment of an occlusion device, and endograft deployment from the common to the external iliac artery. Complications of either approach include buttock claudication and/or sexual dysfunction.

4. Thoracic and Thoracoabdominal Aneurysms

Thoracic and thoracoabdominal aneurysms (TAA), similar to AAA, are most commonly seen in men (male:female, 2–4:1) and patients that are over 65 years old. Associated risk factors include hypertension, atherosclerotic occlusive disease, coronary artery disease, and cerebrovascular disease. Chronic obstructive pulmonary disease is present in more than 30% of patients. Similar to abdominal aortic aneurysms, approximately 20% of patients will have a first-degree relative with a history of aortic aneurysm.

Most thoracic and TAAs are degenerative. Other etiologies include infection and trauma. Inherited connective tissue disorders, such as Marfan's syndrome, Turner's syndrome, Ehlers-Danlos syndrome, and polycystic kidney disease, are associated with the development of thoracic and thoracoabdominal aneurysms with or without aortic dissection. Of these, Marfan's syndrome is the most common syndrome and is characterized by skeletal, ocular (ectopia lentis), and cardiovascular abnormalities including aortic insufficiency and mitral valve prolapse or insufficiency. Marfan's syndrome has been linked to a specific mutation (fibrillin-1) that leads to aortic wall degradation. It is inherited in an autosomal dominant manner with variable penetration and clinical manifestations. Family history is absent, however, in 25% of patients presenting with this syndrome because of a spontaneous mutation.

Thoracic aortic aneurysms can be classified according to location into ascending aortic aneurysms, arch aneurysms, and descending thoracic aneurysms. Ascending aortic aneurysms involve dilation of the aortic root with or without aortic valve insufficiency, the latter requiring both graft and aortic valve replacement. Repair is usually recommended in acceptable risk patients and reasonable life expectancy with aneurysms greater than 6 cm. Symptoms may include chest pain, distal embolization, and compression of adjacent structures. Surgical repair is the only option at present and requires cardiopulmonary bypass with or without circulatory arrest. Cardiac surgeons perform this procedure and thus it is outside the scope of this chapter. Arch aneurysms usually presents with similar symptoms with a higher risk of embolization into the cerebrovascular system. Until recently, repair of these aneurysms required cardiopulmonary bypass and in most cases, circulatory arrest. With the evolution of endovascular technology, a less invasive approach can be performed as discussed below.

Descending thoracic aortic aneurysms start at or distal to the left subclavian artery and terminate in the distal descending thoracic aorta, above the celiac axis. Thoracoabdominal aortic aneurysms have been classified in five types.

Type I is a descending thoracic aneurysm with involvement of the proximal visceral segment of the abdominal aorta.
Type II is an aneurysm that starts at or just distal to the left subclavian artery and terminates at the aortic bifurcation.
Type III starts in the mid-descending thoracic aorta and terminates at the aortic bifurcation.
Type IV starts in the distal descending thoracic aorta and terminates at the aortic bifurcation.
Type V starts in the mid-descending thoracic aorta and terminates at or above the renal arteries.

4.1 *Clinical presentation*

Most often these aneurysms are asymptomatic and discovered on routine chest x-ray or other imaging studies performed for evaluation of other pathology. Symptoms can include back pain, hoarseness from compression of the recurrent laryngeal nerve, dyspnea due to compression of the trachea or bronchi, dysphagia from extrinsic compression of the esophagus, and acute paraplegia from embolization into the anterior spinal artery. Distal embolization can occur secondary to dislodgment of thrombus within the aneurysm presenting with acute organ or limb ischemia.

Rupture can be the presenting symptom of the thoracic or TAA in up to 20% of patients. The most important risk factor for rupture is aneurysm size. As with AAA, the risk of rupture increases with increasing aneurysm size. It is estimated that the risk of rupture of aneurysms larger than 8 cm is approximately 80% within one year of diagnosis. The rate of expansion is also an important factor in estimating rupture risk. Average expansion rate is estimated between 0.10 and 0.42 cm per year with expansion over 1 cm per year associated with the extremely high risk of rupture. Considering the difference in hemodynamics between the suprarenal and infrarenal aorta and the added risk involved in repair of thoracic or thoracoabdominal aneurysms, we currently recommend consideration for intervention in acceptable risk patients with aneurysms 6 cm or greater or when the expansion rate is greater than 0.5 cm per year.

4.2 *Management of thoracic and thoracoabdominal aneurysms*

Conservative management for patients with thoracic and TAAs is recommended for patients with aneurysms less than 6 cm who are otherwise asymptomatic. Patients with unacceptable intervention risk or limited life expectancy, in spite of having larger aneurysms, should also be considered for conservative management. Patient preference will also play an important role in this decision. Control of risk factors, particularly aggressive control of hypertension and smoking cessation, is essential in the management of these patients. Similar to abdominal aortic aneurysms, the use of beta-blockers and statins should be routine. When conservative management is elected, follow-up with yearly CT scans will identify patients with increasing risk of rupture who might then consider proceeding with intervention. The use of iodinated contrast for surveillance scans is not necessary.

Mortality after surgical repair of descending thoracic or TAAs has been reported in 4% to 21% of cases. When complications such as renal failure and/or paraplegia occur, mortality is increased significantly. Emergency presentation, congestive heart failure, and history of diabetes have been associated with increased mortality after intervention. Complications after intervention for thoracic or TAAs are similar to repair of abdominal aortic aneurysms but with a significant increase in the incidence of such complications. Several complications, however, deserve specific mention. The risk of stroke is increased in patients undergoing ascending and arch aneurysm repairs. Carotid duplex examination preoperatively is recommended. The risk of paraplegia, the most feared complication, has been estimated in contemporary series between 4% and 15% depending on the extent of the aneurysm. It can be significantly reduced with the use of adjuncts in the operative and perioperative period. In particular, reimplantation of intercostal arteries during surgical repair, selective use of spinal fluid drainage (see below), and maintenance of the mean blood pressure above 80 mm Hg have significantly reduced the risk of paraplegia during thoracic or TAA repair.

4.3 Preoperative management

Overall, the preoperative management of patients with thoracic or TAAs is similar to that of patients with AAA. In addition, consideration for perioperative spinal catheter drainage is an important aspect in patient preparation. Spinal cord ischemia during and after thoracic or thoracoabdominal aortic aneurysm repair is secondary to decreased blood flow to the spinal cord due to the interruption of intercostal arteries that supply the anterior spinal artery. Collateral blood flow to the anterior spinal cord may also be affected depending on the extent of the repair. These collaterals emanate from the vertebral artery, lumbar arteries, and internal iliac arteries. Collateral blood flow to the anterior spinal cord will be the net result of perfusion pressure minus intraspinal pressure. Elevating the blood pressure increases blood flow through these collaterals, whereas draining spinal fluid reduces intraspinal pressure. This combination is intended to augment overall blood flow to the spinal cord. Patients who have had prior infrarenal abdominal aortic surgery (ligation of lumbar arteries), or will have exclusion of the left subclavian artery (decreased flow through vertebral collaterals), and or internal iliac artery interruption and coverage of the critical segments T9 and T12 of the descending thoracic aorta should have intraoperative and perioperative spinal fluid drainages. Spinal canal pressure is maintained at 10 cm H2O using a gravity drain during intervention and for at least 48 hours after repair. We prefer to insert the spinal fluid drain the night before intervention in case a bloody drainage is noted, which may be observed and resolved overnight. Otherwise a bloody tap in the morning of the procedure may necessitate postponing the intervention. In the absence of a neurologic deficit, the drain is removed after raising the pressure to 20 cm H2O for six hours. It is important to recognize that delayed deficits may occur, which may necessitate reinsertion of the spinal drain. Maintaining the blood pressure, even if pressors are necessary, above a mean of 80 mm Hg is also recommended.

4.4 Surgical repair

Surgical repair of thoracic and TAAs involves prosthetic graft replacement of the affected segment with revascularization of critical aortic branches within the aneurysm. Either reimplanting the visceral or intercostal arteries as a Carrel patch onto an appropriate-sized opening in the graft (inclusion technique) or individual bypass grafts can accomplish the latter (Fig. 3). When these vessels are reimplanted as a patch, it is important to keep this as small as possible as aneurysmal degeneration of the implanted patch can occur. The choice of incision will depend on the extent of the aneurysm. A median sternotomy is the incision of choice for ascending and arch aneurysms. Descending thoracic aneurysms are exposed through a

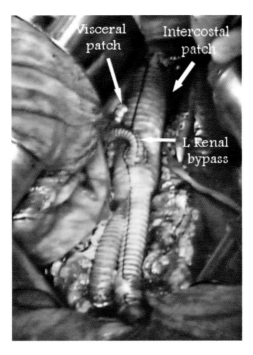

Fig. 3. Surgical repair of a thoracoabdominal aneurysm. Note reimplantation of the visceral vessels and intercostal arteries as a patch.

left thoracotomy with the patient in the right lateral decubitus position. For more extensive aneurysms, involving both the thoracic and abdominal aorta, a thoraco-retroperitoneal incision is made with the patient in the right semi-lateral decubitus position with the hips slightly rotated to the left and hyperextension of the table. This permits simultaneous exposure of the thoracic and abdominal aorta. Division of the diaphragm, when necessary, should be done in a circumferential manner avoiding injury to the phrenic nerve. Preservation of the diaphragm has been associated with a decrease incidence of respiratory complications. Arterial line blood pressure and pulmonary pressure monitoring are routine. The technical aspects of this procedure are beyond the scope of this chapter.

Adjunctive measures intended to decrease the risk of postoperative organ dysfunction have been found to significantly improve outcomes. Maintenance of blood flow to the lower body and viscera during aortic cross-clamping using extracorporal circulatory support decreases the risk of declamping hypotension and helps preserve organ function. In addition, it reduces myocardial strain during high aortic cross-clamping. Most commonly, left atrium to femoral extracorporeal circulation is used. From this circuit, individual cannulas can be used to preserve visceral circulation during repair of this segment of the aneurysm.

Postoperative renal insufficiency is associated with a significant increase in mortality following TAA repair. Thus, preservation of renal function is critical. Several adjuncts have been described including individual catheter perfusion during cross-clamp, renal cooling, and pharmacologic agents. Variable results with these efforts have been reported. We routinely administer intravenous mannitol prior to aortic cross-clamp and continue to use individual catheter perfusion with normothermic blood.

The extensive exposure necessary for these procedures frequently leads to hypothermia. Hypothermia will increase the risk of arrhythmias and coagulopathy. On the other hand, modest systemic cooling can be protective to the viscera and spinal cord. Current practice advocates the use of "permissive hypothermia" where the core temperature is kept around 32°C. A heat exchanger in the extracorporeal circulatory circuit will help maintain adequate body temperature. Coagulopathy can also be secondary to aggressive anticoagulation, intraoperative excessive bleeding with inadequate factor replacement, and visceral ischemia. We use the modest anti-coagulation with an initial dose of 0.5 mg/kg of intravenous heparin, maintaining the ACT around 250 seconds. This allows safe use of the extracorporeal circuit while at the same time reducing intraoperative bleeding. Intraoperative blood loss can be significant given the magnitude of the procedure. We routinely use a cell saver during the operation and monitor serum calcium. Liberal use of coagulation factor and platelets replacement, particularly toward the end of the procedure, is recommended.

The overall results of surgical repair of thoracic and TAAs have improved significantly over the last 10 years. With the use of adjuncts, the incidence of complications has also been reduced. The five-year survival of patients is between 60% and 70%. Advanced age, renal failure, Type II thoracoabdominal aneurysms, and continued cigarette smoking significantly reduce long-term survival.

4.5 *Endovascular repair*

Endovascular repair has emerged as an excellent alternative for repair in high-risk patients with thoracic aneurysms. Similar to endovascular treatment of abdominal aortic aneurysms, the goal of endovascular repair of thoracic aneurysms is to exclude the sac from circulation by deployment of an endovascular graft from within the aorta. Access is usually through the femoral artery although with the size of the deployment systems in current devices, a conduit is not infrequently necessary. Current technology is limited to descending thoracic aneurysms where no critical aortic branch is covered. Rapidly evolving technology, however, is being developed for treatment of thoracoabdominal aneurysms with endovascular grafts that have individual branches to maintain circulation to critical organs.

Since 2005, a number of manufacturers have developed and receive FDA approval for several endovascular grafts that are currently available. Although they differ in construction, materials, and method of deployment, they share, in general, anatomic requirements. A 2–3 cm proximal and distal seal zone for effective exclusion of the aneurysm sac must be present or created. The grafts are usually oversized to this landing zone by 10–15%. Access for deployment will typically require a 7–8-mm artery. In most instances the femoral artery is utilized provided that there is little or no calcification in the external iliac artery and the tortuosity does not interfere with safe deployment. Alternatively, a 10-mm conduit is constructed either to the common iliac artery or in a few instances the aorta using a retroperitoneal approach. Contralateral arterial access is often used for control angiography. Endograft selection and method of deployment are beyond the scope of this chapter.

Indications for endovascular repair of a thoracic aneurysm are the same as for surgical repair. Although initially intended for high-risk patients, given the excellent results that have been reported, the endovascular approach is now preferred. Younger patients who are good operative risks are preferably treated with an open repair. Follow-up after endovascular repair requires continued surveillance with CT scans or MRI. These are usually performed within a month after the procedure, at six months and yearly thereafter. As with endovascular repair of AAA, endoleaks, migration, and aneurysm growth are potential complications. Endoleaks are classified the same as with endovascular abdominal aortic aneurysm repair.

Operative planning is critical. The primary imaging is a CT scan, preferably a 64-slice scan, which provides excellent definition and allows accurate measurements. Patients who have contrast allergy or renal insufficiency can have gated magnetic resonance angiography (MRA) with a noncontrast CT scan. Adequate fixation of the endograft at the landing zone, both proximal and distal, requires careful selection of the appropriate size of the device and the length of the aortic segment to be treated. Often, more than one device will be necessary and in principle, the larger device is deployed within the smaller device with an overlap that varies with the manufacturer.

For purposes of comparison, the aortic arch has been divided into four zones based on the tangential line aligned with the distal sides of each great vessel.

Zone 0 is at the origin of the innominate artery.
Zone 1 is at the origin of the left common carotid artery.
Zone 2 is at the origin of the left subclavian artery.
Zone 3 is at the proximal descending thoracic aorta to the T4 vertebral body.
Zone 4 is at the rest of the descending thoracic aorta.

The ideal landing zone should be relatively straight and the length of treatment the minimum to accomplish exclusion of the aneurysm. This will help prevent spinal cord ischemia.

The proximal landing zone for endovascular repair of a descending thoracic aneurysm often will need to be extended by starting the repair just distal to the left common carotid artery (Zone 2) to provide an adequate proximal landing zone. This requires coverage of the left subclavian artery. The left subclavian artery not only provides circulation to the left upper extremity and the brain but through collaterals, the spinal cord. When planned coverage of the subclavian artery is anticipated, it is critical to assess the patency of the right vertebral artery into the basilar artery, as well as the integrity of the circle of Willis. This identifies patients who cannot tolerate left subclavian artery occlusion in whom mandatory left subclavian revascularization is necessary. This is often accomplished by either left carotid subclavian bypass or transposition. Left subclavian revascularization is essential in patients who have a dominant left vertebral artery, a patent left internal mammary coronary bypass, an occluded or hypoplastic right vertebral artery, or when the left vertebral artery originates from the aortic arch. We also recommend left subclavian revascularization when there is extensive coverage of the thoracoabdominal aorta (see below). On occasion, the patient will become symptomatic during the postoperative period after coverage of the left subclavian artery in which case it should be revascularized as a second procedure. When coverage of the left subclavian artery is necessary, it is best to occlude the artery by either ligation or an endovascular occluder proximal to the left vertebral artery to avoid a Type II endoleak. Preoperative assessment of the vertebral circulation can be accomplished with a duplex scan whereas integrity of the circle of Willis will require either an intracranial CTA or MRA.

The distal landing zone may be extended in some patients by covering the celiac trunk when there is adequate collateral circulation between the celiac axis and superior mesenteric artery. This may be assessed with CTA but should be confirmed with selective angiography. In the absence of adequate collaterals, a bypass to the celiac axis can prevent severe hepatic ischemic complications.

Spinal catheter drainage is indicated in patients who have had prior infrarenal abdominal aortic aneurysm repair and require coverage of the critical T9-L2 segment. We would also recommend spinal catheter drainage in patients that are having the left subclavian artery covered without revascularization, particularly if they have significant internal iliac artery occlusive disease. Management of the lumbar drain is similar to open repair. Similar preventive measures, as with open repair, should include perioperative maintenance of the mean blood pressure at 80 mm Hg or higher.

To date, there have been no randomized clinical trials comparing endovascular repair of descending thoracic aortic aneurysm with open surgical repair. The most valuable information comes from the trials that led to the FDA approval of current devices and the European Registry. Technical success rate averaged 98% in the industry-sponsored trials with a somewhat lower rate in the European Registry, the latter reflecting a less rigorous patient selection. Most failures were related to access. The use of a conduit was necessary in 10–20% of cases. Repairs that started in Zone 2 were required in up to 20% of cases. In the three industry-sponsored trials, there were a total of 495 patients treated by endovascular means compared to 353 patients (nonrandomized or historical controls) in the open cohort. The mortality for the endovascular group was approximately 2% compared to 8.5% in the surgical group. A meta-analysis of 17 studies reported a significant reduction in mortality and major neurologic complications with the endovascular approach. This early advantage translates into an improved five-year survival.

Paraplegia, the most feared complication, is also reduced by the endovascular approach. In the three industry-sponsored trials the endovascular approach average 6.2% versus 13% for the surgical group. The rates of endoleak have ranged between 6.6% and 26% with 4% of patients having an endoleak at five years. Enlargement of the aneurysm sac ranges between 7% and 14% and at five years shrinkage is observed in 50% of patients, with 30% showing no change in size. Clearly longer follow-up is needed. Overall, however, endovascular repair for descending thoracic aortic aneurysms has lower morbidity and mortality than open surgical repair.

4.6 *Combined endovascular and surgical (hybrid) repair of arch and thoracoabdominal aortic aneurysms*

The concept of "debranching" an aortic aneurysmal segment involves extra-anatomic revascularization of critical branches in order to provide an adequate landing zone for an endovascular graft. Once alternative circulation is provided with surgical bypasses, the aneurysm can be treated with an endovascular graft. This has the potential of reducing the magnitude of the repair, avoid aortic cross clamping, and limit the time of ischemia to the particular vascular bed. Intraoperative hypotension is rare, which may further decrease the risk of paraplegia. In the aortic arch, extra-anatomic revascularization may be accomplished with subcutaneous bypasses from an inflow source, usually the right common carotid artery (carotid-carotid bypass, left carotid-subclavian bypass, or transposition). When the innominate artery is involved in the aneurysm, through a median sternotomy, the ascending aorta may serve as the inflow for aorto innominate and carotid bypass. The revascularization would be completed with an extra-anatomic left carotid to left subclavian bypass or transposition. In thoracoabdominal aneurysms, debranching of the visceral segment of the aorta can be accomplished with retrograde grafts originating in the distal aorta or the common iliac arteries. The repair is completed in both instances with the deployment of an endovascular graft excluding the aneurysmal segment (Fig. 4). Many variations to accomplish the "debranching" have been described. In particular to thoracoabdominal aneurysms, the transperitoneal or the retroperitoneal approach

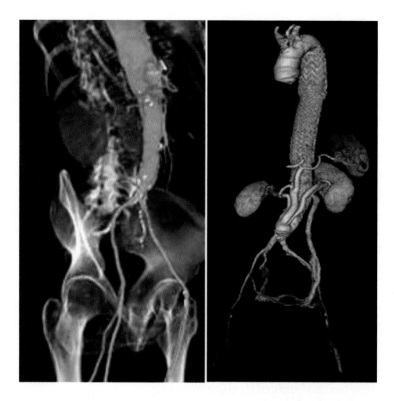

Fig. 4. Combined endovascular and surgical repair of a Type II thoracoabdominal aneurysm.

may be used depending on the visceral branches that require revascularization. The technical aspects of aortic debranching are beyond the scope of this chapter.

The first hybrid approach to treat a thoracoabdominal aneurysm was reported in 1999. Since then, the combined endovascular and surgical approach has emerged as an alternative in high-risk patients. Nevertheless, controversy exists in patient selection, the appropriateness of offering intervention in patients with potentially limited life expectancy because of their comorbidities and whether or not it actually decreases risk. The decision to proceed with a hybrid approach is based on the patient's comorbidities, overall surgical risk, anatomy of the process, and prior surgical intervention. Unstable patients with a contained rupture, or patients with a free rupture, are not candidates for hybrid approach and are best treated with surgical repair. Patients with a prior left thoracotomy, particularly if left heart bypass was used, present significant challenges for reoperative surgery. These patients are good candidates for a combined approach. Similarly, patients who present with a patch rupture after a prior thoracoabdominal aneurysm repair can be considered for a hybrid approach. In patients with significant chronic obstructive pulmonary disease, a frequent risk factor in patients with aortic aneurysms may benefit by avoiding a thoracotomy thus decreasing the risk of pulmonary complications. Similarly, patients with chronic renal insufficiency may benefit by reducing the ischemia time to the kidneys.

The debranching portion of the procedure is a major surgical intervention. It usually takes experienced surgeons anywhere from 6 to 9 hours to accomplish. One potential advantage of the hybrid approach is that it can be performed in two stages. The surgical portion accomplishes the debranching, and the endovascular repair is performed as a second stage. Some investigators have found staging to be beneficial whereas others have found no benefit. A single-stage approach, where the surgical and endovascular portions are completed as one procedure, has the advantage of a single anesthetic and reduction or elimination of the potential for rupture of the aneurysm as can occur in the interval between two stages. This is clearly a better alternative for symptomatic patients. The two-stage approach allows the patient to recover from the more prolonged intervention (surgical portion) thus performing the endovascular repair at a time when there is less risk for hypotension. In addition, it allows the circulatory system to stabilize to the new flow pattern. Our experience to date suggests that patients, who require extensive coverage of the thoracoabdominal aorta, particularly if the infrarenal aorta is involved and to be covered, are candidates for a two-stage approach. Patients who become unstable during the debranching procedure are best treated in two stages. In order to facilitate access for the endovascular portion, patients who are treated in two stages may have a conduit placed at the first stage that can be accessed with a simple cut down and thrombectomy at the second stage. In aortic arch reconstructions, most patients are treated in a single stage. Access for deployment of the endovascular graft is usually retrograde from the femoral or iliac artery when a median sternotomy is not necessary, whereas a conduit can be placed on the hood of the graft for antegrade access when the ascending aorta is the source of inflow.

The results of hybrid repair of thoracoabdominal and arch aortic aneurysms, as published in the literature, have been mixed. Series with 10 or more patients have reported a wide range of mortality from 0% to 31%. The majority of patients treated at Type II or Type III thoracoabdominal aneurysms. A significant factor associated with high mortality has been reported in patients operated emergently or urgently. Overall major morbidity has also been significant (30%). Permanent paraplegia has been observed in approximately 5% of cases and prolonged respiratory support required in 8%. Significant cardiac complications occurred in approximately 5% patients. Renal failure requiring temporary or permanent hemodialysis has averaged 12%. Interestingly, all these complications appear to be reduced when a two-stage approach is used. The most significant complication of the two-stage approach is interval aneurysm rupture, which has occurred in our own experience. Endoleaks on follow-up were seen in approximately 20% of patients with about 40% of these being

Type I. Retrograde graft patency has been excellent. In a review of the literature, with a mean follow-up of 14.5 months, a 97.8% patency was documented. Comparison with the results of open surgical repair seems inappropriate as all patients in these hybrid series were deemed high risk and most were not considered suitable for open surgical repair.

Our own experience with the combined endovascular and surgical approaches to thoracoabdominal aortic pathology has been quite favorable. In our initial report, we have observed no mortality with the permanent paraplegia rate of 5.8% and overall morbidity of 12%. Since then, we have observed two patients with interval aneurysm rupture between stages amongst 35 patients undergoing hybrid repair for a 5.7% 30-day mortality. No additional spinal cord ischemia complication has occurred in patients with thoracoabdominal aneurysm (patients at risk) for an overall paraplegia rate of 3.5%. Cumulative survival at two years is 76%. Our initial patient operated on in 1998, continues to do well 12 years after the procedure. In our opinion, these encouraging results continue to support offering this alternative to high-risk patients with significant thoracoabdominal pathology.

5. Aortic Dissection

Arterial dissection is a condition where an intimal tear leads to separation of the layers of the arterial wall through the media. Blood flow through this separation creates two channels, separated by a septum composed of the intima and part of the media. The process can propagate both distal and or proximal to the intimal tear. The newly created channel of blood flow, within the medial layer, is called the false lumen. Aortic dissection is the most common life-threatening emergency affecting the aorta. It classified as acute when the diagnosis is made within two weeks of the onset of symptoms. When the diagnosis is made after two weeks of the initial symptoms, the aortic dissection is classified as chronic. Anatomic classification is also important and is based on the location of the intimal tear and the extent of the dissection along the aorta. The DeBakey classification uses both the location of the entry tear and the extent of the dissection. According to this scheme, the dissection is classified three types.

Type I: The entry tear originates in the ascending aorta and extends from the aortic arch into the descending or abdominal aorta for varying distances.

Type II: The dissection originates and is confined to the ascending aorta.

Type IIIa: The entry tear is just distal to the left subclavian artery and the extent is limited to the descending thoracic aorta.

Type IIIb: The dissection originates just distal to the left subclavian artery and extends for a variable distance of the abdominal aorta.

The Stanford classification uses the location of the entry tear alone. A Stanford Type A aortic dissection originates in the ascending aorta and, therefore, includes DeBakey Types I and II. A Stanford Type B aortic dissection originates descending thoracic aorta and, therefore, includes DeBakey Types IIIa and IIIb. The Stanford classification, being simpler and clinically relevant, is most commonly used. Patients with Type A aortic dissection require urgent surgical treatment because of the associated high risk for lethal cardiac and aortic complications. Patients with Type B aortic dissection are managed medically unless complications occur (see below).

Two variants of aortic dissection include intramural hematoma and penetrating aortic ulcer. An intramural hematoma is a collection of blood confined to the aortic media. A penetrating aortic ulcer is an intimal tear with a localized disruption of the media and out pouching of the aortic wall. In both instances, there is separation of the media and thus their relationship to aortic dissection. Both tend to resolve spontaneously in 50–80% of patients with progression to either dissection or aneurysmal degeneration in the remainder. Treatment of intramural hematoma is indicated in symptomatic patients or those who show progression of follow-up. In penetrating ulcer, treatment is indicated based on the diameter of the aorta, including the ulcer, with similar indications as aortic aneurysms.

The incidence of acute aortic dissection has been estimated between 2.9 and 3.5 per 100,000 person-years. It is most common in men (4:1 male/female). Type A dissection occurs twice as often as Type B dissection. Patients with Type A dissection tend to be younger than those with Type B aortic dissection. Aortic dissection occurs more often in the morning and in the winter months.

Risk factors for aortic dissection include older age, hypertension, and abnormalities of the aortic wall. Hypertension is present in more than 70% of patients. Structural abnormalities include the presence of a bicuspid aortic valve, aortic coarctation, chromosomal abnormalities (Turner's syndrome and Noonan's syndrome), and arch hypoplasia. Hereditary conditions includes Marfan's syndrome and Ehler Danlos syndrome. The former accounts for over 50% of cases of acute aortic dissection in younger patients. Pregnancy complicated by preeclampsia is a risk factor for aortic dissection particularly in women with Marfan's syndrome. Cocaine abuse has also been associated with acute aortic dissection. Most cases of acute aortic dissection are associated with medial degeneration of the aortic wall or cystic medial necrosis. Hereditary conditions are universally associated with this process. In patients without these syndromes, the degree of this type of medial degeneration is greater than expected, and associated with advanced age and hypertension. Significant atherosclerosis is relatively infrequent in patients with acute aortic dissection. In fact, some have proposed that atheroma may serve to terminate or limit the extent of the dissection. Acute aortic dissection can occur in a patient with a pre-existing aortic aneurysm, which significantly increases the risk of rupture.

Pain is the most common symptom of acute aortic dissection. It is typically of abrupt onset, usually described as sharp, severe, stabbing, and or migratory. Almost 90% of the patients described the pain as "the worst ever". When the pain is in the anterior chest, a Type A aortic dissection is more likely. Patients with Type B aortic dissection more often experience back pain. Syncope may occur secondary to cardiac tamponade and or brachiocephalic vessels involvement. The latter may also be manifested by a stroke. Spinal cord ischemia as a complication of dissection of the descending thoracic aorta can occur in up to 10% of patients. Symptoms of compression of adjacent structures can lead to hoarseness, lower extremity paresthesias from lumbar plexopathy, or Horner's syndrome from compression of the sympathetic ganglia. Pulse deficit with or without extremity ischemia in a patient with severe chest or back pain should raise the suspicion of an acute aortic dissection. When it occurs in the upper extremities, a falsely depressed blood pressure can be misleading. Hypertension is most common, particularly in patients with Type B aortic dissection. Hypotension is rare and most common in Type A aortic dissection complicated by aortic valve dysfunction or cardiac tamponade.

The timely diagnosis of an acute aortic dissection is impeded by the fact that most patients with chest pain do not have acute dissection. The diagnosis is most often established during the evaluation for a different suspected condition such as myocardial ischemia. On chest x-ray, widening of the cardiac or aortic silhouette, displacement of aortic calcification, and/or the presence of a pleural effusion should raise suspicion of an acute aortic dissection. CT angiography and trans-esophageal echocardiography are the best studies to establish the diagnosis. Typical findings on CT are the presence of a true and false lumen with the true lumen typically being the smaller of the two in 90% of cases. Most commonly the celiac, superior mesenteric artery, and right renal artery originate from the true lumen whereas the left renal artery originates from the false lumen. Many variations occur, including any of these critical branches coming from both lumens. The dissection flap or septum tends to be concave toward the true lumen in acute dissection and flat in chronic dissection. MRI has a high sensitivity and specificity but the lack of immediate availability, difficulty in monitoring critically ill patients, and the presence of implants, which contraindicate the study, presents limitations. Angiography is not indicated unless it is being used as part of the treatment strategy.

5.1 *Medical management of acute aortic dissection*

The goal of medical management is intended to reduce the hemodynamic forces that can lead to propagation of the intimal tear with branch vessel compromise and or rupture. Except in hypotensive patients, all patients with acute aortic dissection should receive antihypertensive medication first with a beta-blocker and once effectively blocked (decreased heart rate), with a direct vasodilator (sodium nitroprusside). Instituting the latter first, may actually increase the stress on the aortic wall by the release of catecholamines. Hypotensive patients should undergo rapid evaluation to exclude cardiac tamponade or rupture and institute appropriate surgical intervention. Patients should have invasive monitoring including an arterial line, central line, and central pressure monitoring. Mortality in the early stages of an acute Type A aortic dissection can exceed 1% per hour secondary to tamponade, involvement of the coronary arteries, and or acute aortic valvular insufficiency. Therefore, surgical repair of acute Type A aortic dissection should proceed without delay.

Continued medical therapy is indicated in patients with acute Type B aortic dissection not complicated by malperfusion or rupture. Malperfusion is the result of aortic branch compromise by the dissecting process. It leads to end organ ischemia by one of two mechanisms. A static obstruction occurs when the dissection enters a critical aortic branch resulting in thrombosis or hypoperfusion of the end organ. More commonly, however, a dynamic obstruction occurs because of the compressed true lumen restricting flow or by prolapse of the septum during systole into the branch. The concept of dynamic obstruction is important to understand as patency of a branch on angiography or static imaging can be misleading. The presence of clinical symptoms of malperfusion is most critical in decision making. Symptoms of malperfusion include severe abdominal pain (mesenteric ischemia), refractory hypertension (renal ischemia), hepatic insufficiency (celiac artery compromise with inadequate collaterals), and lower extremity ischemia. The latter may be resolved initially with extra-anatomic revascularization but implies an extensive process, which warrants careful evaluation of other territories.

In the absence of malperfusion, a concomitant aortic aneurysm, increasing size of the false lumen, leak, or rupture, continued medical therapy is indicated. In patients with stable noncomplicated acute Type B aortic dissection, surgical treatment has not been shown to improve results. Therefore, a complication-specific approach to select patients for surgical or endovascular treatment is recommended.

Patients, who are managed medically, will require serial monitoring with CT scans every six months until a stable process is documented and then yearly thereafter. Continued patency of the false lumen, in the chronic stage, is an independent risk factor for aneurysmal degeneration. Aneurysmal degeneration of a chronic dissection is estimated to occur in 25–40% of cases. Three-year survival of patients treated medically is between 68% and 77%.

5.2 *Surgical repair of acute aortic dissection*

The goals of surgical treatment of an acute aortic dissection is to close the intimal tear, eliminate flow through the false lumen leading to false lumen thrombosis, reestablish adequate flow to compromised critical aortic branches, and prevent rupture. Surgical repair is indicated in all patients with Type A aortic dissection and patients with complicated Type B aortic dissection. Ascending aortic graft replacement, with or without aortic valve repair or replacement, and reconstruction of the distal aortic wall to exclude the false lumen is the procedure of choice for patients with Type A aortic dissection. In most instances, malperfusion of critical aortic branches in the abdomen resolves with this procedure. Otherwise, revascularization by alternative means (fenestration and surgical bypass) is necessary. Poor outcomes are associated with unstable patients at presentation and those with significant neurologic deficit. Mortality for surgical intervention in Type A aortic dissection in a large registry was reported at 23.9%. The technical aspects of this intervention are beyond the scope of this chapter.

Surgical repair of Type B aortic dissection most often involves repair of the intimal tear with graft replacement of the proximal descending thoracic aorta. Repair of the aortic layers at the distal anastomosis is performed to obliterate the false lumen. This can be done with either Teflon pledgets or more recently with glue aortoplasty. Resolution of malperfusion either by the procedure itself, or by the use of bypass or fenestration when necessary, is critical. Mortality of surgical treatment of Type B aortic dissection has ranged from 6% to 69% with those requiring surgery within 24 hours of admission having the highest mortality. Three-year survival rate for patients with acute Type B aortic dissection treated surgically is around 80%. The technical aspects of surgical repair of Type B aortic dissection are beyond the scope of this chapter.

5.3 *Endovascular repair of Type B aortic dissection*

Endovascular repair seems a logical alternative to surgical repair in patients with Type B aortic dissection (Fig. 5). It can accomplish obliteration of the entry tear and reestablishment of adequate flow into the true lumen while avoiding aortic cross-clamping and a thoracotomy in a critically ill patient. The technical aspects of this approach are beyond the scope this chapter. Although multiple reports have suggested improved outcomes, a randomized multicenter trial comparing stent grafting with surgical treatment for uncomplicated chronic Type B aortic dissection failed to show any significant benefit. By not including in these trial patients in the acute stage, with a complicated dissection, the issue remains unsolved. A potential advantage of the endovascular approach is timely assessment of patency of critical branches in the abdominal aorta. In the presence of malperfusion, revascularization may be performed by stent grafting or endovascular fenestration. In some cases, surgical fenestration may be necessary, which still leads to a smaller procedure than complete surgical approach. Obliteration of the entry tear may prevent aneurysmal

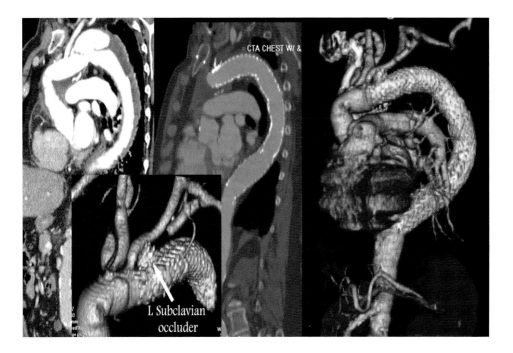

Fig. 5.   Endovascular repair of chronic aortic dissection with aneurysmal degeneration.

degeneration in long term. Continued false lumen patency has been associated with poorer outcomes. Further experience and followup is clearly needed. When false lumen thrombosis occurs, there is remodeling of the aorta. Long-term survival after an endovascular approach is similar to medical treatment and surgical repair. Ongoing clinical trials will help establish the role of endovascular therapy for acute Type B aortic dissection.

References

Adriaensen ME, Bosch JL, Halpem EF, *et al.* Elective endovascular versus open surgical repair of abdominal aortic aneurysms: Systematic review of short-term results. *Radiology* 2002; **224**:739–747.

Alcorn HG, Wolfson SK Jr, Sutton-Tyrrell K, *et al.* Risk factors for abdominal aortic aneurysms in older adults enrolled in the Cardiovascular Health Study. *Arterioscler Thromb Vasc Biol* 1996; **16**:963.

Auer J. Aortic dissection: Incidence, natural history and impact of surgery. *J Clin Basic Cardiol* 2002; **3**:151–154.

Bengtsson H, Bergqvist D. Ruptured abdominal aortic aneurysm: A population-based study. *J Vasc Surg* 1993; **18**:74–80.

Bernard Y, Zimmermann H, Chocron S, *et al.* False lumen patency as a predictor of late outcome in aortic dissection. *Am J Cardiol* 2001; **87**:1378–1382.

Bernhard VM, Mitchell RS, Matsumura JS, *et al.* Ruptured abdominal aortic aneurysm after endovascular repair. *J Vasc Surg* 2002; **35**:1155–1162.

Biasi L, Ali T, Loosemore T, *et al.* Hybrid repair of complex thoracoabdominal aortic aneurysms using applied endovascular strategies combined with visceral and renal revascularization. *J Thorac Cardiovasc Surg* 2009.

Bickerstaff LK, Hollier LH, Van Peenen HJ, *et al.* Abdominal aortic aneurysms: The changing natural history. *J Vasc Surg* 1984; **1**:6.

Bickerstaff LK, Pairolero PC, Hollier LH, *et al.* Thoracic aortic aneurysms: A population-based study. *Surgery* 1982; **92**:1103.

Bickerstaff LK, Pairolero PC, Hollier LH, *et al.* Thoracic aortic aneurysms: A population-based study. *Surgery* 1982; **92**:1103.

Biddinger A, Rocklin M, Coselli J, *et al.* Familial thoracic aortic dilatations and dissections: A case control study. *J Vasc Surg* 1997; **25**:506.

Bockler D, Kotelis D, Geisbusch P, Hyhlik-Durr A, Klemm K, Tengg-Kobligk HV, Kauczor HU, Allenberg JR. Hybrid procedures for thoracoabdominal aortic aneurysms and chronic aortic dissections — A single center experience in 28 patients. *J Vasc Surg* 2008; 724–732.

Brady AR, Thompson RW, Greenhalgh RM, Powell JT. Cardiovascular risk factors and abdominal aortic aneurysm expansion: Only smoking counts [abstract]. *Br J Surg* 2003; **90**:492.

Brunkwall J, Hauksson H, Bengtsson H, *et al.* Solitary aneurysms of the iliac arterial system: An estimate of their frequency of occurrence. *J Vasc Surg* 1989; **10**:381.

Buth J, Laheji RJ. Early complications and endoleaks after endovascular abdominal aortic aneurysm repair: Report of a multicenter study. *J Vasc Surg* 2000; **31**:134–146.

Cambria RA, Gloviczki P, Stanson AW, *et al.* Outcome and expansion rate of 57 thoracoabdominal aortic aneurysms managed nonoperatively. *Am J Surg* 1995; **170**:213.

Cambria RP, Clouse WD, Davison JK, *et al.* Thoracoabdominal aneurysm repair: Results with 337 operations performed over a 15-year interval. *Ann Surg* 2002; **236**:471.

Cambria RP, Brewster DC, Moncure AC, *et al.* Spontaneous aortic dissection in the presence of coexistent or previously repaired atherosclerotic aortic aneurysm. *Ann Surg* 1988; **208**:619–624.

Cho JS, Haider S, Makaroun MS. US multi-center trials of endoprostheses for the endovascular treatment of descending thoracic aneurysms. *J Vasc Surg* 2006; **43**(Suppl A):12A–19A.

Cho JS, Haider S, Makaroun MS. Endovascular therapy of thoracic aneurysms: Gore TAG trial results. *Semin Vasc Surg* 2006; **19**:18–24.

Cina CS, Lagana A, Bruin G, *et al.* Thoracoabdominal aortic aneurysm repair: A prospective cohort study of 121 cases. *Ann Vasc Surg* 2002; **16**:631.

Clouse WD, Hallett Jr JW, Schaff HV, *et al.* Acute aortic dissection: Population-based incidence compared with degenerative aortic aneurysm rupture. *Mayo Clin Proc* 2004; **79**:176–180.

Coady MA, Davies RR, Roberts M, *et al.* Familial patterns of thoracic aortic aneurysms. *Arch Surg* 1999; **134**:361.

Coady MA, Rizzo JA, Hammond GL, *et al.* What is the appropriate size criterion for resection of thoracic aortic aneurysms? *J Thorac Cardiovasc Surg* 1997; **113**:476.

Conrad MF, Crawford RS, Davison JK, Cambria RP. Thoracoabdominal aneurysm repair: A 20-year perspective. *Ann Thorac Surg* 2007; **83**:S856–S861.

Coselli JS, Bozinovski J, LeMaire SA. Open surgical repair of 2286 thoracoabdominal aortic aneurysms. *Ann Thorac Surg* 2007; **83**:S862–S864.

Coselli JS, LeMaire SA, Conklin LD, Adams GJ. Left heart bypass during descending thoracic aortic aneurysm repair does not reduce the incidence of paraplegia. *Ann Thorac Surg* 2004; **77**:1298–1303.

Coselli JS. Thoracoabdominal aortic aneurysms: Experience with 372 patients. *J Card Surg* 1994; **9**:638–647.

Daily PO, Trueblood HW, Stinson EB, *et al.* Management of acute aortic dissection. *Ann Thorac Surg* 1970; **10**:237–246.

Daniel JC, Huynh TT, Zhou W, *et al.* Acute aortic dissection associated with use of cocaine. *J Vasc Surg* 2007; **46**:427–433.

Dapunt OE, Galla JD, Sadeghi AM, *et al.* The natural history of thoracic aortic aneurysms. *J Thorac Cardiovasc Surg* 1994; **107**:1323.

Dardik A, Burleyson GP, Bowman H, *et al.* Surgical repair of ruptured abdominal aortic aneurysms in the state of Maryland: Factors influencing outcome among 527 recent cases. *J Vasc Surg* 1998; **28**:413–420.

Dardik A, Krosnick T, Perler BA, *et al.* Durability of thoracoabdominal aortic aneurysm repair in patients with connective tissue disorders. *J Vasc Surg* 2002; **36**:696.

Darling RC, III, Mehta M, Roddy SP, *et al.* Coverage of celiac artery during thoracic endovascular aneurysm repair: Outcomes of a prospective analysis. Paper presented at the Society for Vascular Surgery Annual Meeting, June 5, 2008, San Diego, CA.

Darling RCD, Brewster DC, Darling RC, *et al.* Are familial abdominal aortic aneurysms different? *J Vasc Surg* 1989; **10**:39.

Datillo JB, Brewster DC, Fan C-M, *et al.* Clinical failures of endovascular abdominal aortic aneurysm repair: Incidence, cause and management. *J Vasc Surg* 2002; **35**:1137–1144.

Davies RR, Goldstein LJ, Coady MA, *et al.* Yearly rupture or dissection rates for thoracic aortic aneurysms: Simple predication based on size. *Ann Thorac Surg* 2002; **73**:17.

DeBakey ME, Henly WS, Cooley DA, *et al.* Surgical management of dissecting aneurysms of the aorta. *Thorac Cardiovasc Surg* 1965; **49**:130–149.

Dent TL, Lindenauer SM, Ernst CB, Fry WJ. Multiple arteriosclerotic arterial aneurysms. *Arch Surg* 1972; **105**:338.

Dietz HC. New insights into the genetic basis of aortic aneurysms. *Monogr Pathol* 1995; **37**:144.

Dimick JB, Cowan JA Jr, Stanley JC, *et al.* Surgeon specialty and provider volumes are related to outcome of intact abdominal aortic aneurysm repair in the United States. *J Vasc Surg* 2003; **38**:739.

Donas KP, Czerny M, Guber I, Teufelsbauer H, Nanobachvili J. Hybrid open endovascular repair for thoracoabdominal aortic aneurysms: Current status and level of evidence. *Eur J Vasc Endovasc Surg* 2007; **34**:528–533.

Drinkwater SL, Bockler D, Eckstein H, *et al.* The visceral hybrid repair of thoracoabdominal aortic aneurysms — A collaborative approach. *Eur J Vasc Endovasc Surg* 2009; **38**(5):578–585.

Eggebrecht H, Nienaber CA, Neuhauser M, *et al.* Endovascular stent-graft placement in aortic dissection: A meta-analysis. *Eur Heart J* 2006; **27**:489–498.

Elefteriades JA, Hartleroad J, Gusberg RJ, *et al.* Long-term experience with descending aortic dissection: The complication-specific approach. *Ann Thorac Surg* 1992; **53**:11.

Elkayam U, Ostrzega E, Shotan A, Mehra A. Cardiovascular problems in pregnant women with the Marfan syndrome. *Ann Intern Med* 1995; **123**:117–122.

Engle J, Safi HJ, Miller CC 3rd, *et al.* The impact of diaphragm management on prolonged ventilator support after thoracoabdominal aortic repair. *J Vasc Surg* 1999; **29**:150.

Englund R, Hudson P, Hanel K, Stanton A. Expansion rates of small abdominal aortic aneurysms. *Aust N Z J Surg* 1998; **68**:21.

Erbel R, Alfonso F, Boileau C, *et al.* Diagnosis and management of aortic dissection. *Eur Heart J* 2001; **22**:1642–1681.

Estrera AL, Miller CC 3rd, Huynh TT, *et al.* Neurologic outcome after thoracic and thoracoabdominal aortic aneurysm repair. *Ann Thorac Surg* 2001; **72**:1225.

Estrera AL, Rubenstein FS, Miller CC 3rd, *et al.* Descending thoracic aortic aneurysm: Surgical approach and treatment using the adjuncts cerebrospinal fluid drainage and distal aortic perfusion. *Ann Thorac Surg* 2001; **72**:481.

Estrera AL, Miller CC 3rd, Chen EP, *et al.* Descending thoracic aortic aneurysm repair: 12-year experience using distal aortic perfusion and cerebrospinal fluid drainage. *Ann Thorac Surg* 2005; **80**:1290–1296.

Fairman RM, Farber M, Kwolek CJ, *et al.* Pivotal results of the Medtronic Vascular Talent Thoracic Stent Graft System for patients with thoracic aortic disease: The VALOR trial. *J Vasc Surg* 2008; **48**:546–554.

Gillum RF. Epidemiology of aortic aneurysm in the United States. *J Clin Epidemiol* 1995; **48**:1289.

Greenwood WR, Robinson MD. Painless dissection of the thoracic aorta. *Ann Emerg Med* 1986; **4**:330–333.

Hagan PG, Nienaber CA, Isselbacher EM, *et al.* The International Registry of Acute Aortic Dissection (IRAD): New insights into an old disease. *JAMA* 2000; **283**:897–903.

Hallin A, Bergqvist D, Holmberg L. Literature review of surgical management of abdominal aortic aneurysm. *Eur J Vasc Endovasc Surg* 2001; **22**:197.

Harris PL, Vallabhaneni SR, Desgranges P. Incidence and risk factors of late rupture, conversion and death after endovascular repair of infrarenal aortic aneurysms: The EUROSTAR experience. *J Vasc Surg* 2000; **32**:739–749.

Hasham SN, Willing MC, Guo DC, *et al.* Mapping a locus for familial thoracic aortic aneurysms and dissections (TAAD2) to 3p24–25. *Circulation* 2003; **107**:3184.

Hollier LH, Symmonds JB, Pairolero PC, *et al.* Thoracoabdominal aortic aneurysm repair. Analysis of postoperative morbidity. *Arch Surg* 1988; **123**:871–875.

Huynh TT, Miller CC 3rd, Estrera AL, *et al.* Determinants of hospital length of stay after thoracoabdominal aortic aneurysm repair. *J Vasc Surg* 2002; **35**:648.

Januzzi JL, Isselbacher EM, Fattori R, *et al.* Characterizing the young patient with aortic dissection: Results from the International Registry of Aortic Dissection (IRAD). *J Am Coll Cardiol* 2004; **43**:665–669.

Jimenez, JC, Moore WS, Quinones-Baldrich WJ. Acute and chronic open conversion after endovascular aortic aneurysm repair: A 14-year review. *J Vasc Surg* 2007; **46**(4):642–647; Epub Aug 30, 2007.

Johansen K, Koepsell T. Familial tendency for abdominal aortic aneurysms. *JAMA* 1986; **256**:1934.

Johansen K, Kohler TR, Nicholls SC, *et al.* Ruptured abdominal aortic aneurysm: The Harborview experience. *J Vasc Surg* 1991; **13**:240–245.

Johnston KW, Rutherford RB, Tilson MD, *et al.* Suggested standards for reporting on arterial aneurysms. Subcommittee on Reporting Standards for Arterial Aneurysms, Ad Hoc Committee of Reporting Standards, Society for Vascular Surgery and North American Chapter, International Society for Cardiovascular Surgery. *J Vasc Surg* 1991; **13**:452.

Juvonen T, Ergin MA, Galla JD, *et al.* Prospective study of the natural history of thoracic aortic aneurysm. *Ann Thorac Surg* 1997; **63**:1533.

Kabbani LS, Criado E, Upchurch GR, Jr., *et al.* Hybrid repair of aortic aneurysms involving the visceral and renal vessels. *Ann Vasc Surg* 24(2):219–224.

Kashyap VS, Cambria RP, Davison JK, *et al.* Renal failure after thoracoabdominal aortic surgery. *J Vasc Surg* 1997; **26**:949.

Katz DJ, Stanley JC, Zelenock GB. Operative mortality rates for intact and ruptured abdominal aortic aneurysms in Michigan: An eleven-year statewide experience. *J Vasc Surg* 1994; **19**:804.

Khan IW, Wattanasauwan N, Ansari AW. Painless aortic dissection presenting as hoarseness of voice: Cardiovocal syndrome, Ortner's syndrome. *Am J Emerg Med* 1999; **17**:361–363.

Kouchoukos NT, Daily BB, Rokkas CK, *et al.* Hypothermic bypass and circulatory arrest for operations on the descending thoracic and thoracoabdominal aorta. *Ann Thorac Surg* 1995; **60**:67.

Kouchoukos NT, Masetti P, Murphy SF. Hypothermic cardiopulmonary bypass and circulatory arrest in the management of extensive thoracic and thoracoabdominal aortic aneurysms. *Semin Thorac Cardiovasc Surg* 2003; **15**:333–339.

Krupski WC, Selzman CH, Florida R, *et al.* Contemporary management of isolated iliac aneurysms. *J Vasc Surg* 1998; **28**:1.

Laheji RJ, Buth J, Harris PL, *et al.* Need for secondary interventions after endovascular repair of abdominal aortic aneurysm: Intermediate-term follow up results of a European collaborative registry (EUROSTAR). *Br J Surg* 2000; **87**:166–173.

Larson EW, Edwards WD. Risk factors for aortic dissection: A necropsy study of 161 patients. *Am J Cardiol* 1984; **53**:849–855.

Lawrence PF, Gazak C, Bhirangi L, *et al.* The epidemiology of surgically repaired aneurysms in the United States. *J Vasc Surg* 1999; **30**:632–740.

Leach SD, Toole AL, Stern H, *et al.* Effect of beta-adrenergic blockade on the growth rate of abdominal aortic aneurysms. *Arch Surg* 1988; **123**:606.

Lederle F, Johnson G, Wilson S, *et al.* The aneurysm detection and management study screening program validation cohort and final results. *Arch Intern Med* 2000; **160**:1425.

Lederle FA, Johnson GR, Wilson SE, *et al.* Prevalence and associations of abdominal aortic aneurysm detected through screening. Aneurysm Detection and Management (ADAM) Veterans Affairs Cooperative Study Group. *Ann Intern Med* 1997; **126**:441.

Lederle FA, Johnson GR, Wilson SE, *et al.* The aneurysm detection and management study screening program: Validation cohort and final results. Aneurysm Detection and Management Veterans Affairs Cooperative Study Investigators. *Arch Intern Med* 2000; **160**:1425.

Lederle FA, Simel DL. The rational clinical examination: Does this patient have abdominal aortic aneurysm? *JAMA* 1999; **281**:77.

Lee WA, Brown MP, Martin TD, *et al.* Early results after staged hybrid repair of thoracoabdominal aortic aneurysms. *J Am Coll Surg* 2007; **205**(3):420–431.

Lefebvre V, Leduc JJ, Choteau PH. Painless ischemic lumbosacral plexopathy and aortic dissection. *J Neurol Neurosurg Psychiatry* 1995; **58**:641.

LePage MA, Quint LE, Sonnad SS, *et al.* Aortic dissection: CT features that distinguish true lumen from false lumen. *AJR Am J Roentgenol* 2001; **177**:207–211.

Leurs LJ, Bell R, Degrieck Y, *et al.* Endovascular treatment of thoracic aortic diseases: Combined experience from the EUROSTAR and United Kingdom thoracic endograft registries. *J Vasc Surg* 2004; **40**:670–679.

Loughran CF. A review of the plain abdominal radiograph in acute rupture of abdominal aortic aneurysms. *Clin Radiol* 1986; **37**:383–387.

Maher MM, McNamara AM, MacEneaney PM, *et al.* Abdominal aortic aneurysms: Elective endovascular repair versus conventional surgery-evaluation with evidence-based medicine techniques. *Radiology* 2003; **228**:647–658.

Makaroun MS, Chaikof EL, Naslund T, Matsumura JS. Efficacy of a bifurcated endograft versus open repair of abdominal aortic aneurysms: A reappraisal. *J Vasc Surg* 2002; **35**:203–210.

Makaroun MS, Dillavou ED, Kee ST, *et al.* Endovascular treatment of thoracic aortic aneurysms: Results of the phase II multicenter trial of the GORE TAG thoracic endoprosthesis. *J Vasc Surg* 2005; **41**:1–9.

Makaroun MS, Dillavou ED, Wheatley GH, Cambria RA. Five-year results of endovascular treatment with the Gore TAG device compared to open repair of thoracic aortic aneurysms. *J Vasc Surg* 2008; **47**:912–918.

Marsalese DL, Moodie DS, Lytle BW, *et al.* Cystic medial necrosis of the aorta in patients without Marfan's syndrome: Surgical outcome and long-term follow-up. *J Am Coll Cardiol* 1990; **16**:68–73.

Matsumura JS, Cambria RP, Dake MD, *et al.* International controlled clinical trial of thoracic endovascular aneurysm repair with the Zenith TX2 endovascular graft: 1-year results. *J Vasc Surg* 2008; **47**:247–257.

McCready RA, Pairolero PC, Gilmore JC, *et al.* Isolated iliac artery aneurysms. *Surgery* 1983; **93**:688.

McMillan WD, Tamarina NA, Cipollone M, *et al.* Size matters: The relationship between MMP-9 expression and aortic diameter. *Circulation* 1997; **96**:2228.

Mehta RH, Manfredini R, Bossone E, *et al.* The winter peak in the occurrence of acute aortic dissection is independent of climate. *Chronobiol Int* 2005; **22**:723–729.

Mehta RH, Manfredini R, Hassan F, *et al.* Chronobiological patterns of acute aortic dissection. *Circulation* 2002; **106**:1110–1115.

Meszaros I, Morocz J, Szlavi J, *et al.* Epidemiology and clinicopathology of aortic dissection. *Chest* 2000; **117**:1271–1278.

Mitchell RS, Ishimaru S, Ehrlich MP, *et al.* First International Summit on Thoracic Aortic Endografting: Roundtable on thoracic aortic dissection as an indication for endografting. *J Endovasc Ther* 2002; **9**(Suppl 2):II98–II105.

Moore WS, Rutherford RB. Transfemoral endovascular repair of abdominal aortic aneurysms: Results of the North-American EVT phrase 1 trial. *J Vasc Surg* 1996; **23**:543–553.

Muluk SC, Kaufman JA, Torchiana DF, *et al.* Diagnosis and treatment of thoracic aortic intramural hematoma. *J Vasc Surg* 1996; **24**:1022–1029.

Murphy EH, Beck AW, Clagett GP, *et al.* Combined aortic debranching and thoracic endovascular aneurysm repair (TEVAR) effective but at a cost. *Arch Surg* 2009; **144**(3):222–227.

Nallamothu BK, Saint S, Kolias TJ, Eagle KA. Clinical problem-solving. Of nicks and time. *N Engl J Med* 2001; **345**:359–363.

Nevitt MP, Ballard DJ, Hallett JW Jr. Prognosis of abdominal aortic aneurysms: A population-based study. *N Engl Med* 1989; **321**:1009.

Neya K, Omoto R, Kyo S, *et al.* Outcome of Stanford Type B acute aortic dissection. *Circulation* 1992; **86**(5 Suppl):II1–II7.

Nienaber CA, Rousseau H, Eggebrecht H, *et al.* Randomized comparison of strategies for Type B aortic dissection: The investigation of STEnt Grafts in Aortic Dissection (INSTEAD) trial. *Circulation* 2009; **120**:2519–2528.

Nienaber CA, Eagle KA. Aortic dissection: New frontiers in diagnosis and management: Part II. Therapeutic management and follow-up. *Circulation* 2003; **108**:772–778.

Ohki T, Veith FJ, Shaw P, *et al.* Increasing incidents of mid-term and long term complications after endovascular graft repair of abdominal aortic aneurysms: A note of caution based on a 9-year experience. *Ann Surg* 2001; **234**:323–335.

Ohmi M, Tabayashi K, Moizumi Y, *et al.* Extremely rapid regression of aortic intramural hematoma. *J Thorac Cardiovasc Surg* 1999; **118**:968–969.

Olsen PS, Schroeder T, Agerskov K, *et al.* Surgery for abdominal aortic aneurysms: A survey of 656 patients. *J Cardiovasc Surg* (Torino) 1991; **32**:636.

Panneton JM, Hollier LH. Dissecting descending thoracic and thoracoabdominal aortic aneurysms: Part II. *Ann Vasc Surg* 1995; **9**:596–605.

Patel MI, Hardman DT, Fisher CM, Appleberg M. Current views on the pathogenesis of abdominal aortic aneurysms. *J Am Coll Surg* 1995; **181**:371.

Patel R, Conrad MF, Paruchuri V, *et al.* Thoracoabdominal aneurysm repair: Hybrid versus open repair. *J Vasc Surg* 2009; **50**(1):15–22.

Perko MJ, Norgaard M, Herzog TM, *et al.* Unoperated aortic aneurysm: A survey of 170 patients. *Ann Thorac Surg* 1995; **59**:1204.

Peterson BG, Eskandari MK, Gleason TG, Morasch MD. Utility of left subclavian artery revascularization in association with endoluminal repair of acute and chronic thoracic aortic pathology. *J Vasc Surg* 2006; **43**:433–439.

Pleumeekers H, Hoes A, van der Does E, *et al.* Aneurysms of the abdominal aorta in older adults. *Am J Epidemiol* 1995; **142**:1291.

Powell JT, Greenhalgh RM. Multifactorial inheritance of abdominal aortic aneurysm. *Eur J Vasc Surg* 1987; **1**:29.

Pressler V, McNamara JJ. Thoracic aortic aneurysm: Natural history and treatment. *J Thorac Cardiovasc Surg* 1980; **79**:489.

Pyeritz RE, McKusick VA. The Marfan syndrome: Diagnosis and management. *N Engl J Med* 1979; **300**:772.

Quinones-Baldrich W. Descending thoracic and thoracoabdominal aortic aneurysm repair: 15 year results using a uniform approach. *Ann Vasc Surg* 2004; **18**:335–342.

Quinones-Baldrich WJ, Jimenez JC, DeRubertis B, Moore WS. Combined endovascular and surgical approach (CESA) to thoracoabdominal aortic pathology: A 10-year experience. *J Vasc Surg* 2009; **49**:1125–1134.

Quinones-Baldrich WJ, Panetta TF, Vescera CL, Kashyap VS. Repair of Type IV thoracoabdominal aneurysm with combined endovascular and surgical approach (CESA). *J Vasc Surg* 1999; **30**(3):555–560.

Quiñones-Baldrich WJ, Nene SM, Gelabert HA, Moore WS. Rupture of the perivisceral aorta: Atherosclerotic versus mycotic aneurysm. *Ann Vasc Surg* 1997; **11**:331–341.

Rampoldi V, Trimarchi S, Eagle KA, *et al.* Simple risk models to predict surgical mortality in acute type A aortic dissection: The International Registry of Acute Aortic Dissection score. *Ann Thorac Surg* 2007; **83**:55–61.

Reece TB, Gazoni LM, Cherry KJ, *et al.* Reevaluating the need for left subclavian artery revascularization with thoracic endovascular aortic repair. *Ann Thorac Surg* 2007; **84**: 1201–1205.

Reed D, Reed C, Stemmerman G, *et al.* Are aortic aneurysms caused by atherosclerosis? *Circulation* 1992; 205–211.

Resch TA, Greenberg RK, Lyden SP, *et al.* Combined staged procedures for the treatment of thoracoabdominal aneurysms. *J Endovasc Ther* 2006; **13**(4):481–489.

Richardson, JW, Greenfield LJ. Natural history and management of iliac aneurysms. *J Vasc Surg* 1988; **8**:165.

Riesenman PJ, Farber MA, Mendes RR, *et al.* Coverage of the left subclavian artery during thoracic endovascular aortic repair. *J Vasc Surg* 2007; **45**:90–94.

Rizzo JA, Coady MA, Elefteriades JA. Procedures for estimating growth rates in thoracic aortic aneurysms. *J Clin Epidemiol* 1998; **51**:747.

Safi HJ, Bartoli S, Hess KR, *et al.* Neurologic deficit in patients at high risk with thoracoabdominal aortic aneurysms: The role of cerebral spinal fluid drainage and distal aortic perfusion. *J Vasc Surg* 1994; **20**:434.

Safi HJ, Campbell MP, Ferreira ML, *et al.* Spinal cord protection in descending thoracic and thoracoabdominal aortic aneurysm repair. *Semin Thorac Cardiovasc Surg* 1998; **10**:41.

Safi HJ, Hyunh TT, Hassoun HT, *et al.* Preventing renal failure in thoracoabdominal aortic aneurysm repair. *Perspect Vasc Surg Endovasc Ther* 2004; **16**:3.

Safi HJ, Miller CC 3rd, Huynh TT, *et al.* Distal aortic perfusion and cerebrospinal fluid drainage for thoracoabdominal and descending thoracic aortic repair: Ten years of organ protection. *Ann Surg* 2003; **238**:372.

Schepens M, Dossche K, Morshusi W, *et al.* Introduction of adjuncts and their influence on changing results in 402 consecutive thoracoabdominal aortic aneurysm repairs. *Eur J Cardiothorac Surg* 2004; **25**:701.

Scott RA, Tisi PV, Ashton HA, Allen DR. Abdominal aortic aneurysm rupture rates: A 7-year follow-up of the entire abdominal aortic aneurysm population detected by screening. *J Vasc Surg* 1998; **28**:124.

Shah PK. Inflammation, metalloproteinases, and increased proteolysis: An emerging pathophysiological paradigm in aortic aneurysm. *Circulation* 1997; **96**:2115.

Spittell PC, Spittell Jr JA, Joyce JW, *et al.* Clinical features and differential diagnosis of aortic dissection: Experience with 236 cases (1980 through 1990). *Mayo Clin Proc* 1993; **68**:897–903.

Starnes WS, Quiroga E, Hutter C, *et al.* Management of ruptured abdominal aortic aneurysm in the endovascular era. *J Vasc Surg* 2010; **51**:9–18.

Steyerberg EW, Kievit J, Alexander de Mol Van Otterloo JC, *et al.* Perioperative mortality of elective abdominal aortic aneurysm surgery: A clinical prediction rule based on literature and individual patient data. *Arch Intern Med* 1995; **155**:1998.

Sunder-Plassmann L, Orend KH. Stent-grafting of the thoracic aorta — complications. *J Cardiovasc Surg* (Torino) 2005; **46**:121–130.

Sundt TM. Intramural hematoma and penetrating atherosclerotic ulcer of the aorta. *Ann Thorac Surg* 2007; **83**:S835–S841.

Svensson LG, Coselli JS, Safi HJ, *et al.* Appraisal of adjuncts to prevent acute renal failure after surgery on the thoracic or thoracoabdominal aorta. *J Vasc Surg* 1989; **10**:230.

Svensson LG, Crawford ES, Hess KR, *et al.* Experience with 1509 patients undergoing thoracoabdominal aortic operations. *J Vasc Surg* 1993; **17**:357.

Svensson LG, Crawford ES, Hess KR, *et al.* Dissection of the aorta and dissecting aortic aneurysms. Improving early and long-term surgical results. *Circulation* 1990; **82**(5 Suppl):IV24–IV38.

Syed MA, Fiad TM. Transient paraplegia as a presenting feature of aortic dissection in a young man. *Emerg Med J* 2002; **19**:174–175.

Tasoglu I, Imren Y, Iriz E, *et al.* Rectal obstruction attributable to bilateral iliac aneurysms. *Surgery* 2007; **141**:279–280.

Trimarchi S, Nienaber CA, Rampoldi V, *et al.* Contemporary results of surgery in acute Type A aortic dissection: The International Registry of Acute Aortic Dissection experience. *J Thorac Cardiovasc Surg* 2005; **129**:112–122.

Trimarchi S, Nienaber CA, Rampoldi V, *et al.* Role and results of surgery in acute Type B aortic dissection: Insights from the International Registry of Acute Aortic Dissection (IRAD). *Circulation* 2006; **114**(1 Suppl):I357–I364.

Tsai TT, Evangelista A, Nienaber CA, *et al.* Long-term survival in patients presenting with Type A acute aortic dissection: Insights from the International Registry of Acute Aortic Dissection (IRAD). *Circulation* 2006; **114**(1 Suppl):I350–I356.

Tsai TT, Fattori R, Trimarchi S, *et al.* Long-term survival in patients presenting with Type B acute aortic dissection: Insights from the International Registry of Acute Aortic Dissection. *Circulation* 2006; **114**:2226–2231.

van de Mortel RH, Vahl AC, Balm R, *et al.* Collective experience with hybrid procedures for suprarenal and thoracoabdominal aneurysms. *Vascular* 2008; **16**(3):140–146.

Vardulaki K, Walker N, Day N, *et al.* Quantifying the risks of hypertension, age, sex, and smoking in patients with abdominal aortic aneurysm. *Br J Surg* 2000; **87**:195.

Verdant A, Cossette R, Page A, *et al.* Aneurysms of the descending thoracic aorta: Three hundred sixty-six consecutive cases resected without paraplegia. *J Vasc Surg* 1995; **21**:385–390.

Verloes A, Sakalihasan N, Koulischer L, Limet R. Aneurysms of the abdominal aorta: Familial and genetic aspects in three hundred thirteen pedigrees. *J Vasc Surg* 1995; **21**:646.

Vogt PR, von Segaesser LK, Goffin Y, Pasic M, Turina MI. Cryopreserved arterial homografts for *in situ* reconstruction of mycotic aneurysms and prosthetic graft infection. *Eur J Cardiothorac Surg* 1995; **9**(9):502–506.

Vollmar JF, Paes E, Pauschinger P, *et al.* Aortic aneurysms as late sequelae of above-knee amputation. *Lancet* 1989; **2**:834.

Wahlberg E, Dimuzio PJ, Stoney RJ. Aortic clamping during elective operations for infrarenal disease: The influence of clamping time on renal function. *J Vasc Surg* 2002; **36**:13.

Wakefield TW, Whitehouse Wm Jr, Wu SC, *et al.* Abdominal aortic aneurysm rupture: Statistical analysis of factors affecting outcome of surgical treatment. *Surgery* 1982; **91**:586–596.

Walsh SR, Tang TY, Sadat U, *et al.* Endovascular stenting versus open surgery for thoracic aortic disease: Systematic review and meta-analysis of perioperative results. *J Vasc Surg* 2008; **47**: 1094–1098.

Webster MW, Ferrell RE, St Jean PL, *et al.* Ultrasound screening of first-degree relatives of patients with an abdominal aortic aneurysm. *J Vasc Surg* 1991; **13**:9.

Whalgren CM, Larsson E, Magnusson PKE, *et al.* Genetic and environmental contributions to abdominal aortic aneurysm development in a twin population. *J Vasc Surg* 2010; **51**:3–8.

Wills A, Thompson MM, Crowther M, *et al.* Pathogenesis of abdominal aortic aneurysms-cellular and biochemical mechanisms. *Eur J Vasc Endovasc Surg* 1996; **12**:391.

Zarins CK, White RA, Moll FL, *et al.* The AneuRx stent-graft: Four-year results and worldwide experience 2000. *J Vasc Surg* 2001; **33**:S135–S145.

Zarins CK, White RA, Schwarten D, *et al.* AneuRx stent–graft versus open surgical repair of abdominal aortic aneurysms: Multicenter prospective clinical trial. *J Vasc Surg* 1999; **29**:292–308.

Zierer A, Voeller RK, Hill KE, *et al.* Aortic enlargement and late reoperation after repair of acute Type A aortic dissection. *Ann Thorac Surg* 2007; **84**:479–486.

Chapter 8

Management of Aneurysms of the Peripheral Arteries

Juan Carlos Jimenez and Ali Alktaifi

———————

Learning Objectives

- Learn and understand the natural history, causes, and incidences of peripheral artery aneurysms.
- Learn to identify patients at risk for peripheral artery aneurysms and the principles of the focused vascular examination for diagnosis.
- Learn the indications for repair of peripheral artery aneurysms.
- Be familiar with the various approaches to open operative repair of peripheral artery aneurysms.
- Be familiar with the various approaches to endovascular repair of peripheral artery aneurysms.
- Understand the potential complications of repair, both open and endovascular.

1. Introduction

An aneurysm is defined as dilatation of a vessel to 1.5 times greater than its normal diameter. True arterial aneurysms involve dilatation of all layers of the vessel wall. False aneurysms or pseudoaneurysms involve a defect in the arterial wall secondary to either trauma or infection. Peripheral artery aneurysms are diagnosed less commonly than aneurysms of the abdominal aorta but present with significant patient morbidity when complications arise. Because of their anatomic location in a relatively small, contained space when compared with abdominal aortic aneurysms (AAA), rupture, shock, and exsanguination are less frequent. Complications typically arise following thrombosis and embolization of peripheral artery aneurysms and patients most commonly present with symptoms of limb ischemia, nerve compression, and compartment syndrome. Although the most common cause of most peripheral artery aneurysms is atherosclerosis, certain key exceptions exist with aneurysms of the distal subclavian-axillary artery and peripheral aneurysms of

157

mycotic origin. An understanding of the underlying cause is imperative for proper management of these potentially complex patients.

2. Aneurysms of the Lower Extremities

2.1 *Popliteal artery aneurysms*

Popliteal artery aneurysms (PAA) are the most common peripheral artery aneurysm and the second most common aneurysm treated following AAA. Although the true prevalence is not known exactly, they are believed to present in 1–3% of the general population. They are more common in men and infrequently seen in women. The most common cause of PAA is atherosclerosis, although rare causes include Marfan's, Ehlers-Danlos, and Bechet's syndromes. There is a well-recognized association between PAA and both AAA and contralateral PAA. Patients with AAA should be examined and screened for PAA and vice-versa during the initial vascular surgery assessment.

Diagnosis of PAA's is made following palpation of the popliteal artery pulse during the vascular examination. Abnormally strong pulsation, especially in patients with known AAA, should be imaged with duplex ultrasonography (Figs. 1 and 2). Both legs should be screened once the unilateral diagnosis of PAA is made. Computed tomography and conventional angiography are useful for preoperative

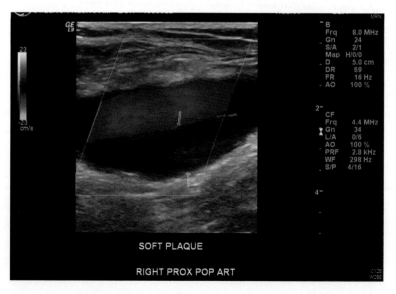

Fig. 1. Duplex ultrasound demonstrating extensive mural thrombus within the arterial lumen of a popliteal aneurysm.

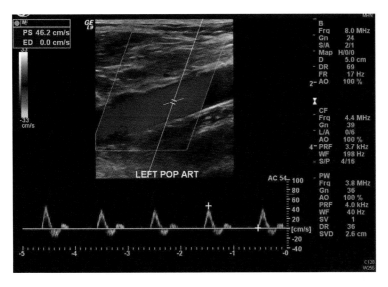

Fig. 2. Duplex ultrasound in the same patient highlighted in Fig. 1 demonstrates a normal contralateral popliteal artery. Patients should always be screened for bilateral popliteal aneurysms.

planning and for assessment of proximal superficial femoral artery diameter and tibial artery patency and runoff (Figs. 3 and 4).

Embolization and thrombosis are the most common complications encountered with PAAs. They are associated with a high rate of critical limb ischemia and

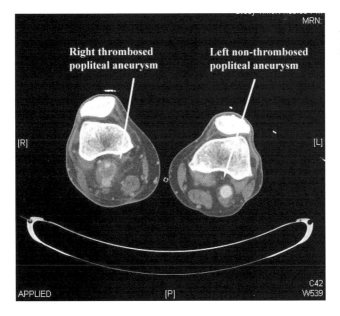

Fig. 3. Computed tomography angiography demonstrating a thrombosed right popliteal aneurysm and a non-thrombosed left popliteal aneurysm in the same patient.

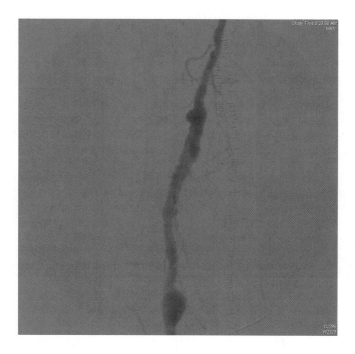

Fig. 4.   Digital subtraction angiography performed during prior to endovascular repair of a popliteal aneurysm.

amputation when they become symptomatic and outcomes are generally poor compared with elective repair of nonthrombosed PAAs. Amputation rates as high as 67% have been reported with patients with thrombosed PAAs. The expansion rate of the PAA in asymptomatic patients has been reported to be around 1.5 mm per year with aneurysm diameters less than 2.0 cm. PAA growth increases to 3.0 mm per year at sizes 2.0–3.0 cm and 3.7 mm per year at sizes greater than 3.0 cm in recent population-based studies. We recommend treatment of PAAs $\geq$ 2 cm due to the increased risk of complications with larger diameters. Symptomatic PAAs should be treated immediately regardless of size. Options for treatment include both open surgical and endovascular techniques. Principles of these techniques are discussed below.

2.1.1 *Surgical repair of the non-thrombosed popliteal artery aneurysm*

The central principle behind surgical treatment of PAAs is exclusion of the aneurysm both proximally and distally with restoration of luminal patency. The traditional approach to open PAA repair involves of exposure of normal caliber artery proximal and distal to the PAA. The patient is placed in the supine position on the operating table and incisions are made in the medial leg both above and below the knee. Reversed saphenous vein graft is the preferred conduit for this approach because

160

of significantly improved long-term patency in below knee bypasses and decreased risk of infection compared with prosthetic graft (PTFE, Dacron, *etc.*). The proximal anastomosis must originate from nonaneurysmal artery and, occasionally, the proximal superficial femoral and common femoral arteries are used. The vein graft is then tunneled anatomically (along the course of the native artery) and anastomosed to normal caliber below-knee popliteal artery. The distal anastomosis should be made to the most proximal normal caliber artery due to decreased patency in the smaller and more distal tibial arteries.

In our clinical experience at UCLA, we have demonstrated good patient outcomes using a posterior approach with the patient in prone position. This approach is efficacious in patients with focal PAAs located within the popliteal fossa. Aneurysms, which extend proximal to the adductor hiatus should be repaired using the medial approach. The tibioperoneal trunk and the origins of the tibial arteries can be readily exposed using the posterior approach by extending the dissection distally between the two heads of the gastrocnemius muscle. Once adequate exposure is obtained, the popliteal artery is clamped proximally and distally. The aneurysm is opened, resected, and debrided proximally and distally to normal caliber artery. We routinely use an interposition knitted Dacron (polyester) graft of either 6.0 mm or 8.0 mm diameter to restore luminal patency. Care is taken to keep the graft length as short as possible, but not under tension.

In our series of posterior PAA repair, our 30-day primary patency was 100% and the mean length of hospital stay was 3.3 days. Using the Kaplan–Meier life-table method, primary, assisted primary, and secondary patencies were 92.2%, 95.8%, and 95.8%, respectively. Limb salvage was 100%.

Potential complications of open PAA repair include risks of general anesthesia, graft failure, lymphocele, wound and/or graft infection, postoperative bleeding, worsening of ischemia, and limb loss.

2.1.2 *Endovascular repair of the nonthrombosed popliteal artery aneurysm*

With the recent and rapid development of improved stent-graft technology, outcomes following endovascular exclusion of PAAs have improved and this technique offers a less invasive alternative to open surgical repair. Endovascular PAA repair may offer an advantage in patients without available saphenous vein or high-risk surgical candidates. The technique involves accessing either the ipsilateral or contralateral common femoral artery either percutaneously or *via* cutdown. A sheath is introduced and a guidewire is placed into the arterial lumen *via* Seldinger technique. We prefer the use of polytetrafluoroethylene (e-PTFE) lined nitinol stents (Fig. 5). We most commonly use the Gore Viabahn endoprosthesis (Gore Medical, Flagstaff, Az).

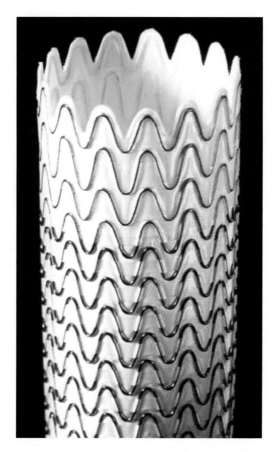

Fig. 5.   Endovascular exclusion of peripheral aneurysms has become a feasible treatment option in recent years to improved stent-graft technology.

These devices are available in sizes ranging from 5 to 13 mm. This device requires a sheath size, which ranges from 7 F to 12 F and the stent graft is sized approximately 10–15% larger than the diameter of the target vessel. A seal zone of normal artery proximally and distally of at least 2 cm is required. Deployment of the stent graft is performed using intraoperative fluoroscopy and following placement, a completion angiogram is performed to ensure technical success.

Although no randomized trials comparing this technique to open repair have been performed, good short-term and mid-term outcomes have been reported. Long-term patency is relatively unknown. Primary and secondary patency rates at two years have been reported between 80% and 90% in recent studies with limb salvage rates approaching 100%. Potential complications include access site complications, early and late graft thrombosis, distal embolization, vessel perforation, graft infection, and limb loss.

2.1.3 *Management of the thrombosed popliteal artery aneurysm*

Acute thrombosis of a PAA is a limb and life-threatening emergency. Patients may present with symptoms ranging from mild claudication to rest pain. Patients with critical ischemia typically present with signs ("5 Ps") of acute limb threat including: pain, pallor, poikilothermia, pulselessness, and paralysis. Urgent revascularization with either thrombolysis or thromboembolectomy and bypass should be performed. Debate exists regarding which approach is preferred in patients presenting with thrombosed PAA. A recent review of 895 cases by Kropman *et al.* demonstrated that thrombolysis prior to surgery did not result in a significant reduction in the number of amputations in these patients. However, the presence of two or three patent tibial arteries for runoff is associated with improved long-term graft patency and thromboembolectomy in these smaller arteries can be technically challenging. At UCLA, patients presenting with mild to moderate ischemia symptoms (claudication) undergo conventional angiography and intraarterial thrombolysis with the purpose of clearing acute thrombus from the runoff arteries to improve outflow for our bypass graft. Patients presenting with acute limb-threatening symptoms undergo surgical exploration with urgent thromboembolectomy and bypass. Intraoperative thrombolysis has also been used with moderate success immediately either before or after the placement of our bypass graft. Care must be taken to monitor the patient postoperatively for symptoms of ischemia-reperfusion syndrome. These include rhabdomyolysis, metabolic acidosis, compartment syndrome, hyperkalemia, and arrhythmia.

Reported amputation rates in the literature are significantly higher for patients presenting with thrombosed PAAs compared with elective repair. Symptomatic aneurysms have also been associated with decreased graft patency, increased post-operative complications (wound infection, foot drop, AV fistula, *etc.*), and increased 30-day mortality. In a recent review of the Swedish Vascular Registry, Ravn *et al.* reported the results of 571 patients undergoing surgical repair of PAA. The overall amputation rate within one year of operation was 8.8%. The limb loss rates for nonthrombosed and thrombosed PAAs was 1.8% and 12.0%, respectively.

2.2 *Femoral artery aneurysms*

The majority of femoral artery aneurysms (FAA) are false aneurysms related to trauma or iatrogenic complications following percutaneous femoral cannulation and catheterization. The estimated incidence of iatrogenic femoral pseudoaneurysm is 3% in modern series. True femoral aneurysms are rare and their true incidence is not known. The main cause of FAA is atherosclerosis. Their natural history is believed to be similar to popliteal aneurysms; however, few published studies of

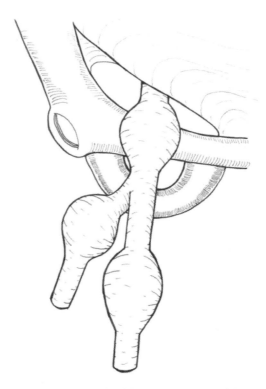

Fig. 6. Sketch of true femoral artery aneurysms involving the common, superficial, and profunda femoris arteries.

true FAAs exist and most were written prior to 1980. Femoral artery aneurysms are frequently bilateral and associated with other aneurysms in the majority of patients. They are rarely seen in women. They most are frequently present in the common femoral artery but the superficial femoral and profunda femoris arteries may also be aneurysmal (Fig. 6).

Two large studies published by Cutler *et al.* and Graham *et al.* advocated conflicting approaches to treatment. In Cutler's series, 18 asymptomatic patients had excellent early and late graft patency. However, the 45 symptomatic patients had high rates of amputation and recurrent symptoms. Graham *et al.* reported the results of 172 atherosclerotic femoral aneurysms in 100 male patients over a 22-year period. Only three of 105 aneurysms followed nonoperatively were associated with later major limb-threatening complications. The most frequent complications were thrombosis and embolization; however, a significant percentage of patients also had synchronous popliteal artery aneurysms making the source of emboli unclear.

The most common symptom associated with FAA is localized pain with large aneurysms causing compression of the femoral vein and nerve. Patients with arterial thrombosis and embolization may present with symptoms ranging from claudication to rest pain and gangrene. Duplex ultrasound is a good initial screening test and provides information regarding the absolute size, the amount of intraluminal thrombus, and involvement of arterial branches (profunda femoris, superficial femoral artery, *etc.*). Computed tomography is an accurate diagnostic test for further characterization and preoperative planning.

In our practice at UCLA, all rapidly enlarging (≥ 3 mm in six months) and symptomatic FAAs are recommended for treatment. Because the average diameter of a normal common femoral artery is approximately 8 mm and the natural history is largely unknown, we currently recommend treatment for asymptomatic FAAs greater than 2.5 cm or extensive intraluminal thrombus at any size.

2.2.1 *Surgical management of true FAAs*

At our institution, we prefer to expose the femoral artery *via* a vertical incision extending from the level of the inguinal ligament to the distal extent of the aneurysm. If the FAA is large and a groin incision is insufficient to obtain proximal control, a separate transverse retroperitoneal incision can be used to expose the external iliac artery for clamping. Distal control of the femoral artery is also obtained including the superficial femoral and profunda femoris arteries if needed. Following systemic heparinization, the proximal and distal arteries are clamped and the aneurysm is opened longitudinally. Removal of intraluminal thrombus and aneurysm resection is performed. We prefer the use of a Dacron interposition graft (8 or 10 mm) to restore luminal patency (Fig. 7). A separate bypass graft to the profunda femoris artery may be required if this vessel is involved with the aneurysm. Potential complications of surgical repair include systemic risks of general anesthesia, graft thrombosis, embolization, postoperative bleeding, and limb loss. Because of the location of FAAs at the hip joint, we recommend the use of endovascular stent graft repair to only high-risk surgical patients who cannot undergo an open operation due to significant medical comorbidities.

When a mycotic FAA is suspected, the use of prosthetic graft material should be strictly avoided and appropriate intravenous antibiotic therapy should be instituted. Frequently, retroperitoneal exposure of the external iliac artery is required for proximal control, prior to exposure of the aneurysm itself. Surgical treatment involves resection of the pseudoaneurysm and aggressive debridement of all infected tissue. Reconstruction with patch angioplasty or interposition graft with autogenous tissue (saphenous vein, cadaveric homograft, *etc.*) should be performed.

3. Aneurysms of the Upper Extremities

3.1 *Subclavian and axillary artery aneurysms*

True subclavian artery aneurysms (SAA) are rare and comprise only 0.13% of all atherosclerotic aneurysms (Fig. 8). Syphilis and tuberculosis were the most common

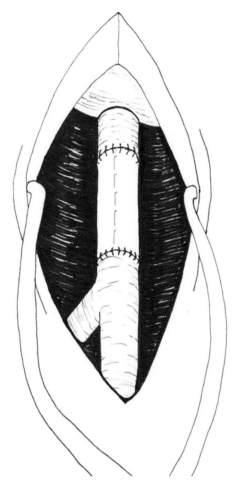

Fig. 7. Sketch of completed open repair of a common femoral artery aneurysm with an interposition prosthetic graft.

causes in the early 20th century and comprise 15% and 10% of reported cases, respectively. Fibromuscular dysplasia has also been implicated as a cause. More distal SAAs, which also involve the proximal axillary artery, are usually the result of poststenotic dilatation due to thoracic outlet compression. A cervical rib is frequently encountered in these patients contributing to arterial thoracic outlet syndrome. Chest and shoulder pain is a common presenting symptom. Digital ischemia and gangrene are symptoms of distal embolization. Brachial plexopathy and Horner's syndrome have also been reported. In a series by Pairolero *et al.*, 31 patients with subclavian-axillary artery aneurysms were treated. Eight patients were asymptomatic and 23 presented with upper extremity pain. Ruptured SAAs can present with severe chest pain, respiratory distress, and shock. Large intrathoracic SAAs can be detected

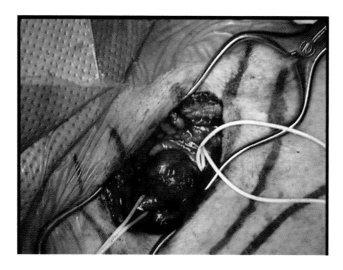

Fig. 8.   Subclavian artery aneurysm in a patient with thoracic outlet syndrome.

on chest radiography as a superior mediastinal mass. Computed tomography and magnetic resonance angiography are useful in planning repair, both endovascular and surgical.

Axillary artery aneurysms are usually the result of post-stenotic dilatation in the presence of thoracic outlet compression. These are usually an extension of aneurysmal disease of the distal subclavian artery as described above. Other causes include blunt or penetrating trauma, occupational and crutch-induced injuries, and iatrogenic complications.

3.2 *Principles of endovascular treatment*

Due to the difficult surgical exposure of the proximal subclavian artery, endovascular repair of SAAs is the preferred method of treatment at our institution. Because of the small diameter of the brachial artery and the relatively large sheath (7f–12f) sizes requires for stent-graft deployment, we perform an ipsilateral brachial cutdown for access. Femoral approach is an alternative choice for access. A guidewire is used to traverse the lumen of the aneurysm and a destination sheath placed. Two centimeters of proximal and distal seal are preferred for proper aneurysm exclusion. The patency of both vertebral arteries is established with preoperative duplex ultrasound and computed tomography. We prefer not to cover the ipsilateral vertebral artery if it appears dominant on preoperative imaging. Aneurysms of the distal subclavian artery located at the thoracic outlet are surgically repaired due to concern for graft kinking and compression. Endovascular management of axillary artery aneurysms has been described but studies are limited to case reports with short-term follow up.

3.3 *Principles of surgical repair*

Left-sided intrathoracic SAAs usually require a left thoracotomy for proximal exposure. Right-sided intrathoracic SAAs require a median sternotomy with right supraclavicular extension to achieve proximal and distal control. Treatment includes aneurysm ligation or excision with or without arterial reconstruction. Approximately 25% of patients without arterial reconstruction develop arm claudication. Aneurysms of the distal subclavian-axillary artery in patients with suspected thoracic outlet syndrome usually require decompression of the thoracic outlet with resection of cervical (usually present) and first ribs. Arterial reconstruction is performed once the external compression is relieved. Potential complications of repair include: bleeding, infection, delayed limb ischemia, brachial plexus injury, stroke, and amputation.

4. Brachial Artery Aneurysms

The majority of brachial artery aneurysms (BAA) are pseudoaneurysms (false aneurysms) following trauma or iatrogenic injury. The increased use of the brachial artery for cardiac catheterization and endovascular procedures puts it at particular risk for injury. In a recent review of 323 procedures performed requiring brachial artery access, the complication rate was 6.5%. Eleven patients developed brachial artery pseudoaneurysms with five requiring operative repair. Other causes of false BAA include orthopedic fractures, penetrating trauma, occupational injuries, and crutch-induced trauma. Of note, mycotic aneurysms following intravenous drug use can occur and are frequently located at the antecubital fossa. True aneurysms of the brachial artery are rare and are usually idiopathic in nature. Association with collagen vascular disorders such at Ehler-Danlos or Marfans syndromes. Other associated disorders include Type I Neurofibromatosis, Kawasaki's disease, Giant-cell arteritis, and cystic adventitial disease.

Most BAAs require surgical excision with arterial reconstruction. Options include resection of the aneurysm with primary anastomosis, patch angioplasty, or placement of an interposition vein graft. The conduit of choice is greater saphenous vein due to its comparable diameter and ease of harvest. Generally, only short segments of artery require reconstruction. Iatrogenic false aneurysms secondary to vessel trauma usually require primary suture repair. In the presence of a mycotic BAA, all infected tissue must be debrided to normal artery proximally and distally. Reconstruction should be performed with autogenous tissue and prosthetic materials should be strictly avoided.

5. Hypothenar Hammer Syndrome

Hypothenar Hammer syndrome (HHS) was first described in 1970 by Conn. Patients present with finger ischemia from embolization from the palmar ulnar artery. It is associated with repetitive trauma to the hand and striking of the palm. Findings include aneurismal degeneration of the ulnar artery with distal embolization, segmental occlusions, and elongation of the ulnar artery with a corkscrew appearance. Patients present with a range of symptoms including pain, cold intolerance, cyanosis, and gangrene. Arteriography remains the gold standard for radiological diagnosis.

Treatment for HHS includes thrombolysis for segmental arterial thrombosis. Treatment of symptomatic ulnar artery aneurysms includes resection with either primary anastomosis or placement of an interposition vein graft. Asymptomatic patients should be treated conservatively with avoidance of trauma and antiplatelet therapy.

References

Beseth BD, Moore WS. The posterior approach for repair of popliteal artery aneurysms. *J Vasc Surg* 2006; **43**:940–945.

Curi MA, Geraghty PJ, Merino OA, Veeraswamy RK, Rubin BG, Sanchez LA, *et al.* Mid-term outcomes of endovascular popliteal artery aneurysm repair. *J Vasc Surg* 2007; **45**:505–510.

Chue CD, Hudsmith LE, Stumper O, De Giovanni J, Thorne SA, Clift P. Femoral vascular access complications in adult congenital heart disease patients: audit from a single tertiary center. *Congenit Heart Dis* 2008; **3**:336–340.

Cutler BS, Darling RC. Surgical management of arteriosclerotic femoral aneurysms. *Surgery* 1973; **74**:764–773.

Dent TL, Lindenauer SM, Ernest CB, Fry W. Multiple arteriosclerotic arterial aneurysms. *Arch Surg* 1972; **105**:338–344.

Dougherty MJ, Calligaro KD, Savarese RP, DeLaurentis DA. Atherosclerotic aneurysm of the intrathoracic subclavian artery: a case report and review of the literature. *J Vasc Surg* 1995; **21**:521–529.

Galland RB. Popliteal aneurysms: from John Hunter to the 21st century. *Ann R Coll Surg Engl* 2007; **89**:466–471.

Graham LM, Zelenock GB, Whitehouse WM, Erlandson EE, Dent TL, Lindenauer M, Stanley JC. Clinical significance of arteriosclerotic femoral artery aneurysms. *Arch Surg* 1980; **115**:502–507.

Johnson ON, Slidell MB, Macsata RA, Faler BJ, Amdur RL, Sidaway AN. Outcomes of surgical management for popliteal artery aneurysms: an analysis of 583 cases. *J Vasc Surg* 2008; **48**:845–851.

Kropman RHJ, Schrijver AM, Kelder JC, Moll FL, deVries JPPM. Clinical outcome of acute leg ischaemia due to thrombosed popliteal artery aneurysm: systematic review of 895 cases. *Eur J Vasc Endovasc Surg* 2010; In press.

Lovegrove RE, Javid M, Magee TR, Galland RB. Endovascular and open approaches to non-thrombosed popliteal aneurysm repair: a meta-analysis. *Eur J Vasc Endovasc Surg* 2008; **36**: 96–100.

Midy D, Berard X, Ferdani M, Alric P, Brizzi V, Ducasse E, *et al.* A retrospective multicentric study of endovascular treatment of popliteal artery aneurysms. *J Vasc Surg* 2010; In press.

Pittathankal AA, Dattani R, Magee TR, Galland RB. Expansion rates of asymptomatic popliteal aneurysms. *Eur J Vasc Endovasc Surg* 2004; 382–384.

Pairolero PC, Walls JT, Payne WS, Hollier LH, Fairbalm JF. Subclavian-axillary artery aneurysms. *Surgery* 1981; **90**:757–763.

Ravn H, Bergqvist D, Bjorck M. Nationwide study of the outcome of popliteal artery aneurysms treated surgically. *Br J Surg* 2007; **94**:970–977.

Stahl RD, Lawrence PF, Bhirangi K. Left subclavian artery aneurysm: two cases of rare congenital etiology. *J Vasc Surg* 1999; **29**:715–718.

Sarkar R, Coran AG, Cilley RE, Lindenauer SM, Stanley JC. Arterial aneurysms in children: clinico-pathologic classification. *J Vasc Surg* 1992; **15**:585–586.

Chapter 9
Vascular Surgical Emergencies and Trauma

Peter F. Lawrence

———————

Learning Objectives

- Learn the common symptoms and signs and the treatment of acute limb-threatening ischemia.
- Become familiar with the diagnosis and management of patients presenting with ruptured arterial aneurysms and dissection.
- Learn the common signs, symptoms, and treatment of cerebrovascular vascular surgical emergencies.
- Become familiar with the principles in the management of vascular trauma.

1. Acute Limb-Threatening Ischemia

Acute limb ischemia can occur in patients with or without prior history or evidence of arterial insufficiency. Diseases of the vessels to the limb, such as direct trauma, atherosclerosis, peripheral aneurysms, dissection, popliteal entrapment, and adventitial cystic disease, can all cause acute arterial ischemia when *in-situ* thrombosis of an artery abruptly closes it. Clinical severity is especially severe if there has not been a gradual reduction in the vessel lumen over time, with concomitant development of collateral vessels.

Acute arterial occlusion may also occur due to embolization from another source, such as atrial fibrillation, mural thrombus, atrial myxoma with embolization, and even atheroembolization from a proximal aortic source. In all cases of embolization, the key determinant of the degree of ischemia is the location of the embolus, the degree of occlusion of the vessel, and the adequacy of the collateralization around the vessel. When the ischemia is severe, it may cause any or all of the "six Ps": pulselessness, poikilothermia, pain, pallor, paresthesias, and paralysis. The degree of each of these findings determines the degree of urgency in the treatment of acute ischemia (Table 1).

Table 1. The six signs of acute extremity ischemia (6 Ps) (in increasing order of severity of ischemia).

Pulselessness
Poikilothermia (cool)
Pallor
Pain
Paresthesias
Paralysis

1.1 *Diagnosis of acute ischemia*

The initial history and physical examination can immediately make the diagnosis in most patients, particularly when the patient has been evaluated and examined previously. The combination of physical findings of ischemia, combined with the pulse pattern and Doppler signals in the distal vessels, usually results in a correct diagnosis. Findings that suggest advanced ischemia include limb paralysis and muscle rigor.

1.2 *Imaging in acute arterial ischemia*

1.2.1 *Duplex ultrasound scanning*

Duplex ultrasound scanning can often extend the physical examination and eliminate the need for angiography, particularly in patients with acute ischemia who are near the critical time for tissue loss. When there is an absence of pulses in the limb by physical examination that indicates a site below the inguinal ligament, a duplex scan can identify the site of occlusion, determine if the vessel is patent below that level, and assess the quality of the artery. In particular, it is important to determine whether the patient had pre-existing chronic ischemia or if the problem is an acute embolus or thrombus. When the occlusion is caused by an acute embolus or thrombus, without the presence of extensive atherosclerotic disease, there is a high likelihood of successful revascularization with simple thrombectomy. If the vessel has pre-existing disease and will likely need thrombolysis or distal bypass in addition to embolectomy or thrombectomy.

1.2.2 *Arteriography (CTA, MRA, catheter angiography)*

Arteriography should be performed in every patient with acute ischemia, either prior to revascularization, to help determine the site of occlusion and coexisting disease, or after revascularization, to determine whether or not there is residual intraluminal disease that requires further therapy. Each institution has different equipment, staff, and physician expertise that affects the choice of imaging. Catheter angiography, CT angiography, and MR angiography all are capable of assessing the arterial vessels and they provide a roadmap for further therapy. If all are available, then the intra-operative approach with catheter angiography is the fastest. CT angiography is usually the best approach for disease above the knee. Magnetic resonance angiography is usually best below the knee, although is does not visualize calcification and, therefore, cannot always accurately assess the underlying status of the artery.

1.3 *Initial therapy in acute ischemia*

The initial approach in patients with acute ischemia is prevention of further embolus with anticoagulation, imaging to determine the extent of the disease, thrombectomy or thrombolysis to remove the clot and plaque from the artery (see Table 1).

1.4 *Definitive therapy*

Once the extent of the disease and degree of ischemia have been determined, therapy moves to the definitive stage with revascularization, fasciotomy to allow swelling of ischemic limb, and management of the metabolic effects of the ischemia on the overall status of the patient.

1.4.1 *Anticoagulation*

Unless there are contraindications to anticoagulation such as recent hemorrhagic stroke, patients should be immediately anticoagulated with heparin (70–100 mg/kg). If patients have a history of heparin-induced thrombocytopenia, an alternative, such as argatroban or lepirudin, should be used. Following initial bolus anticoagulation, patients should receive a continuous infusion of heparin, based on APTT or ACT measurements

1.4.2 *Thrombolysis*

Thrombolysis is indicated in the patient who has ischemia that is not immediately limb threatening, or in patients who have more extensive disease that is not limited to a localized embolus. When a surgically accessible embolus is present with a patent distal vessel, surgical embolectomy is usually the best option. However, when there is preexisting disease or an embolus is associated with thrombus of the diseased vessel, then thrombolysis, sometimes followed by embolectomy, endarterectomy, or bypass, increases the probability of limb survival.

1.4.3 *Reconstructive procedures*

1.4.3.1 Embolectomy

Embolectomy is particularly useful when an embolus is limited in length and often is lodged at a bifurcation. When an embolectomy can be performed before the embolus causes extensive distal thrombosis, the revascularization is rapid and the reperfusion often precludes the need for fasciotomy and the risk of limb loss is lessened.

1.4.3.2 Angioplasty/stenting

When thrombolysis is complete, there is often underlying disease that threatens the long-term likelihood of success. In this circumstance, angioplasty and stenting of the residual disease will increase the likelihood of vessel patency and reduce the likelihood of late occlusion

1.4.3.3 Bypass

Although angioplasty and stenting is the first choice in most patients, occasionally, bypass is required to revascularize the patient, particularly with the underlying chronic occlusive disease is extensive. Patients with TASC D occlusive disease, which is extensive, often require a surgical bypass for limb salvage.

1.4.3.4 Aneurysm repair

When acute distal thrombosis is due to acute or chronic aneurysm occlusion, thrombolysis prior to aneurysm repair has been shown to improve limb salvage, but once the distal and proximal vessels have been cleared of clot, repair of the aneurysm is indicated to prevent recurrence and rethrombosis. This can be done with a covered stent, surgical bypass, or surgical interposition graft.

1.4.4 *Fasciotomy*

Patients who have had ischemia for >3 hours prior to revascularization are candidates for surgical fasciotomy. Those who undergo gradual revascularization with thrombolysis often do not need fasciotomy, but those who undergo thrombectomy or surgical bypass often need concomitant fasciotomy.

1.4.5 *Amputation*

Amputation is reserved for patients with acute ischemia who were not ambulatory prior to the acute ischemic event, patients who have such advanced ischemia that revascularization risks death from acidosis and hyperkalemia or renal injury, due to rhabdomyolysis, and those who have such advanced signs as muscle rigor, limb anesthesia and paralysis, and irreversible skin changes, such that survival and limb salvage are highly unlikely. When immediate amputation is indicated, the least stressful amputation is a physiologic cryo-amputation, with dry ice, which can be done at the bedside. In some patients who are more stable, a guillotine amputation removes the source of toxicity and makes the patient easier to handle than a patient who has undergone a physiologic amputation.

1.5 *Post-procedure management*

1.5.1 *Treatment of rhabdomyolysis*

Rhabdomyolysis (skeletal muscle death) is evident in patients who develop brown urine, acidosis and hyperkalemia, and an elevated serum CPK level. Although serum myoglobin levels can be obtained, there is a direct parallel between the CPK and serum myoglobin, so many do not wait for the outcome of this test. When rhabdomyolysis is suspected or occurs, the best approach is to provide a high volume of fluids, diurese the patient, and alkalinize the urine. With this approach, as well as controlling further ischemia, there is a good likelihood of preventing further renal injury. Occasionally, dialysis is required in order to salvage renal function. Since the impact of rhabdomyolysis is mostly from mechanical obstruction of the collecting tubule, once dialysis has removed all remaining myoglobin, there is a good possibility of renal function improvement.

1.5.2 *Treatment of gangrene*

Once gangrene is present, whether manifested by blistering of the skin, muscle rigor, or irreversible nerve injury, evidenced by paralysis and anesthesia of the limb, amputation will be required of at least some portion of the limb. If possible, the amputation should be delayed until the level of irreversible ischemia has been determined.

1.5.3 *Treatment of neuropathy*

Ischemic neuropathy can lead to anesthesia of the limb, hypoesthesia, or severe burning pain. Over time, ischemic neuropathy often improves, particularly when the length of ischemic time was limited and the patient does not have underlying neuropathy. Time and nerve-stabilizing drugs can be used until the limb stabilizes or recovers.

1.5.4 *Long-term anticoagulation*

When patients develop limb-threatening ischemia, those who developed it due to emboli need long-term anticoagulation. Those who had underlying vascular disease that has been corrected may not need long-term anticoagulation, but often require it until the limb stabilizes and maximum perfusion has been gained.

2. Acute Deep Venous Thrombosis

2.1

Most patients with DVT develop gradual swelling and leg pain and do not have limb-threatening ischemia. A small subset, though, develop such massive swelling that the leg viability is threatened. This becomes a vascular emergency and need to be treated with more than traditional anticoagulation and elevations, although both of these are initial steps. Most patients with massive swelling, or phlemasia cerulea dolens, have occlusion of the iliofemoral venous system that often extends into the femoral popliteal venous system.

2.1.1 *Diagnosis*

Duplex ultrasound is the most accurate, rapid, and cost-effective method of diagnosing iliofemoral venous thrombosis, although it is often suspected after the initial physical examination.

2.1.2 *Treatment*

All patients with DVT should be treated with heparin anticoagulation as an inpatient or outpatient, unless there is a contraindication such as recent surgery or high bleeding risk. Low molecular weight heparin has been increasingly used for patients because it can be dosed based on body weight, does not need monitoring, and can be given as an outpatient, often by the patient or a family member. For those patients with DVT above the level of the popliteal vein who have a contraindication to heparin, a vena caval filter should be placed. For those patients with massive swelling and limb threat, after initial leg elevations and anticoagulation with heparin, treatment should begin immediately with catheter-directed thrombolysis and/or mechanical thrombectomy. Techniques that deliver high concentrations directly into the thrombus can rapidly clear the thrombus within hours and reduce the risk of limb threat. The access for catheter direct thrombolysis is often the popliteal vein from the prone position. Specific training in each of the infusion catheters and mechanical devices is required to achieve optimal results.

3. Ruptured Aneurysms

Rupture of an aneurysm is associated with a high mortality, although new approaches are reducing the mortality to more acceptable levels. The ubiquitous CT and MRI scans have led to many aneurysms being diagnosed and treated before they present with rupture, although there continues to be patients with undiagnosed or untreated aneurysms whose initial presentation is rupture. The presence of "fast ultrasound" in many ERs and CT scan immediately available to the ER has reduced the number of patients who require treatment with free rupture. There is often a period of hemodynamic stability before a leaking aneurysm converts to a ruptured aneurysm, where the diagnosis can be confirmed by CT scan and the patients treated prior to hemodynamically instability and free rupture.

3.1 *Thoracic aortic aneurysms*

Thoracic aneurysms rupture in three groups of patients — young patients with traumatic transection, older patients with type B aortic dissections who develop aneurysmal degeneration, and patients with primary thoracic aneurysms — either due to atherosclerotic degeneration or due to a collagen vascular disorder such as Marfans syndrome. The traditional approach to ruptured TA with open repair, either with a clamp and sew technique, left heart bypass, or distal perfusion from an aorto-aortic shunt is associated with a significant risk of paraplegia, renal failure, and visceral ischemia, as well as a high mortality. Recently, several types of thoracic aortic endografts have become available that can provide an endovascular solution with a lower risk of death and paraplegia. In aortic transection, the improved results have been dramatic; although not all manufacturers have endograft with a small enough profile to be used in the nonaneurysmal thoracic aorta.

3.2 *Thoracoabdominal aneurysms*

A ruptured TAA is currently among the highest risk patient population, since there is not an endograft commercially available in the United States for this problem. Therefore, open repair is currently the only option and has the best outcome when performed by a surgical team with experience with elective TAA repair

3.3 *Abdominal aortic aneurysm*

Ruptured AAA has a high mortality with many patients dying before arrival at the hospital, some dying prior to repair, many dying in the OR, and an equal number dying post operatively of multi-organ system failure. The recent introduction of repair using an endograft has significantly reduced the surgical mortality, particularly when the patient has optimal anatomy with a cuff of normal aorta below the renal arteries that measures 1.5 cm. Having endografts in stock that can be taken off the shelf, which is necessary to provide immediate care is paramount.

3.4 *Mesenteric*

Of mesenteric aneurysms, splenic artery aneurysms are the most vulnerable to rupture, although celiac, SMA and renal aneurysms also rupture. Splenic aneurysms are more prevalent in women and particularly prone to rupture in women during pregnancy, where the operative mortality is very high. Splenic aneurysm can be repaired electively with laparoscopic repair, open repair, or with coil embolization or covered stents, although when ruptured, these should primarily be repaired surgically.

3.5 *Peripheral*

Peripheral aneurysms occasionally rupture. They most commonly embolize or thrombose. When they rupture, it is usually contained and cause severe pain and compression on surrounding structures, rather than hypotension.

3.5.1 *Principles of treatment of ruptured aneurysms*

Irrespective of site, a ruptured aneurysm is a surgical emergency and should be treated immediately, often bypassing the CT scanner if the patient is profoundly hypotensive. In most patients, there is time to place larger bore IVs, crossmatch blood, and prepare the OR. If a patient is hemodynamically stable, a CT scan with IV contrast is preferred. GI contrast is contraindicated because it delays treatment. Permissive hypotension, where the blood pressure is allowed to settle at below normal levels as long as the patient is mentating and perfusing critical organs, is the best approach to prevent a contained rupture from becoming a free rupture as the blood pressure is raised to normal or supranormal levels.

4. Thrombosed/Embolizing Aneurysms

It is a rare event that a central aortic or iliac aneurysm embolizes or thromboses; however, it does occur occasionally. Smaller aneurysms and particularly, peripheral lower extremity aneurysms are the ones that typically embolize or thrombose. The reason for these differences is not known. Historically, when a peripheral aneurysm thrombosed or embolized, causing acute limb ischemia, an emergency operation was performed, with repair of the aneurysm and thrombo-embolectomy with a balloon catheter. Using this approach, there was a very high limb loss, even when flow was reestablished, but the distal thrombus that could not be completed removed with the balloon catheter. Over the past 20 years, since thrombolysis has been available, a different approach, with initial thrombolysis, followed by aneurysm repair once the

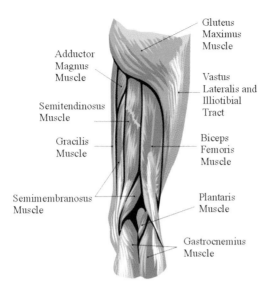

Adductor
Magnus
Muscle

Semitendinosus
Muscle

Gracilis
Muscle

Semimembranosus
Muscle

Gluteus
Maximus
Muscle

Vastus
Lateralis and
Illiotibial
Tract

Biceps
Femoris
Muscle

Plantaris
Muscle

Gastrocnemius
Muscle

Fig. 1. Posterior approach to the popliteal artery. When there is a knee dislocation without other associated injuries, the best visualization of the popliteal injury is posterior, and the recovery is more rapid, because no ligamentous or muscle structures need to be divided. The proximal limit of this dissection is the adductor canal. Distally, the two heads of the gastrocnemius muscle can be divided down to the Achilles tendon.

limb has been revascularized, has resulted in a much better limb salvage rate and much better outcomes (Fig. 1).

5. Angioaccess

5.1 *New access requirements*

Despite efforts to identify patients and provide an access site prior to the need for dialysis, over 50% of patients who require dialysis for chronic renal disease do not have a functioning access site when they first need dialysis. Consequently, the ability to provide immediate access is often required of vascular surgeons. Uncuffed and cuffed catheters are usually the technique to provide access, but occasionally an AV prosthetic graft with good hemostatic qualities can be placed urgently and used immediately for dialysis. For most patients, though a central double lumen dialysis catheter is the initial step when immediate dialysis is needed. Although many sites can be used, including femoral veins, subclavian veins, and internal jugular veins, the most durable central access site with a low risk of bleeding complications, infection, and pneumothorax with good long-term patency is the internal jugular vein, with the right being preferred to the left for anatomic reasons. All central access should be placed under ultrasound guidance to reduce the risk of inadvertent arterial stick, pneumothorax, distal positioning, *etc.* Similar

Table 2.   Signs of inadvertent arterial placement of an intended central venous catheter.

1. Absence of wire visualization in the central vein below the puncture site when advancing it
2. Arterial pressure tracings
3. Arterial blood gas parameters
4. Abnormal path of catheter on chest x-ray (should be seen passing directly into the SVC/right atrium without tortuosity)

techniques are employed when thrombosis or failure of existing AV access occurs (Table 2).

6. Aortic Dissection

6.1 *Thoracic aorta*

Thoracic aortic dissection is an event that is managed based on the location of the dissection, the status of the aorta in the dissected region, and the perfusion of the vessels distal to the dissection. Stanford Type A dissections involve the ascending aorta and require immediate repair to prevent the dissection from causing retrograde pericardial tamponade or acute coronary artery occlusion. Although aortic stent grafts are currently being used experimentally, they will take an increasing role in the management of acute ascending aortic dissection in the future. Stanford Type B dissections begin in the descending aorta and usually progress distally to the visceral vessels and extremity vessels, although they may also dissect proximally into the aortic arch. The decision about treatment of Type B dissection is based on the extent of pain and whether or not it can be controlled, the size of the aorta at the site of dissection, whether it is at risk for rupture or has already ruptured, and the adequacy of perfusion of the vessels distal to the site of the dissection

6.1.1 *Diagnosis*

CT angiography is the best initial test to both diagnose aortic dissection and determine optimal therapy. It helps determine the extent of the dissection, the status of branch vessels, and helps determine whether the branches come off the true or false lumen. Sometimes, malperfusion cannot be seen easily on static CT angiography, and either dynamic CT angiography or intravascular ultrasound (IVUS) is required to determine whether the visceral and renal vessels arise from the true or false lumen.

Catheter angiography should be reserved for fenestrations (connecting the true and false lumens with a catheter and balloon) and delivering stent grafts to treat the dissection.

6.1.2 *Medical management*

All patients require blood pressure control with agents that reduce cardiac contractility, such as Beta blockers. If blood pressure is well controlled and the patient still has pain, then this is one indication for treatment of the dissection. For patients with Marfan's syndrome, treatment with the angiotensin reduction blocking (ARB) agent, Losartan, is associated with reduced chronic enlargement of aneurysms.

6.1.3 *Surgical management*

6.1.3.1 Surgery

Surgery is still the "gold standard" for Type B aortic dissection, although endovascular approaches are increasingly being used. Principles in surgery are to replace the aorta at the site of the aortic tear, to reestablish blood flow to any distal vessel that is associated with organ malperfusion, and to replace the aorta if is has resulted in rupture. Surgical procedures for acute aortic dissection are high risk, due to the fragile aortic tissue, difficulty in correcting all of the dissection, risk of spinal cord ischemia, and malperfusion of critical vessels, which is often associated with coagulopathy.

6.1.3.2 Endovascular management of Type B aortic dissection

Although not yet FDA approved for treatment of acute aortic dissection, endografts have been successfully used in other countries for treatment and are currently undergoing FDA-approved clinical trials to determine their appropriate place in the treatment of acute aortic dissection.

6.2 *Abdominal/visceral dissections*

Abdominal/visceral dissections that originate in the abdominal aorta or its branches are much less common than those that originate in the thoracic aorta; however, with the increased use of CT angiography and MR angiography, patients with both asymptomatic and symptomatic abdominal aortic dissections are being identified and treated. Although experiences are much smaller with these patients, the same principles apply regarding diagnosis and treatment. Unless there is evidence of malperfusion, control of blood pressure is critical, followed by invasive treatment only if there is uncontrolled pain or evidence of malperfusion.

7. Stroke/TIA

7.1 *Carotid thrombosis/embolization*

Acute stroke is most commonly due to intracerebral hemorrhage from aneurysms or hypertension, intracerebral thrombosis from intracerebral vascular disease, or acute dissection. The vascular surgeon becomes involved in patients with acute transient ischemia attacks (TIA) and stroke when the source of their acute event is in the extracranial carotid system or aortic arch vessels.

7.1.1 *Imaging*

Imaging of the arch and carotid vessels is critical to decision making and should be done as rapidly as feasible, since thrombolysis must be started within four hours of the event to achieve maximum value. CT angiography is the best diagnostic modality, since it not only defines the disease in these vessels accurately, but also shows calcification that may influence therapy. MRA can also be useful and is particularly good at defining the intracerebral damage, which also may guide therapy and the timing of any revascularization efforts.

7.1.2 *Treatment of carotid occlusion, string sign, and free-floating thrombus*

When the internal carotid artery becomes acutely occluded, is the source of emboli, or has impending closure, the vascular surgeon is often consulted to determine the feasibility of carotid stenting or endarterectomy. The decisions regarding these problems are complex, since recanalization of the ischemic brain penumbra may be associated with worsening of the stroke. The neurologic stability of the patient is critical, and patients with worsening neurologic deficit, after 4–6 hours, are poor candidates for recanalization. Once the patient has stabilized or improved neurologically, the risk of treatment lessens and they should then be considered for revascularization. These are among the most difficult decisions and should be made in conjunction with a stroke neurologist and neurointerventional radiologist if available. MRI blood flow studies are often used to determine areas of infarction, ischemia, and low flow in patients with deficits and to help guide further therapy. If patients require surgery, all antiplatelet and anticoagulation therapy should be continued through surgery and bleeding in the OR should be controlled with meticulous technique, topical thrombin therapy, and neck drainage.

7.2 *Subclavian/innominate acute occlusion*

The subclavian or innominate artery may thrombose due to emboli from the heart, thrombosis of a pre-existing atherosclerotic plaque, or occlusion due to coverage of a thoracic aortic aneurysm. In all of these situations, an assessment of the impact on the distal limb is critical, since many patients will tolerate proximal subclavian artery occlusion without severe ischemic symptoms. When ischemia does occur, as manifested by hand and arm pain, associated with absent pulses, then revascularization is indicated. When a treated thoracic aneurysm is the cause, then carotid-subclavian bypass is the optimal therapy. When a subclavian aneurysm thromboses, thrombolysis with aneurysm repair is often the best treatment. When emboli occlude the subclavian artery, thrombolysis, thrombectomy, and bypass are all options and the choice is dependent on the experience of the vascular surgeon.

8. Vascular Trauma

8.1 *Thoracic vascular trauma*

Blunt thoracic aortic injuries are associated with high morbidity and mortality. Autopsy studies have estimated that thoracic aortic injuries account for approximately one-third of blunt traumatic fatalities, with the majority of deaths occurring at the scene of the trauma. Thirty percent of patients are found to have associated major head injuries. There is also a high association between thoracic and intra-abdominal injuries in these patients. In hemodynamically stable patients, CT Angiography is the diagnostic study that will evaluate the location and extent of the injury and determine the appropriate approach. Although thoracic aortic transection is the most frequently diagnosed blunt thoracic vascular injury, subclavian artery, innominate artery, and major venous injuries may also occur and require different approaches.

Endovascular repair has been increasingly used for patients with blunt thoracic aortic transection who are stable enough to survive the time needed for CTA and then can reach the operating room following trauma. A recent review of the National Trauma Databank demonstrated, however, that two-thirds of patients are unable to undergo attempts at aortic repair due to instability and additional comorbidities. Thoracic endovascular aortic repair (TEVAR) has been associated with lower postoperative mortality and ischemic spinal cord complication rates than open repair. The most common location for an aortic injury following blunt trauma is the isthmus, which is located just distal to the origin of the left subclavian artery. Because the site of blunt aortic trauma frequently approximates the left subclavian artery, coverage of this vessel is sometimes required to extend the length of the proximal seal zone for the stent-graft. Revascularization of the left subclavian artery following TEVAR coverage with carotid-subclavian bypass is sometimes required. Indications for revascularization include: vertebrobasilar ischemia, development of left upper extremity ischemic symptoms, hypoplastic right vertebral artery, a patent left internal mammary graft, and a functioning dialysis fistula in the left arm.

A brachial approach for catheter access, sometimes preceded with a femoral angiogram and proximal balloon control, can provide access for covered stent placement of blunt subclavian and innominate artery injuries, whether the problem is occlusion, transection, or pseudoaneurysm.

Full-thickness penetrating injuries to the thoracic aorta, associated with hemodynamic instability, usually require emergent aortic cross-clamping to prevent exsanguination and are associated with an extremely high patient mortality. Although TEVAR repair has been reported, the majority of these injuries require open repair through a median sternotomy or left anterolateral thoracotomy, depending on the location of the injury. Circulatory support and arrest is often required for proximal ascending aortic injuries.

8.2 *Abdominal vascular trauma*

8.2.1 *Blunt abdominal vascular trauma*

Blunt abdominal vascular trauma is among the most commonly diagnosed either after a FAST ultrasound scan of the abdomen in the emergency department or after a CT scan of the abdomen. Occasionally, patients are so unstable that they require immediate celiotomy and the vascular injury is discovered at that time. All actively bleeding major arteries require repair, but the treatment is dependent on the site of the injury; surgery can often worsen the situation.

8.2.1.1 Pelvic vascular injuries

Pelvic vascular injuries, which may be either arterial or venous, are usually associated with a pelvic fracture, and are best managed nonoperatively, unless there is exsanguinating hemorrhage. Stabilization of the fracture with external fixation will often reduce or eliminate bleeding. Catheter embolization of arterial and venous bleeding sites is usually the best and most effective means of controlling pelvic bleeding. In the OR, if a patient has a rapidly expanding pelvic hematoma, ligation of the hypogastric arteries and pelvic packing may control hemorrhage, but this is often futile.

8.2.1.2 Other vascular injuries

There are many other vascular injuries that can occur from blunt trauma. Exposure of the retroperitoneum is often required to identify and repair these vessels. The "Mattox maneuver" is an excellent way to visualize the entire aorta and its

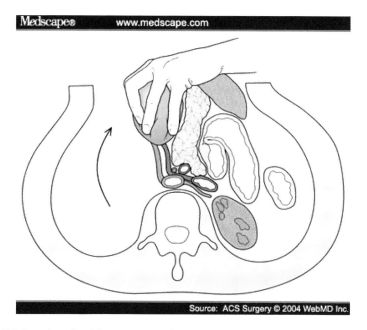

Fig. 2. Medial visceral rotation (Mattox maneuver) for proximal control of the visceral portion of the aorta. The peri-visceral aorta is very difficult to approach anteriorly due to the presence of the pancreas, but medial rotation of the spleen, left colon, and left kidney allow exposure of the entire abdominal aorta. If more proximal control is needed, division of the diaphragm is also possible with this approach.

branches and gain proximal control before entering the hematoma (Fig. 2). Renal artery injuries are often notorious for failure to salvage the kidney and, therefore, can be graded by the extent to the parenchyma injury and the location of the bleeding. Although major renal artery bleeding should be repaired, kidney function is unlikely to be salvaged due to the sensitivity of the renal parenchyma to renal ischemia.

8.2.2 *Penetrating abdominal vascular trauma*

Penetrating abdominal vascular trauma is generally due to either gunshot wounds or stab wounds, although there are certainly other mechanisms of injury. When a penetrating injury occurs, vascular injury is only one concern of many and these patients are often cared for by trauma surgeons who have extensive experience in the comprehensive management of this type of patient. The specific management of vascular injuries is beyond the scope of this chapter, although general principles can be outlined.

8.2.2.1 Resuscitation and angioaccess

When a vascular injury is suspected, patients should be resuscitated only to the point of critical organ perfusion and "permissive hypotension" permitted to prevent resuscitation hemorrhage, which may be life threatening. In addition, large bore central lines and several IVs for resuscitation are routine. Trauma surgeons will also order blood components for transfusion of red cells and coagulation factors, and set up a warming system for blood and fluids if the blood loss becomes excessive. A volume resuscitation system for the delivery of large fluid volume is also part of the routine care of these patients.

8.2.2.2 Incisions for penetrating abdominal trauma

The best exposure for abdominal trauma is a midline incision, which provides access to the entire abdomen. Once the abdomen is opened, exposure of vascular injuries will depend on the location of the injury. The principle of proximal and distal control prior to exploring the hematoma and vascular injury is a good practice in virtually all circumstances. When the injury involves the chest and abdomen, occasionally a single thoracoabdominal incision is preferable to separate chest and abdominal incisions. Although previous recommendations were to only expose certain penetrating abdominal injuries, with current techniques to provide exposure, virtually all large vessel injuries, except for pelvic vascular injuries that are not expanding, should be exposed, examined, and repaired. When a complex vascular injury is anticipated, most ORs are now equipped with angiography and an angiogram/venogram will not only identify the injury, but be used to place balloon catheters for endovascular control, when needed. Occasionally, embolization is the only therapy needed for vascular injuries that occur in vessels not feeding critical organs.

8.3 *Extremity*

Signs that a vascular injury is associated with an extremity injury, whether it is due to blunt or penetrating trauma, are loss of distal pulses, pulsatile or massive hemorrhage from a wound, proximity of the injury to major vessels, and adjacent bone fracture or major nerve injury. When these findings are present, a high index of suspicion for arterial or venous injury should prompt imaging to determine whether or not an injury is present. Initial imaging can often be performed with duplex ultrasound, but, if not clear-cut, should advance to CT angiography. Catheter-directed angiography, which has been the gold standard in the past, is now reserved primarily for delivery of endovascular therapy, since the diagnosis can be made more rapidly and as accurately with a combination the ultrasound and CT angiography.

8.3.1 *Blunt trauma*

The mechanism of injury can often help determine the severity of the injury and associated injuries to nerves, long bones, and soft tissue. Often, the associated injury to soft tissues is more severe than the vascular injury and determines the likelihood of limb survival, assuming that hemorrhage can be controlled. The principles of vascular repair of acute venous and arterial injuries are that they should be repaired in certain locations such as the popliteal artery and that autogenous tissue, with primary anastomosis, vein, or arterial conduits are preferable to prosthetic tissue for resistance to infection and long-term patency. However, the larger the vessel injured, the greater the patency and better that prosthetic grafts perform. Occasionally, large vessel injuries have a very high anticipated risk of infection and cadaveric cryopreserved vein is a better conduit than either prosthetic graft or autogenous tissue.

8.3.1.1 Popliteal artery injury post-knee dislocation

This is one of the most common blunt injuries post-knee dislocation from a dashboard injury. In an automobile accident, the knee injury may not be obvious, but the absence of pulses and the abrupt cutoff at the joint space of the knee are clear indications of this injury. The diagnosis can be confirmed by duplex ultrasound in minutes and, in a patient without underlying vascular disease, precludes the need for an angiogram. With a limited time of 2–4 hours for reperfusion, immediate repair, before the knee stabilization, is critical to salvaging the leg. Fasciotomies are often necessary, since the ischemic period often approaches 3–4 hours, even with immediate repair. The repair can best be accomplished with the patient in the prone position, and can often be accomplished with mobilization of the artery and resection of the injured vessel with primary anastomosis. If the repair would be under tension, then an interposition vein graft should be used. If the popliteal vein is also injured, then the vein conduit should be harvested from the contralateral leg.

8.3.2 *Penetrating trauma*

Penetrating trauma to the extremities with major vascular injury is often life threatening and, yet can often be repaired without limb loss. Increasingly, endovascular approaches are being used for control of hemorrhage and repair of vascular defects. As opposed to blunt trauma, mortality is higher in penetrating limb trauma with vascular injury, due to exsanguination. Therefore, control of hemorrhage takes a high priority in these patients. Occasionally, the injury is distal enough in the limb to allow a tourniquet to be placed on the limb in the field or ER, and the control of hemorrhage can be addressed in the OR, although injuries are often more proximal and, therefore, cannot be controlled with pressure or proximal control. In these scenarios, endovascular balloon control, usually in the OR with either fixed imaging equipment or high resolution fluoroscopy, is used to prevent hemorrhage until surgical control can be obtained.

In the extremities, major penetrating vascular injuries are invariably associated with long bone injuries and major motor and sensory nerve injuries, due to their proximity.

8.4 *Cerebrovascular injuries*

Cerebrovascular injuries are most common with penetrating injuries due to both stab and gunshot wounds of the neck and upper chest, although vascular injuries may also occur with blunt injuries. Zones of the neck have been used historically to manage these injuries, when endovascular approaches were not available. Currently, an endovascular approach preceded by angiography is being increasingly used in the primary management of many of these patients.

8.4.1 *Penetrating neck injuries*

Penetrating neck injuries are classified based on the location of the injury, the extent of bleeding, associated injuries, and the neurologic status of the patient. The zones of the neck are seen in Fig. 3.

8.4.1.1 Diagnosis

If the patient is hemodynamically stable, the best approach is to precede definitive vascular repair with endoscopic assessment of the aerodigestive tract by an otolaryngologist. If the injury is in Zone 2 and, therefore, surgically accessible, and is associated with an aerodigestive injury that requires open repair, then a direct vascular

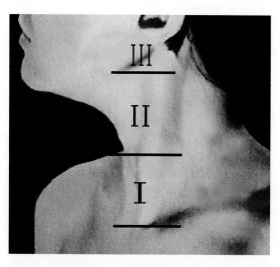

Fig. 3. Zones of the neck. There are three neck zones in trauma, as demonstrated in this figure. The significance of this classification is that Zones 1 and 3 are less surgically accessible and require different diagnostic and surgical approaches, while Zone 2 can be approached surgically with proximal and distal control.

repair is indicated and no further diagnostic vascular workup is required. For patients who are hemodynamically stable and have Zone 1 and 3 injuries, a CT angiogram will help both define the injury and determine the appropriate technique for repair. When the patient is not stable and has either active bleeding or expanding hematoma, then angiography in the OR is the best approach to both control hemorrhage with a balloon catheter, define the location and extent of the injury, and often can be used to provide definitive repair. For proximal Zone 1 injuries, the patient should also be prepped for open surgery, in case he or she deteriorates hemodynamically.

8.4.1.2 Treatment

The basic approach to all vascular injuries is to obtain proximal and distal control before exploring the site of the injury. A hybrid approach is occasionally required, where proximal control is obtained surgically, but distal control is not possible and, therefore, an endovascular balloon must be placed in the OR for distal control. Once control is obtained, the options for repair include direct "lateral" repair or primary resection with reanastomsis for stab wounds without arterial injury. Interposition vein grafts are preferred for arterial injuries associated with GI injury and/or contamination. Prosthetic grafts for preferred in uncontaminated wounds, although there are situations in which a prosthetic graft must be used in the face of contamination due to better size match or to minimize operative time when other life-threatening injuries are present.

Neurologic status is not a major consideration in acute injuries. Although there is a possibility of making a neurologically impaired patient worse with revascularization, due to reperfusion of previously ischemic areas of the brain, most series have shown that many patients benefit from revascularization and regain some, if not all of their prior function. When the injury is not acute, the decision for revascularization is more difficult and requires a more extensive workup with brain perfusion scans. Venous injuries are usually repaired if technically feasible, although ligation may be used for almost any venous injury in the neck.

8.4.2 *Cerebrovascular blunt injuries*

Cerebrovascular blunt injuries are not immediately life threatening due to hemorrhage, but they are often associated with other injuries to the head and chest that may require immediate repair for survival.

8.4.2.1 Diagnosis

If the patient is hemodynamically stable, CT angiography or catheter-based angiography may be used, depending on availability. The advantage of catheter angiography in the OR is that definitive treatment can often be provided after diagnosis, while

CT angiography is limited to diagnosis. However, many emergency rooms have CT scanners immediately available and there is less delay in establishing the diagnosis than with catheter angiography in the operating room. An angiography suite or catheterization lab is suboptimal for trauma patients who often require other open procedures simultaneously or sequentially.

8.4.2.2 Treatment

Although many blunt injuries require open repair, a significant number of injuries can be treated with endovascularly placed covered stents and, therefore, do not require open surgery. In addition, proximal balloon catheter control can often be useful prior to surgery when the access is difficult or when there is a significant risk of hemorrhage with open repair due to lack of proximal control. Most blunt arterial injuries have extensive damage to the artery and require resection of the damaged artery and interposition grafting to prevent rethrombosis or development of anastomotic pseudoaneurysms.

References

Arthurs ZM, Starnes BW, Sohn VY, Singh N, Martin MJ, Andersen CA. Functional and survival outcomes in traumatic blunt thoracic aortic injuries: an analysis of the National Trauma Databank. *J Vasc Surg* 2009; **49**: 988–94.

Compton C, Rhee R. Peripheral vascular trauma, *Perspect Vasc Surg Endovasc Ther* 2005; **17**(4): 297–307.

Estrera AL, Gochnour DC, Azizzadeh A, Miller CC 3rd, Coogan S, Charlton-Ouw K, Holcomb JB, Safi HJ. Progress in the treatment of blunt thoracic aortic injury: 12-year single-institution experience. *Ann Thorac Surg* 2010; **90**: 64–71.

Goaley TJ, Dente CJ, Feliciano DV. Torso vascular trauma at an urban Level I trauma center, *Perspect Vasc Surg Endovasc Ther* 2006; **18**(2):102–112.

Gossage JA, Ali T, Chambers J, Burnand KG. Peripheral arterial embolism: prevalence, outcome, and the role of echocardiography in management, *Vasc Endovasc Surg* 2006; **40**(4):280–286.

Kauvar DS, Sarfati MR, Kraiss LW. Mortality and limb loss in isolated lower extremity vascular trauma: analysis of the National Trauma Data Bank, *J Vasc Surg* 2010; **52**(2):532.

Li W, D'Ayala M, Hirshberg A, Briggs W, Wise L, Tortolani A. Comparison of conservative and operative treatment for blunt carotid injuries: analysis of the National Trauma Data Bank, *J Vasc Surg* 2010; **51**(3):593–599.e2.

Meissner MH, Wakefield TW, Ascher E, Caprini JA, Comerota AJ, Eklof B, Gillespie DL, Greenfield LJ, He AR, Henke PK, Hingorani A, Hull RD, Kessler CM, McBane RD, McLafferty R. Acute venous disease: venous thrombosis and venous trauma, *J Vasc Sur* 2007; **46**(6):S25–S53.

Patel HJ, Hemmila MR, Williams DM, Diener AC, Deep GM. Late outcomes following open and endovascular repair of blunt thoracic aortic injury. *J Vasc Surg* 2010 [Epub ahead of print].

Rahimi SA, Clement Darling R, Mehta M, Roddy SP, Taggert JB, Sternbach Y. Endovascular repair of thoracic aortic traumatic transections is a safe method in patients with complicated injuries, *J Vasc Surg* 2010; in press.

Starnes BW, Arthurs ZM. Endovascular management of vascular trauma, *Perspect Vasc Surg Endovasc Ther* 2006; **18**(2):114–129.

Teixeira PG, Inaba K, Barparas G, Georgiou C, Toms C, Noguchi TT, *et al.* Blunt thoracic aortic injuries: an autopsy study. *J Trauma* 2011; **70**: 197–202.

Trivedi PS, Sachs T, Pomposelli FB, Wyers MC, Hamdan AD, Schermerhorn ML. National outcomes of open and endovascular repair of traumatic transection of the thoracic aorta, *J Vasc Surg* 2010; **51**(6):63S.

Chapter 10

Management of Visceral and Renovascular Occlusive and Aneurysmal Disease

Juan Carlos Jimenez and Darin Saltzman

Learning Objectives

- Learn the natural history, presentation, and diagnosis of acute mesenteric ischemia and become familiar with available treatment options.
- Learn the natural history, presentation, and diagnosis of chronic mesenteric ischemia and become familiar with available treatment options.
- Understand typical symptoms and optimal medical management in patients with renal artery stenosis.
- Familiarize yourself with benefits and limitations of endovascular and surgical treatments for renal artery stenosis based on recent medical literature.
- Understand the common characteristics, diagnostic methods, indications, and options for treatment of visceral artery aneurysms.

1. Visceral Occlusive Disease

1.1 *Acute mesenteric ischemia*

Acute mesenteric ischemia (AMI) is a life-threatening condition that may result in profound and irreversible intestinal ischemia if not recognized early and treated appropriately. AMI has been found to carry a relative risk for death of 3.0 in patients who are greater than 60 years of age. The most common cause of AMI is an embolus to the superior mesenteric artery (SMA), which results in acutely diminished intestinal perfusion. The proximal source of the embolism can derive from many anatomic locations; however, an intracardiac mural thrombus exacerbated by cardiac arrhythmias, myocardial infarction, or structural heart defects are the most common inciting factors. Mural thrombi from proximal aneurysms can also dislodge and embolize distally to the SMA. Paradoxical venous thromboemboli can embolize into the arterial system through a patent foramen ovale and any other anatomic right to left shunt. Septic emboli from endocarditis are a less common etiology yet can occur. The SMA arises from a narrow angle relative to the other visceral arteries and this anatomic configuration is the reason why emboli terminate in the SMA more frequently. The embolus usually lodges several centimeters from the vessel's origin just distal to the middle colic artery. Visceral angiograms typically demonstrate an abrupt occlusion of the SMA distal to the middle colic artery with minimal collateralization. This is virtually diagnostic of AMI originating from an acute embolus.

Arterial thrombosis is the next most common cause of AMI and is usually seen in patients with preexisting atherosclerotic lesions at the origins of all three visceral vessels (celiac artery, SMA, and inferior mesenteric artery). Hypercoaguable states can also lead to acute thrombosis. Acute thrombosis of an arterial plaque usually occurs at the level of the aorta. On visceral angiogram, the occlusion is usually seen at the origin of the SMA as opposed to more distally, as is seen with embolic causes. Because of its more proximal location, a larger percentage of arterial branches are occluded and more extensive intestinal ischemia is seen over a broader anatomic area.

Another cause of AMI is nonocclusive mesenteric ischemia (NOMI). In this syndrome, arterial perfusion of the intestine occurs in the absence of thromboembolic occlusion. Extensive atherosclerotic plaque, without the presence of a discrete hemodynamically significant visceral artery occlusion, is usually found throughout the mesenteric circulation. NOMI is exacerbated by low cardiac output particularly associated with congestive heart failure. Cardiac arrhythmia, such as atrial fibrillation, may induce acute intestinal ischemia in the setting of hypotension, hypovolemia, and low cardiac output. Other risk factors include: vasoactive drugs (*i.e.* beta blockers, cocaine, Digoxin, *etc.*) or systemic vasopressors (*i.e.* levophed, dopamine, neosynephrine, *etc.*).

Thrombosis of the superior mesenteric vein (SMV), portal vein, and inferior mesenteric vein (IMV) can also cause AMI. Hypercoaguable states are most frequently implicated in this disease process. Other causes include malignancy, trauma, abdominal surgery, pancreatitis, and liver failure. Frequently, patients with this disorder are hospitalized for other causes and the diagnosis is made due to poor feeding or deterioration in the patient's overall condition. Many require systemic vasopressors, which worsens the degree of intestinal ischemia due to splanchnic vasoconstriction. The progression of bowel ischemia is less rapid than with acute arterial occlusion and treatment involves immediate systemic anticoagulation. Edema and hemorrhage of the intestinal wall correlate with the extent of mesenteric venous thrombosis. Mucosal sloughing is usually a late finding.

1.1.1 *Clinical presentation and diagnosis*

Patients with acute mesenteric ischemia frequently present with a sudden onset of severe abdominal pain. Other signs include diarrhea, nausea, vomiting, and abdominal distension. The classic finding is "pain out of proportion" to findings on physical examination. Thus, early in the presentation, tenderness is not elicited with deep palpation; however, the patient has complains of constant and severe abdominal pain. Rebound and guarding are absent in the early period of AMI. As bowel ischemia and infarction progress, peritoneal signs develop. In this disease process, rebound and guarding are considered late findings and their absence should not delay diagnosis and treatment. Other signs may include tachycardia, fever, dehydration, disorientation, decreased urine output, and shock. Typical findings on laboratory studies include metabolic acidosis, leukocytosis, increased lactic acid levels, elevated amylase levels, and elevated liver function tests.

Following the history and physical examination, the initial diagnostic test of choice for AMI is computed tomography. Advantages include the relative ease and speed of performance, infusion of contrast through peripheral intravenous lines, and the ability to image simultaneously the mesenteric arteries, veins, and the visceral organs. Findings in the bowel wall related to acute mesenteric ischemia may include bowel wall thickening, dilatation, and attenuation that can be easily detected using this imaging modality. Pneumatosis intestinalis (air within the bowel wall) as well as mesenteric edema and ascites can also be detected. During the arterial phase of contrast infusion, the visceral vessels can also be evaluated for thrombosis, embolus, dissection, and aneurysm.

1.1.2 *Treatment*

Patients presenting with signs and symptoms of AMI require urgent abdominal exploration, assessment of bowel viability, and revascularization. Because exploratory laparotomy is the fastest and most accurate method of examining the integrity of the small and large bowel, it is recommended over endovascular therapy for patients with AMI. Several techniques are available to assist the vascular surgeon with assessment of bowel viability. We routinely administer 1–2 ampules (500 mg to 1000 mg) of intravenous fluorescein followed by evaluation of the bowel with an ultraviolet Wood's lamp. A "patchy" pattern of fluorescein distribution is frequently seen in nonviable areas, which require resection. Doppler evaluation of the mesenteric arteries should also be performed by the surgeon. Intraoperative angiography may also be performed to reassess restoration of mesenteric flow following revascularization. Assessment of bowel viability and intestinal resection should be made only after revascularization of the SMA. We frequently perform a "second-look" laparotomy within 24 hours to reassess bowel viability and the need for further resection.

The most common operation for revascularization of the SMA in patients with AMI is open embolectomy. Exposure of the SMA is performed and silastic vessel loops are placed around the vessel for proximal and distal control. If the artery feels relatively soft and free of plaque, a transverse arteriotomy is performed distal to the area of obstruction and the arterial lumen is assessed for thrombus. Balloon-tipped embolectomy catheters are passed gently proximally and distally until no further clot can be removed. The transverse incision is then closed primarily with simple interrupted prolene sutures. If the cause of ischemia is acute thrombosis of a visceral plaque, endarterectomy with patch angioplasty or aorto-mesenteric bypass may be required. Details of these procedures are beyond the scope of this chapter.

1.2 *Chronic mesenteric ischemia*

Atherosclerosis of the visceral arteries is the most common underlying etiology in patients presenting with chronic mesenteric ischemia. Asymptomatic occlusive disease of the mesenteric arteries is a common finding in elderly patients. Studies have reported that approximately 18% of patients over the age of 65, examined with duplex ultrasonography, have a critical stenosis of at least one visceral vessel. The extensive collaterals present within the mesenteric arterial circulation allow most patients to maintain adequate visceral perfusion and remain symptom free. Stenosis or occlusion of all three visceral arteries is usually required for symptoms to develop.

1.2.1 *Clinical presentation and diagnosis*

The variability of symptoms in patients with chronic abdominal pain often makes diagnosis challenging, resulting in the increases of treatment delay and morbidity. These patients usually have several risk factors for atherosclerosis and a heavy smoking history is common. Patients with CMI present with postprandial pain and weight loss, which progresses over a period of weeks to years. "Food fear" and anxiety surrounding the development of pain following meals is a common feature in patients with this disease. Patients typically complain of pain for about 30–45 minutes after eating. Other symptoms may include diarrhea, nausea, and bloating. Findings on physical examination are usually nonspecific. Hyperactive bowel sounds are common. Rebound and guarding are usually absent, except in the late stages of the disease, when intestinal necrosis or perforation has occurred.

In patients with CMI, duplex ultrasound is a useful diagnostic modality for diagnosis. Typically, these patients are thin and cachectic, which facilitates imaging with this technique. Color Doppler scanning can be used to assess luminal flow velocities and resistance index in the visceral arteries and their beds as well as evaluate end organ perfusion. The accuracy of visceral ultrasound studies is influenced by the skill of the ultrasound technician, patient body habitus, excessive intraluminal bowel gas, and the effects of respiration.

Computed tomography is a fast and accurate imaging modality, which is useful in visualizing the visceral arteries and the bowel in patients with suspected CMI. The benefits of CT with regard to the diagnosis of mesenteric ischemia are described earlier in this chapter. Disadvantages include the use of nephrotoxic contrast agents and the possibility of allergic and anaphylactic reactions to iodinated contrast. Magnetic resonance angiography provides detailed images of visceral artery and end organ anatomy; however, disadvantages include long scan times and nonvisualization of arterial calcification. Although the gadolinium contrast used with MRA is used in smaller volumes, recent concerns over nephrogenic systemic fibrosis associated with renal failure have limited its use in these patients.

Angiography remains the gold standard radiologic modality for visualizing occlusive disease of the visceral arteries. Disadvantages include increased risk of access site complications, thrombosis, embolization, and dissection secondary to intraarterial catheter placement and manipulation.

1.2.2 *Treatment*

New developments and advances in technology have greatly expanded the role of endovascular therapy for patients with mesenteric ischemia in recent years. Percutanous access for wire cannulation of the mesenteric arteries can be performed either through the femoral or through the brachial arteries. Balloon angioplasty and stenting are the most common interventions for symptomatic visceral arterial occlusive disease and recent studies have documented excellent technical results with low patient morbidity (Fig. 1).

Endovascular therapy is the treatment of choice in high-risk patients with CMI at our institution (Fig. 2). High technical success rates and decreased patient morbidity and mortality rates in these patients have been reasonably well established and are supported by the current literature. However, in younger patients who are good surgical candidates, the advantage of visceral angioplasty and stenting is not so well established. Restenosis and symptomatic recurrence rates remain relatively high as documented in recent studies with long-term followup and often require earlier reintervention than traditionally reported with open surgical revascularization.

Exploratory laparotomy with revascularization of the occluded visceral arteries is the traditional method of treating patients with CMI. Several different operations are used for reperfusion of the chronically ischemic viscera and have been used for many

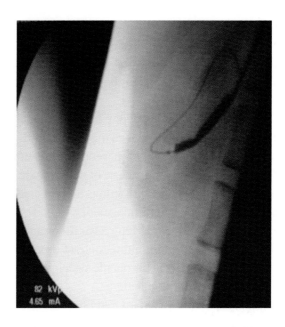

Fig. 1. Balloon angioplasty of a hemodynamically significant celiac artery stenosis.

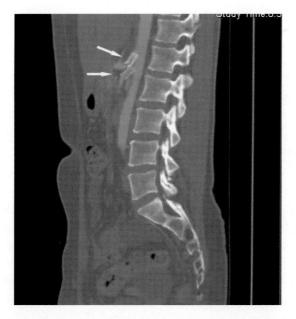

Fig. 2. CT angiogram demonstrates patent celiac and superior mesenteric artery stents following treatment for chronic mesenteric ischemia.

years with acceptable patient morbidity and mortality. These include transaortic endarterectomy, antegrade mesenteric bypass, and retrograde mesenteric bypass. Antegrade bypass techniques include the supraceliac aorta as the source of inflow for the proximal anastomosis. Examples include aorto-celiac and aorto-SMA bypass with either autogenous conduit (*i.e.* saphenous vein, cryopreserved femoral artery) or prosthetic graft. In the setting of extensive bowel necrosis or perforation, autogenous conduit is preferred. Retrograde bypass can also be performed using the iliac artery as the inflow source with similar conduits. Detailed descriptions of these techniques are beyond the scope of this book.

1.3 *Renovascular occlusive disease*

1.3.1 *Presentation and diagnosis*

Atherosclerosis is the underlying cause of renal artery stenosis (RAS) in most patients. Fibromuscular dysplasia (FMD) is another less common etiology and is more common in females. The incidence of RAS has been estimated to be 0.5% of the Medicare population and 5.5% of patients with chronic renal failure. Renal artery stenosis from atherosclerotic disease is associated with a death rate of approximately 16% per year, mostly from associated cardiovascular morbidity. Although patients with RAS develop severe and refractory hypertension and renal failure, it is difficult to predict which patients will respond to revascularization and which benefit from medical management alone. Other negative effects of RAS include flash pulmonary edema, congestive heart failure, and unstable angina pectoris.

Renovascular hypertension should be suspected when blood pressure values rise above the ranges usually associated with essential hypertension. Refractory hypertension in children and young adults should prompt investigation for RAS. Previously normotensive individuals, above the age of 55, with a rapid onset of hypertension should also be suspected. Activation of the renin-angiotensin system is believed to be the main inciting factor leading to refractory hypertension in patients with RAS. Sodium retention is increased by both increased levels of Angiotensin II and Aldosterone, which, in turn, reduce sodium secretion in the post-stenotic kidney. However, the pathophysiology of the disorder is not completely understood, leading to difficulties in predicting clinical response to treatment.

1.3.2 *Imaging*

Recent advances in vascular imaging allow for enhanced visualization of occlusive lesions of the renal arteries. Duplex ultrasound is the initial test choice for initial identification of renal artery lesions. It is also useful to evaluate characteristics of the kidney itself including asymmetry, cortical thickness, and overall perfusion. It is relatively inexpensive and noninvasive. There is no radiation exposure to the patient and no exposure to nephrotoxic contrast agents. Disadvantages include operator dependence and artifact due to bowel gas or patient body habitus. Although standards vary depending on the vascular laboratory where the study is performed, increased blood flow velocities are associated with higher-grade renal artery stenoses. Duplex ultrasound can also be used for surveillance following renal artery angioplasty and stenting to monitor for in-stent restenosis (Fig. 3).

Improved multi-detector computed tomography allows for rapid image acquisition and excellent visualization of the renal arteries. This modality, however, provides an anatomic and not a physiologic assessment of RAS. A major limitation of this technique in these patients is the increased nephrotoxicity of iodinated contrast agents required to obtain images in the arterial phase. Other disadvantages include radiation exposure and artifact from severely calcified arteries.

Magnetic resonance angiography allows for high-resolution images of the renal arteries without the radiation exposure associated with computed tomography (Fig. 4). It is noninvasive and large volumes of nephrotoxic contrast are not required. Because of concerns over nephrogenic systemic fibrosis due to gadolinium exposure, its role in patients with chronic renal failure has been questioned. Other limitations include nonvisualization of calcification, longer imaging times, and increased relative costs.

Catheter angiography is rarely used prior to CTA or MRA but is still considered the "gold standard" for the diagnosis of renal artery stenosis (Figs. 5A and 5B). Functional assessments of RAS can be performed by measuring pressure gradients

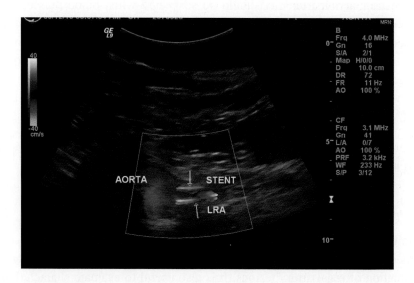

Fig. 3.   Duplex ultrasound demonstrates in-stent restenosis within a previously placed stent in the renal artery.

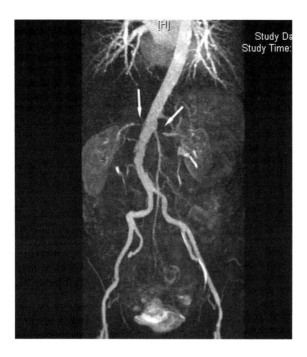

Fig. 4. Magnetic resonance angiography demonstrating bilateral renal artery stenoses.

proximal and distal to the suspected lesion. The amount of iodinated contrast and radiation can also be controlled and limited by the operator. It is, however, an invasive procedure with risks from arterial embolization, thrombosis, dissection, bleeding, and pseudoaneurysm formation. Because of its invasiveness, increased cost, and risk of complication, catheter angiography should only be used on an intent-to-treat basis and not as a screening modality.

1.3.3 *Treatment*

Optimizing medical management of renovascular hypertension must be performed prior to either endovascular or surgical revascularization. The cornerstone of this treatment is antihypertensive drug therapy, primarily by blockade of the renin-angiotensin system. These medications include angiotensin-converting enzyme inhbitors (ACE) and angiotensin receptor blockers (ARB). Other agents include calcium channel blockers, diuretics, and alpha and beta-blockers, *etc*. Lipid-lowering agents, smoking cessation, and tight blood sugar control in diabetics should also be used in patients with known RAS.

The benefits of endovascular revascularization of hemodynamically significant renal artery lesions with balloon angioplasty and stenting are unclear, despite a recent sharp increase in their use in patients with RAS. Between 1996 and 2005,

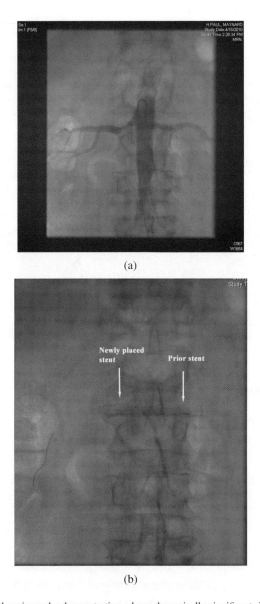

Fig. 5. (a) Conventional angiography demonstrating a hemodynamically significant right renal artery stenosis. Note the presence of a previously placed stent in the left renal artery. (b) Bilateral renal stent placement for renal artery stenosis.

a four-fold increase in the number of these procedures was noted in the Medicare population. The results of three recent randomized trials comparing renal artery stenting with medical management alone have not demonstrated any difference in clinical outcomes between the two groups.

The largest of these, the ASTRAL trial, randomly assigned 806 patients with atherosclerotic renal disease to either revascularization in addition to medical therapy or medical therapy alone. The median followup period was 34 months. No significant improvements in blood pressure or reductions in renal or cardiovascular events were noted. Thirty-eight periprocedural (less than 24 hours) complications were seen in 31 patients (9%). They included pulmonary edema, myocardial infarction, renal artery embolization, renal artery occlusion, and three cases of cholesterol embolization leading to limb amputation. Complications at one month included two deaths from cardiac causes and four patients with groin hematoma requiring rehospitalization. Thus, there were significant risks associated with percutaneous renal artery stenting with no worthwhile clinical benefit.

The role of surgical revascularization for RAS has diminished in the endovascular era. It is largely limited to patients requiring simultaneous aortic reconstruction; younger patients requiring a more durable repair, unfavorable renal artery anatomy for endovascular treatment, and restenosis following prior renal stenting. A recent randomized trial compared operative *vs.* interventional treatment for renal artery ostial occlusive disease and found that mortality was not higher in the surgical group and procedure-related morbidity was higher in the endovascular group. Another recent retrospective study from the Massachusetts General Hospital compared open renal revascularization (endarterectomy and bypass) with angioplasty and stenting. Both groups had similar outcomes in blood pressure improvement; however, the open group achieved better outcomes with stable or improved renal function.

2. Visceral Artery Aneurysms

Visceral artery aneurysms are rare. Associated risk factors include atherosclerosis, hypertension, systemic inflammation, trauma, collagen vascular disease, infection, fibromuscular dysplasia, and cirrhosis. Most of the literature regarding this disease process consists of single-center retrospective series with small numbers or isolated case reports. Because of their low incidence and frequency, the natural history of VAAs is not clearly known and indications for treatment can vary widely. Although their estimated incidence is only 0.1–2%, VAAs may present with rupture in 30–40% of patients, with elevated mortality rates.

The most common locations for VAAs are splenic (60%), hepatic (20%), superior mesenteric (5%), and celiac (4%) arteries. Gastroduodenal, renal, pancreatic-duodenal, jejunal, ileocolic, and inferior mesenteric artery aneurysms are less common. Rupture is believed to occur more frequently when the maximum diameter exceeds 2 cm. We recommend treating asymptomatic VAAs greater than or equal to 2 cm and symptomatic ones regardless of size.

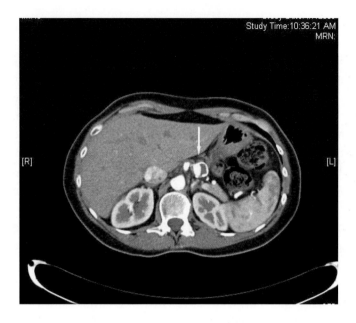

Fig. 6. Computed tomography demonstrates a large and calcified splenic artery aneurysm.

2.1 *Splenic artery aneurysms*

Splenic artery aneurysms (SAA) constitute approximately 60% of all visceral artery aneurysms (Fig. 6). The majority of patients remain asymptomatic and they are often discovered incidentally by abdominal computed tomography for unrelated conditions. While the overall rupture risk is actually quite low, rupture is associated with high mortality in patients with SAA. Associated risk factors for rupture include pregnancy, portal hypertension, and liver transplantation. Acute rupture may occur into the lesser sac or freely into the peritoneum leading to a life-threatening hypovolemia and hemorrhagic shock. Therapy is indicated for aneurysms 2 cm or greater. All patients with symptomatic or rapidly expanding aneurysms should also be treated. All young females of childbearing age with SAA should be surgically treated. Smaller aneurysms require close outpatient observation with serial imaging with either CTA or MRA to monitor aneurysm growth.

The most commonly described endovascular therapy for SAA is coil embolization (Figs. 7A and 7B). Because the spleen has a rich collateral network from several different arterial beds, the removal of inline flow through the main splenic artery does not always compromise splenic viability. Saccular aneurysms with a discrete neck can be embolized without disrupting this direct splenic artery flow. Other options include injection of fibrin or thrombin glue and exclusion of the aneurysm with a covered stent graft if the anatomy is favorable.

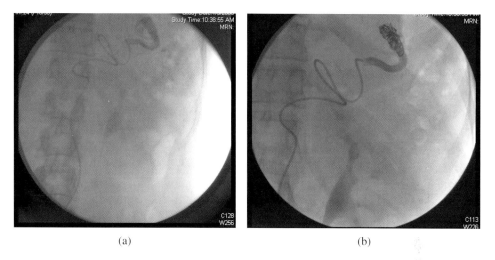

(a)   (b)

Fig. 7. (a) Splenic artery aneurysm prior to coil embolization and (b) thrombosis of splenic artery aneurysm following coil embolization.

Limitations of this technique include the tortuosity, frequently encountered in the splenic artery, small vessel size, and splenic infarction. In our experience, 25% of these patients develop symptomatic splenic infarction. A high index of suspicion for this complication should be maintained following coil embolization of SAAs. Aneurysms closer to the splenic hilum are associated with increased splenic ischemia. Patients typically complain of postprocedural abdominal pain and may present with fevers and elevated white blood cell counts. Refractory abdominal pain in the setting of splenic infarction usually requires either laparoscopic or open splenectomy, which should be done during the same hospitalization if symptoms are severe.

Surgical management of SAAs can be achieved with several techniques depending on the characteristics of the aneurysm. Resections with primary repair, patch angioplasty, or placement of an interposition saphenous vein graft are the most common methods. Ligation and splenectomy is a less desirable but available option.

2.2 Hepatic artery aneurysms

Hepatic artery aneurysms (HAA) are the second most common VAA. The majority of occurs in males, are solitary, and located in an extrahepatic location. Most patients are asymptomatic. Symptomatic patients may present with hemobilia, jaundice, and right upper quadrant pain. A large number of HAAs are pseudoaneurysms. This can be attributed to the increased use of interventional procedures of the biliary tract in recent years. True aneurysms occur four times more frequently in the extrahepatic arteries, usually involve the common hepatic artery, and are associated mainly with atherosclerosis or acquired medial degeneration. Mycotic aneurysms are rare (<5% of hepatic artery aneurysms). Other causes may include polyarteritis nodosa, pancreatitis, liver transplantation, neurofibromatosis, Wegener granulomatosis, and tuberculosis. Mortality rates of greater than 50% have been reported following acute rupture.

An endovascular option for therapy is exclusion of the aneurysm with a covered stent graft. This has been described in multiple case reports. Success of this technique depends on the presence of proximal and distal "landing zones" with normal diameters for adequate seal. Care must be taken to avoid coverage of the gastroduodenal artery due to its close proximity to the common hepatic artery. Surgical repair can usually be achieved with aneurysm resection and reconstruction of the artery with primary repair, patch angioplasty, or placement of an interposition graft. If infection is suspected, prosthetic materials should be avoided (covered stent grafts, PTFE, Dacron, *etc.*).

2.3 *Renal artery aneurysms*

Renal artery aneurysms (RAAs) are the third most common visceral aneurysm with a reported incidence of 0.6–1%. Most are asymptomatic. The most common cause of RAAs is fibromuscular dysplasia. Other etiologies include collagen vascular disorders, trauma, iatrogenic injury, Kawasaki's disease, and vasculitis. Both true and false (pseudoaneurysms) may occur. Symptomatic patients can present with hypertension, flank pain, hematuria, renal infarct, and rupture. Obstruction of the collecting system has been reported in patients with larger aneurysms. Treatment is generally recommended for any RAA greater than 2 cm. However, other factors such as age of the patient, related symptoms and comorbidities, gender, and combined renovascular hypertension. Pregnant females tend to have a particularly high rupture risk. Because the mortality for rupture in pregnancy is reported to be 60–80%, all women of childbearing age contemplating pregnancy should undergo RAA repair regardless of size.

Although endovascular techniques have been described in small retrospective series and case reports, the favored method of repair in low risk patients is surgical. Techniques include aneurysm resection with primary repair, patch angioplasty, or placement of an interposition bypass graft. In a recent series from our institution, 14 open RAA repairs were performed over a five-year period. In patients with concurrent hypertension, operative repair was associated with lower medication requirements. No ruptures, renal failure, nephrectomies, or deaths occurred in the treatment group.

2.4 *Celiac artery and superior mesenteric artery aneurysms*

Celiac artery aneurysms (CAAs) comprise approximately 4% of all visceral artery aneurysms. They are believed to occur in approximately 0.2% in the overall population. The most common underlying etiology is atherosclerosis and medial degeneration. Other causes include infection, trauma, connective tissue disorders, or vasculitis (Takayasu arteritis, polyarteritis nodosa, fibro-muscular dysplasia, and Bechet's disease). Syphilitic aneurysms occur less commonly in the modern era but have been reported. CAAs can present with epigastric pain or upper gastrointestinal hemorrhage. Worsening abdominal pain usually indicates a rapidly expanding aneurysm or rupture. Patients may also present with dysphagia which may occur from mechanical compression of the adjacent esophagus. Endovascular repair has been reported, including coil embolization of the hepatic artery and exclusion of the CAA with a covered stent graft. Because of the collateral blood supply between the celiac artery and the SMA, coverage of the celiac may be achieved in selected patients without end-organ ischemia. However, prediction of success following celiac artery coverage is difficult and preservation of flow following aneurysm repair should be attempted.

Superior mesenteric artery aneurysms (SMAA) represent approximately 5% of all visceral artery aneurysms. The most common etiology is infectious or mycotic. Other causes include trauma, dissection, atherosclerosis, polyarteritis nodosa, pancreatitis, and neurofibromatosis. Patients with symptomatic SMAAs present with intermittent upper abdominal pain. Symptoms may be caused by both thrombosis and distal embolization. Open surgical intervention is the recommended treatment for this type of aneurysm due to multiple side branches frequently encountered on the main SMA trunk. Embolization is not an option in these patients. Direct inline flow must be restored following aneurysm resection due to the risk of acute intestinal infarction resulting from disruption of the SMA circulation. Exclusion with a covered stent graft has also been reported.

2.5 *Less common visceral artery aneurysms*

True aneurysms of the gastroduodenal (GDA) and pancreaticoduodenal (PDA) arteries are often degenerative while pseudoaneurysms are often complications from acute and chronic pancreatitis. Patients may present with either intrabdominal or retroperitoneal bleeding. Coil embolization is the endovascular treatment of choice for these aneurysms due to the presence of extensive end organ collaterals. When treating aneurysms in the pancreaticoduodenal distribution, collateral supply to these aneurysms is extensive. Endovascular approaches to aneurysms of the GDA and/or PDA should be considered first-line treatment whenever possible because surgical exposure of these aneurysms is very difficult. Descriptions in the surgical literature are limited to case reports and beyond the scope of this chapter.

References

Acosta S, Ogren M, Sternby NH, *et al.* Clinical implications for the management of acute thromboembolic occlusion of the superior mesenteric artery: autopsy findings in 213 patients. *Ann Surg* 2005; **241**:516–522.

ASTRAL investigators, Wheatley K, Ives N, Gray R, *et al.* Revascularization versus medical therapy for renal artery stenosis. *N Engl J Med* 2009; **361**:1953–1962.

Bax L, Woittiez AJ, Kouwenberg HJ, *et al.* Stent placement in patients with atherosclerotic renal artery stenosis and impaired renal function: a randomized trial. *Ann Intern Med* 2009; **150**:840–848.

Chandra A, O'Connell JB, Quinones-Baldrich W, Lawrence PF, *et al.* Open surgical repair of renal artery aneurysms in the endovascular era: a safe, effective treatment for both aneurysm and associated hypertension. *Ann Vasc Surg* 2010; **24**:503–510.

Jimenez JC, Quinones-Baldrich WJ. Mesenteric vascular disease: general considerations. In: Cronenwett JL and Johnston KW (Eds.), Rutherford's Vascular Surgery, 7th Edition. WB Saunders, Elsevier, 2010.

Kasirajan K, O'Hara PJ, Gray BH, *et al.* Chronic mesenteric ischemia: open surgery versus percutaneous angioplasty and stenting. *J Vasc Surg* 2001; **33**:63–71.

Mateo RB, O'Hara PJ, Hertzer NR, *et al.* Elective surgical treatment of symptomatic chronic mesenteric occlusive disease: early results and late outcomes. *J Vasc Surg* 1999; 821–832.

Messina LM, Shanley CJ. Visceral artery aneurysms. *Surg Clin North Am* 1997; **77**:425–441.

Park WM, Gloviczki P, Cherry Jr. KJ, *et al.* Contemporary management of acute mesenteric ischemia: factors associated with survival. *J Vasc Surg* 2002; **35**:445–452.

Sarac TP, Altinel O, Kashyap V, *et al.* Endovascular treatment of stenotic and occluded visceral arteries for chronic mesenteric ischemia. *J Vasc Surg* 2008; **47**:485–491.

Schwartz LB, Gewertz BL. Mesenteric ischemia. *Surg Clin North Am* 1997; **77**:275–507.

Shanley CJ, Shah NL, Messina LM. Common splanchnic artery aneurysms: splenic, hepatic, and celiac. *Ann Vasc Surg* 1996; **10**:315–322.

Sharafuddin MJ, Olson CH, Sun S, *et al.* Endovascular treatment of celiac and mesenteric arteries stenosis: applications and results. *J Vasc Surg* 2003; **38**:692–698.

Textor SC. Current approaches to renovascular hypertension. *Med Clin North Am* 2009; **93**:717–732.

Tulsyan, N. *et al.* The endovascular management of visceral artery aneurysms and pseudoaneurysms. *J Vasc Surg* 2007; **45**:276–283.

Chapter 11
Chronic Venous Insufficiency and Venous Thrombo-Embolic Disease

Allan W. Tulloch and David A. Rigberg

Learning Objectives

- The reader should be able to describe the anatomy of the venous system of the legs and the interaction between the deep and superficial systems.
- Describe the pathophysiology of chronic venous insufficiency (CVI).
- Describe the workup for CVI and the contemporary treatments available for this condition.
- Understand the pathophysiology of deep venous thrombosis (DVT).
- Understand the rationale of modern treatment algorithms for DVT and pulmonary embolism (PE), as well as the consequences of these conditions.

1. Chronic Venous Insufficiency

1.1 *Background*

The treatment of chronic venous insufficiency (CVI) and varicose veins has undergone a radical transformation in the last decade. The rapid adoption of endovenous ablation, utilizing heat generated by either a radiofrequency generator or a laser, has led to the movement away from operating room management of these conditions to a treatment paradigm with office-based techniques. As the techniques for dealing with venous insufficiency have evolved and become less invasive, there has also been increased awareness of the frequently disabling symptoms associated with this condition. Cramping, heaviness, and "tiredness" of the limbs are just a few of the frequent complaints associated with CVI. In addition, there are a number of signs that occur, including leg swelling, large varicosities, hyperpigmentation, and eventually venous ulceration (Table 1). A working knowledge of the pathophysiology of CVI is useful in understanding the treatments available.

Table 1. Classification of CVI. The CEAP system considers the clinical class, etiology (congential, primary, and secondary), anatomy (superficial, perforator, or deep), and pathophysiology (reflux, obstruction, or both). The clinical classes are listed above.

C-Clinical Class	Characteristics
0	No clinical findings or symptoms
1	Telangiectasia/spider veins
2	Varicose veins
3	Edema
4	Pigmentation, lipodermatosclerosis
5	Prior ulceration, now healed
6	Active ulceration
A,S	Asymptomatic, symptomatic

1.2 Pathophysiology

It is important to remember that venous pressure is a fraction of arterial pressure under normal conditions, and that venous valves essentially control this pressure. A functioning valve allows the return of blood from the legs to the heart, while preventing retrograde flow, or reflux. When there is valvular dysfunction, it allows this back pressure to be reflected down the extremity, and when the patient assumes an upright position, the change in venous pressure can be considerable. In addition, the increased pressure can lead to dilation of the venous segment below the malfunctioning valve, and subsequent failure of the valve at this level. This simple pathology explains why CVI patients consistently report that their symptoms are at their best first thing in the morning, before they get out of bed. When the legs are elevated, there is essentially no clinically significant reflux. This phenomenon can also be readily observed in many CVI patients. Their large varicosities, essentially branches of refluxing veins that have been chronically under high pressure, may all but disappear when their legs are elevated. Treatment is generally aimed at removing the source of reflux and this can be done as long as there is enough function to the remainder of the venous system in the affected extremity.

1.3 Anatomy

There are essentially three systems of veins in the lower extremities. The superficial veins are usually involved with CVI and include the greater and small saphenous veins, as well as some other named branches (Figs. 1a and 1b). The greater saphenous vein connects to the femoral vein at the saphenofemoral junction and this is the most common site for clinically significant reflux. The small saphenous vein runs along the calf and although the anatomy has much variation, it usually connects to the deep system at the popliteal vein (saphenopopliteal junction).

The deep veins run with their similarly named arterial counterparts and are subfascial structures. Deep venous thrombosis can lead to severe CVI in the form of the post-phlebitic syndrome. However, this is not the common form of CVI. Usually, valvular dysfunction in the deep system is somewhat limited, which allows treatment of the superficial system to be effective. Finally, there is a system of perforator veins. These structures penetrate the fascia to connect superficial veins and branches to the deeper structures. In the normal state, flow should always be from superficial to deep, and when these veins fail, the flow is reversed. These refluxing perforators can become large and can be associated with overlying venous ulceration.

If a patient has longstanding saphenofemoral junction reflux, this pressure may dilate the entire saphenous vein, such that the entire vein is refluxing. At this point, the vein is really no longer acting as a dynamic structure but rather as a passive conduit. When the deep system has normal valvular function, the problem can be corrected by interrupting the ability of the vein to allow reflux. As a practical matter, this cannot be done by repairing the valves in the superficial system. Rather, the vein can be either physically removed or "closed," so that it can no longer act as a passive tube. Even in situations where there is some reflux in the deep system, treatment of the superficial reflux can still be helpful. Often, the deep system reflux is limited to the common femoral vein, and as long as the superficial femoral vein (more appropriately called the femoral vein) and profunda femoris vein are competent, removing the path down the saphenous vein essentially removes any path for the deep system reflux to proceed. Indeed, it is frequently helpful to treat superficial reflux even if there is more extensive deep system valvular dysfunction. However, great care must always be exercised to insure that the deep system is of adequate caliber before doing so.

1.4 *Diagnosis*

The workup for CVI starts with a careful history and physical examination. There is a fair amount of variation in the presenting symptoms for the condition, but there are common elements in the history that are of great use in securing the diagnosis. One of the hallmarks is that the symptoms tend to progress during the day, particularly when the patient has been on his or her feet. This is true for subjective

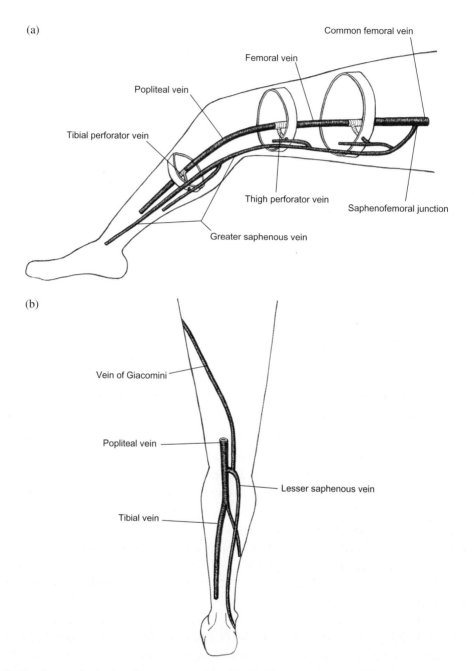

Fig. 1. The superficial veins of the lower extremities include the greater and lesser (short) systems. (a) demonstrates the greater saphenous system, including the named branches at the saphenofemoral junction as well as the anterior and posterior arch (or branch) veins below the knee. The perforator veins (b) provide connections between the deep and superficial systems. Although named, it is usually most useful to describe them in terms of their distance from the ankle.

complaints, such as heaviness and fatigue, as well as more objective complaints, such as swelling and engorged varicosities. Many patients, after determining this for themselves, will report that they have learned to elevate their legs when symptoms occur. Some will have even started wearing compression stockings. Onset of symptoms can also be a great clue. Women frequently can associate the onset of symptoms with pregnancy and many female patients note that their symptoms are tied to their menstrual cycle. A familial tendency is also frequently noted in CVI patients.

The physical examination is useful not only for arriving at the diagnosis of CVI, but frequently in determining the pattern of disease. The presence of leg swelling, varicosities, hyperpigmentation, or even ulceration must be carefully noted. CVI can certainly co-exist with peripheral arterial disease; therefore, the pedal pulses must be checked and documented. There is a specific pattern to the hyperpigmentation seen with CVI, typically in a distribution around the medial malleolus. This represents deposition of hemosiderin in the dermal tissues and usually occurs with long-standing CVI. The saphenous veins themselves should be sought and if they can be seen or felt, their size and depth should be noted. For patients with numerous varicosities, either a diagram can be made, or a digital photograph taken. Swelling is best documented by taking measurements of the leg below the knee and at the ankle. The time of day of the measurements should be recorded as well, for there can be considerable variation as was previously described. Finally, one must record the presence of any varicosities that have eroded, or appear to be on the verge of eroding, through the skin. When this occurs, the bleeding can be impressive and patients should be instructed on how to dress their leg in the event this occurs.

Following the initial patient encounter, most patients are referred for a duplex ultrasound. In a common scenario, patients will have had a venous duplex already performed; however, this study will turn out to be a rule out DVT study, and will lack the material necessary for the diagnosis and treatment of CVI. Many noninvasive vascular laboratories have a protocol for CVI and the clinician should always specify why the venous examination is being ordered. The study should include all of the elements of the DVT study and examination of the greater and lesser (short) saphenous veins. Most laboratories will also seek out the presence of enlarged and refluxing perforator veins. Although reflux is typically defined as reversal of flow for greater 0.5 seconds, many health insurers require greater times; therefore, the actual time should be carefully recorded in the study. These studies should be performed with most patients in a standing position, and notation made whether or not reflux occurs spontaneously (without Valsalva maneuver or squeezing the leg central to the area being studied). The sizes of the saphenous veins are needed as well; these structures should be measured at the level of the saphenofemoral junction, the mid-thigh, just below the knee (GSV), and at the popliteal space and ankle (SSV). Larger varicosities should be examined as well, and reflux reported if present. As with the saphenous veins, the sizes of the branches need to be recorded in the study. Finally, perforator veins need to be noted in the study. Again, it is important to include their size as well as their distance from the ankle.

1.5 *Treatment*

For most patients, the diagnosis of CVI is secured with the history, physical examination, and the venous insufficiency protocol duplex scan. The initial therapy for the vast majority of patients with mild venous insufficiency is conservative treatment with (1) compression stockings (2), leg elevation, and (3) nonsteroidal anti-inflammatory agents (NSAIDs). For compression, most patients with typical CVI symptoms are prescribed 20–30 mm Hg stockings, although there are different pressures available for various indications (Table 2). The length of the garment depends on the patient's pattern of disease and the location of tender varicose branches. Typically, a stocking that is knee-high will suffice and patients are more likely to use garments of this length consistently than longer and more restrictive stockings. Compressive therapy serves a number of important functions. It allows many patients, particularly those with severe and debilitating symptoms, some relief in a prompt manner. It is also important that patients understand that even following treatment, they can still benefit from the garments if they are going to be in a situation with prolonged sitting or standing (*i.e.* travel). This is also true in the post-procedure period if they undergo an intervention for their veins. Finally, almost every insurer requires a trial of compressive therapy, ranging from six weeks to six months prior to coverage.

Table 2.

15–20 mm Hg	Mild edema, mild varicosities, and aching legs
20–30 mm Hg	Advanced aching/fatigue, moderate edema, and DVT prophylaxis
30–40 mm Hg	Established CVI, advanced edema, and post-thrombotic state
40–50 mm Hg	Severe edema and open venous ulceration
50+ mm Hg	Severe edema not responsive to lesser pressures and severe post-thrombotic syndrome

Note: Graded compression stockings are available in a range of pressures. Venous indications for the pressures are listed above. They are also available in various lengths, from knee-high up to panty hose. Consideration should be given to the likelihood that the patient will wear the garments; a knee-high stocking is more beneficial if the patient uses it than a more restrictive appliance that is avoided.

As mentioned previously, many patients determine on their own that elevation is beneficial in alleviating their symptoms. As part of their conservative treatment, the physician should encourage the patient to find time to elevate his/her legs at intervals throughout the day. Many patients find that they are able to continue exercise regimens if they elevate their legs for a period of time directly following these activities. For patients with continued aching and pain, NSAIDs can be helpful and are considered an integral part of first-line conservative therapy. Additional adjuvant conservative therapy may consist of weight loss where appropriate.

Throughout the course of conservative treatment, the physician must follow the progress of the patient and note what, if any, effects the therapy is having. The therapy itself can have diagnostic implications. For example, a patient who has no benefit from compressive therapy may have a different etiology for his/her symptoms. If a patient tries, but is unable to tolerate the compression stockings, this has to be clearly documented in the medical record. Patients are occasionally wary of reporting a beneficial effect of compression, as they may be under the false impression that if their stockings are helpful, they will not receive any further therapy. This is not the case, as most patients will qualify for treatment if there is an appropriate definitive therapy available.

The majority of patients with CVI secondary to GSV incompetence and a number of patients with CVI secondary to SSV incompetence are now well treated with endovenous techniques. These procedures essentially reproduce the effects of high ligation and stripping of the saphenous veins; the incompetent vein is removed from the circulation, so that passive reflux of venous pressure down the leg does not occur. The endovenous procedures are done in a minimally invasive fashion; they are now routinely performed in an office setting with local anesthesia.

All endovenous ablation works by thermal destruction of the vein. The source of heat generation is either a laser fiber (endovenous laser therapy or EVLT) or a radiofrequency generator (RFA). Both of these sources of energy produce high, but focused, temperatures. Thus, within 5 mm of an RFA catheter that is 120°C at its surface or a laser fiber with a temperature of 1000°C, normal body temperature can be maintained. This prevents extended thermal damage to the vein and surrounding tissues (particularly the skin) during treatment. The principles of therapy are the same for both modalities and for treatment of both the GSV and SSV. Initially, there must be confirmation that the vein is refluxing and is enlarged (greater than 4–5 mm with patient standing), not excessively enlarged (greater than 1.5 cm) and not excessively tortuous (which precludes catheter advancement). The vein is accessed under ultrasound guidance, usually 5–10 cm below the knee and a sheath is placed in the vein. A laser fiber or RFA catheter is then advanced through the sheath under ultrasound and positioned 2–3 cm from either the saphenofemoral or saphenopopliteal junction. This portion of the case is done under great care, as inadvertent placement of the catheter too close to the deep system can cause damage to the deep veins. The target vein is then surrounded with tumescent anesthetic, a solution made up of saline, lidocaine, epinephrine, and bicarbonate. This solution accomplishes three goals: (1) anesthesia of the target area, (2) the prevention of thermal injury *via* a "heat sink", and (3) compression of the target vein. The GSV is located between layers of fascia and the fluid can be administered between these layers such that the vein is both surrounded and depressed away from the skin to a minimal depth of 2 cm. The bed is then placed in a steep Trendelenburg position to further empty the target vein and the energy is applied while the physician provides external pressure over the segment of vein that is being treated. For the RFA, 7 cm of vein at a time is treated for 20 seconds and then the catheter is backed up at intervals. For the EVLT, there is continuous pullback of the catheter during treatment. The process of actual thermal ablation is rapid and on the order of 90–120 seconds for both modalities. The sheath and catheter are removed and the patient's leg is wrapped with an ace bandage for 48 hours. The patients are encouraged to ambulate in the immediate post-procedural time, but to elevate their legs following light activities. Strict bed rest is discouraged, as this could theoretically lead to thrombotic complications.

Follow-up in most practices includes physical examination of the treated leg and a duplex ultrasound examination of treated vein and the saphenofemoral junction within 48–72 hours. For the GSV, the ideal finding is an occluded GSV with a maintained epigastric vein (Fig. 2). In our practice, we occasionally see thrombus that extends to the deep system and very rarely protrudes significantly into the common femoral vein. We have devised a recommended treatment paradigm for these situations, including the use of low molecular weight heparin in some cases. This is all done to prevent the formation of a true DVT, although we have not seen this complication.

Most patients recuperate rapidly from their endovenous ablation. Some patients return to work within a day. However, patients are advised to try to arrange 2–3 days off of their usual routine to allow for recovery. Other than the thrombotic complications described above, patients can have bruising and hematoma formation (usually associated with the injection of the tumescent anesthetic), paresthesias secondary to nerve injury, and even the rare case of thermal injury to the skin. Fortunately, all of these complications are rare.

Successful closure of the target vein is achieved in over 90% of cases and several large registries have documented durability of this procedure, with 90% of veins still closed at three years. These results will probably improve, as the new protocols for RFA utilize a higher treatment temperature (older catheters used 80–85°C; new catheters use 120°C). Further refinements in laser fibers, particularly with the treatment wavelength utilized, have also taken place.

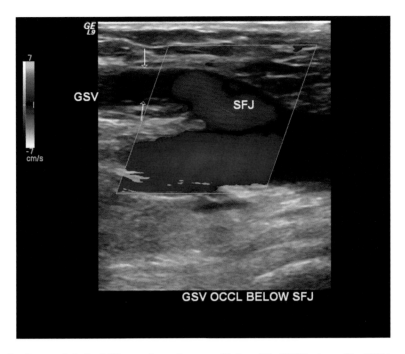

Fig. 2. An ultrasound obtained 48 hours after endovenous ablation of the GSV is shown. The GSV is occluded, as evidenced by the lack of color flow. The saphenofemoral junction is patent, and clearly there is no involvement with the common femoral vein (blue flow on scan).

1.5.1 *Treatment of branches and perforators*

Many CVI patients have large varicosities. These may be a significant source of symptoms themselves and are frequently dealt with along the saphenous vein. During a duplex examination, an astute clinician will note that a large varicosity coming off of the saphenous system can essentially siphon off the majority of the refluxing flow. In this situation, the GSV appears enlarged down the level where the branch joins it. The GSV can all but disappear below this level, while the branch, now running superficial to the saphenous fascia, attains a very large size. These branches, if straight, may be accessed directly and treated with endovenous ablation. However, these branches are usually tortuous and must be treated using an alternate modality. For larger branches, micro-stab phlebectomy works very well. 2–3 mm incisions are made adjacent to the varicosity and a hook-shaped instrument is inserted and used to grasp the vein and to lift it above the level of the skin. The branch is then gently rotated to disrupt the connections to the surrounding tissues and gentle traction is placed on it until it avulses. Pressure is held over the site for several minutes and a compression dressing avoids the formation of a hematoma. This phlebectomies can be done at the same time as the ablation, or in follow-up. Some practitioners prefer the latter, as there are some data to suggest that there is a reduction in the number of branches requiring removal after saphenous ablation.

Another alternative for the treatment of varicose branches is sclerotherapy. In this treatment, the vein is injected with either a detergent solution (such as polidocanol or sodium morrhuate) or osmotic sclerosants such as hypertonic saline. The material damages the endothelium in the target vessel, eventually leading to obliteration. Sclerotherapy can be used for larger branches as an alternative to phlebectomy, although it tends to require multiple sessions for complete success.

Perforator treatment can also be performed with endovenous techniques. The indications are not as clear-cut as for treating the saphenous veins, but recent data support that the closure of refluxing perforators associated with venous ulcers does lead to ulcer healing. Historically, these veins required operations with large operations to get to the subfascial anatomy. More recently, endoscopic surgery with subfascial perforator clipping was favored (SEPS). Currently, endovenous ablation, again with either RFA or EVLT, is performed. Specialized catheters are available to approach this anatomy, and accessing these veins requires advanced ultrasound skills. Careful follow-up with a wound center, combined with perforator closure, has the highest likelihood of success.

1.6 Conclusions

CVI is a common condition with underappreciated clinical sequelae. Newer technologies allow the modern clinician to approach this disorder with an array of minimally invasive therapies that are especially useful in a patient population that is frequently young, working, and active. An understanding of the pathophysiology behind the disorder allows the clinician to appropriately diagnose and treat CVI with techniques that are both acceptable to the patients and successful in correcting the disorder.

2. Venous Thromboembolism

2.1 Background

Venous thromboembolism (VTE) comprising deep venous thrombosis (DVT) and pulmonary embolism (PE) remains a significant health care problem with over 500,000 new cases and an estimated 50,000 deaths in the United States each year. The connection between DVT and PE was first described by Virchow over 150 years ago and his eponymous triad of vessel wall injury, stasis, and hypercoagulability is still the recognized mechanism by which intravascular thrombosis occurs. Of those patients who survive DVT, approximately half will go on to develop chronic venous insufficiency. While treatment has invariably involved anticoagulation in those patients who do not have a contraindication, and in some cases open thrombectomy, endovenous approaches have emerged as a powerful treatment modality in the last decade. In the following sections, the pathophysiology, diagnosis, treatment, prevention, and long-term complications for VTE will be described.

2.2 *Pathophysiology*

Deep venous thrombosis occurs most commonly in the deep veins of the lower extremity, although upper extremity DVT is an increasingly observed clinical entity that deserves some mention. A significant portion of proximal DVTs (iliofemoral) originate in the soleal veins of the calf before breaking off and lodging more proximally. Stasis as a predisposing factor for DVT is seen in patients who have undergone recent trauma, major surgical procedures, patients who are bedridden, as well as patients who have been sitting for long periods of time such as in airplane flights. There are also anatomical considerations that can lead to turbulent and static flow as seen in both May-Thurner Syndrome and Paget-Schroetter Disease. May-Thurner Syndrome is typified by compression of the left common iliac vein by the right iliac artery predisposing to thrombosis while Paget-Schroetter Disease is typified by venous compression in the thoracic outlet, usually between the anterior scalene and the first rib leading to an effort-induced thrombosis of the axillary vein.

Hypercoagulability, in a very general sense, can be divided into hereditary or acquired causes. Hereditary hypercoagulability disorders are relatively common with Factor V Leiden mutations affecting up to 5% of the population. In fact, up to 40% of patients with DVT will have Factor V Leiden mutations. Other hereditary disorders predisposing to DVT include antithrombin III deficiency, protein C or S deficiencies, lupus anticoagulant, antiphospholipid antibody, mutant prothrombin 20201A, non-O blood groups, and hyperhomocysteinemia to name a few. As research in this field continues, more genetic conditions that predispose patients to DVT will certainly be identified. Acquired hypercoagulability is seen in patients who smoke, women who are on oral contraceptives, hormone replacement therapy, or pregnant, obese patients, patients with heart failure, inflammatory bowel disease, cancer, and the elderly. It is believed that inflammation plays a significant role in acquired hypercoagulability and any condition that elevates pro-inflammatory factors may indeed predispose patients to developing DVTs.

2.3 *Diagnosis*

Physical examination findings for patients with DVT can vary from asymptomatic patients, to those who have an iliofemoral DVT and present with unilateral leg swelling, pain, pitting edema, and blanching that can either spare the collateral vessels (*phlegmasia alba dolens*) or compromise the collateral vessels leading to more severe congestion, circulatory compromise, or collapse (*phlegmasia cerulea dolens*). Swelling itself usually occurs one segment below the level of occlusion. Patients may have a palpable cord on examination and some patients may exhibit Homan's sign (pain on passive dorsiflexion), although individual signs are in and of themselves nonspecific with relatively low sensitivity. In 1997, Wells *et al.* developed a pre-test scoring system based on several signs, symptoms, and comorbidities to help determine the likelihood of DVT (Table 3).

Laboratory testing can be a useful way to screen patients deemed to be at low risk of having DVT. D-dimers test for the cross-linked degradation products of fibrin by plasmin and have been reported to have proximal and distal sensitivities of 98.4% and 90.6%, respectively, and negative predictive values of 99.3% and 98.6%, respectively when used in conjunction with clinical judgment.

Duplex ultrasound remains a convenient and easy bedside test to look for DVT, but is limited by the experience of the examiner. In the right hands, the sensitivity of the test can be over 95% when the DVT is located proximally with a slightly lower specificity. However, pelvic and calf DVTs remain challenging to diagnose with ultrasound. Furthermore, caution should be exercised in interpreting the results of a negative test in the presence of suspected thromboembolism, as the thrombus may have already embolized from the extremity. Nonetheless, duplex ultrasound remains the diagnostic test of choice when DVT is suspected.

Table 3.   Wells scoring system to predict DVT.

Finding	Score
Active cancer	+1
Paresis, paralysis, or recent plaster cast immobilization of lower extremity	+1
Bedridden >3 days or major surgery within four weeks	+1
Localized tenderness over distribution of deep veins	+1
Entire leg swollen	+1
Calf swelling >3 cm compared to contralateral side	+1
Pitting edema (greater in symptomatic leg)	+1
Collateral superficial veins (nonvaricose)	+1
Alternative diagnosis as likely or greater than DVT	−2

Note: Score 0 or less — low risk (3% probability DVT); Score 1–2 — moderate risk (17% probability DVT); and Score 3 or more — high risk (75% probability DVT).

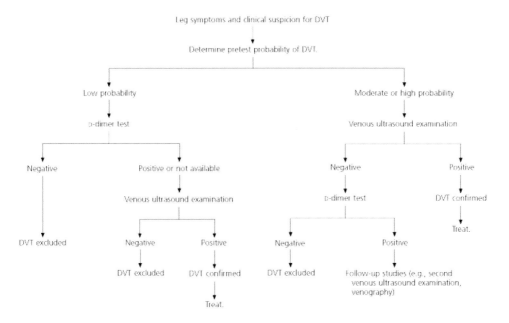

Fig. 3. Algorithm to diagnose DVT.

Contrast venography has classically been considered the gold standard to confirm the diagnosis of DVT. However, the procedure itself is invasive, costly, less readily available, and has potential risks from the contrast including allergic reactions and renal dysfunction. Venography today is reserved for patients in whom ultrasonography is negative or equivocal despite a high index of clinical suspicion for DVT. A suggested diagnostic algorithm is illustrated in Fig. 3.

2.4 *Treatment*

The goals of treatment for DVT include minimizing the risk of pulmonary embolism, preventing the propagation of thrombus, and facilitating the resolution of the clot itself to prevent long-term complications. Anticoagulation remains the first-line treatment for uncomplicated DVT and includes 5–7 days of treatment with parenterally administered unfractionated heparin, low molecular weight heparin (LMWH), or fondaparinux, and a more prolonged course of an oral vitamin K antagonist for 3–6 months. However, certain absolute and relative contraindications to the use of anticoagulants do exist (Table 4).

Heparin and its derivatives inactivate thrombin and activated Factor X through an antithrombin dependent mechanism. By inactivating thrombin, heparin not only prevents fibrin formation, but also inhibits thrombin-induced activation of platelets and Factors V and VIII.

Table 4.   Contraindications to anticoagulant therapy.

Absolute contraindications
Active bleeding
Severe bleeding diathesis or platelet count ≤20,000/mm
Neurosurgery, ocular surgery, or intracranial bleeding within the past 10 days
Relative contraindications
Mild-to-moderate bleeding diathesis or thrombocytopenia
Brain metastases
Recent major trauma
Major abdominal surgery within the past two days
Gastrointestinal or genitourinary bleeding within the past 14 days
Endocarditis
Severe hypertension (*i.e.*, systolic blood pressure >200 mm Hg, diastolic
blood pressure >120 mm Hg, or both) at presentation

Unfractionated heparin is typically administered as an intravenous infusion. Patients should receive 5000 U as a loading dose (or 80 U/kg) and at least 30,000 U every 24 hours. The anticoagulant response of heparin varies among patients, so laboratory monitoring with the activated partial-thromboplastin time (aPTT) is required every six hours with adjustments made based on a validated weight-based normogram to keep the patient in the therapeutic range. Because of differences between the reagents and coagulometers used to measure the aPTT, the therapeutic range will vary from institution to institution. However, as a general rule, the therapeutic aPTT should fall between 1.5 and 2.5 times the patients' normal value. Complications of heparin include hemorrhage in up to 7% of patients, hypersensitivity reactions, heparin-induced thrombocytopenia (HIT), and osteoporosis in long-term users.

Because of the high morbidity and mortality associated with heparin-induced thrombocytopenia (HIT), a brief description is warranted. HIT is an immune-mediated response that occurs when antibodies form to a complex between heparin and platelet Factor 4 (PF4). These antibodies lead to platelet activation, and thus a pro-thrombotic state, despite the fact that the patient is thrombocytopenic by laboratory measures. HIT often presents first with thrombosis and has been reported in both the arterial and venous systems. Mortality is estimated at 20–30% after thrombosis. The development of HIT can be either early or late. In patients receiving heparin for the first time, HIT can develop 5–10 days after first administration, while pre-sensitized patients who already have heparin-PF4 antibodies can develop HIT within hours of use. Conversely, patients may develop late onset of HIT as long as five days after heparin withdrawal. The diagnosis of HIT is made based on: (1) thrombocytopenia (drop in platelet count below 100×10^9 per L or a drop >50% from the patient's baseline), (2) exclusion of other causes of thrombocytopenia, and (3) resolution of thrombocytopenia after heparin cessation. There are also different functional tests and assays looking for HIT antibodies that can be sent to confirm the diagnosis. For suspected or diagnosed HIT, heparin should be stopped immediately. A different anticoagulant should be promptly started as HIT patients are at high risk of thrombosis. Anticoagulants that do not cross-react with HIT antibodies include danaparoid, lepirudin, argatroban, and fondaparinux. LMWH (*i.e.* Lovenox) does cross-react with HIT antibodies and should be avoided. Patients should be transitioned to warfarin over a minimum of five days and remain anticoagulated for 2–3 months to prevent recurrence of thrombosis. Heparin should be avoided in patients with a previous diagnosis of HIT.

LMWH can also be used in the treatment of DVT and has been shown to have a lower incidence of HIT and osteoporosis. Administration is usually subcutaneous once or twice a day by weight per the manufacturer's directions. As an example, enoxaparin dosing is 1 mg/kg twice a day or 1.5 mg/kg once a day to a maximum of 180 mg per day. Generally, patients are not monitored with laboratory studies and LMWH has been shown to be safe and effective as an outpatient therapy to treat uncomplicated DVT. However, outpatient treatment is unsuitable for patients with massive thrombosis, serious coexisting illnesses, or a high risk of hemorrhage (*i.e.* patients who are very old, have recently undergone surgery, have a history of bleeding, or have renal or liver disease).

Long-term treatment and prevention of DVT with warfarin, titrated to an international normalized ratio (INR) of 2.0–3.0, remains a cornerstone of therapy. The antithrombotic effect of Warfarin is not seen for 48–72 hours, so heparin is used as a bridge to therapy. Furthermore, when warfarin is started alone, patients may experience a transient deficiency in protein C, which can cause skin necrosis. Other side effects of warfarin include bleeding, dermatitis, and painful erythema over areas with large amounts of subcutaneous fat. Most changes are reversible with cessation of warfarin or administration of fresh frozen plasma. The metabolism of warfarin is affected by administration of other medications (*e.g.* phenylbutazone, sufinpyrazone, disulfuram, metronidazole, and trimepthorpim-sulfamethoxazole all potentiate warfarin's action), and warfarin itself can alter the metabolism of some medications. Careful monitoring of drug levels is necessary to avoid drug toxicity. Pregnant patients should avoid oral anticoagulants altogether as they are known teratogens. Instead those patients should be placed on heparin.

Length of treatment with warfarin is dependent on several factors, including whether or not this is a first episode of DVT, whether or not there are ongoing risk factors for venous thromboembolic disease, and whether or not there is a known genetic hypercoagulability condition. It is recommended that any patient with a first episode of DVT and a known time-limited or reversible risk factor (trauma, surgery, *etc.*) be treated for at least three months. For those patients with idiopathic VTE, treatment should be at least six months. Patients with recurrent idiopathic VTE or known hypercoagulability may need more extended anticoagulation of at least 12 months and possibly lifelong therapy.

In cases of more severe DVT, the use of fibrinolytic agents such as tissue-type plasminogen activator (tPA), streptokinase, and urokinase have been shown to be effective, but have a high incidence of hemorrhage as well as allergic reactions. With the advent of catheter-based delivery systems that can deliver tPA directly to the thrombus, systemic fibrinolytic therapy is seen less and less. Indications currently used to determine which patients are candidates for pharmacomechanical catheter-directed thrombolysis include symptom duration and severity, the anatomical extent of DVT, the presence of signs of circulatory compromise, and the patient's bleeding risk profile, life-expectancy, and anticipated activity level. Patients with short life expectancy, those who do not ambulate and those with factors predisposing them to bleeding complications are relatively poor candidates for aggressive therapy. In general, patients with circulatory compromise and limb-threatening ischemia as seen in *phlegmasia cerulea dolens* should undergo emergent catheter-directed thrombolysis unless there is a strong contraindication in which case operative thrombectomy should be performed. After thrombus removal and lysis, some practitioners recommend the routine use of venous stents over any areas of residual stenosis to prevent recurrence of DVT, although no controlled trials have been performed to support this practice.

In those patients with a contraindication to anticoagulation, those patients who develop a PE despite anticoagulation and in those patients with chronic PE or post-pulmonary embolectomy, an inferior vena cava filter should be placed (Table 5). These devices can be permanent or retrievable where retrieval is usually through the jugular vein. The patency of IVC filters is over 95% with only 2–4% of patients having recurrent VTE. Of those patients with recurrent VTE, many are from sources outside of the filtered flow including the upper extremity. Complications are rare and can range from a mild hematoma to migration of the device into the pulmonary artery potentially causing death.

2.5 *Prophylaxis*

The rationale for thromboprophylaxis in hospitalized patients has been well validated with DVT rates of 10–40% in general surgical patients and rates up to 80% for critical care patients not receiving thromboprophylaxis. Concerns are often raised regarding the risk of hemorrhage in patients on prophylactic anticoagulation, but randomized studies have shown little or no increase in the incidence of clinically

Table 5.   Definite and relative indications for IVC filter placement.

Definite indications for IVC filter placement

Recurrent VTE despite adequate anticoagulation

DVT or documented VTE in a patient with a contraindication to anticoagulation

Complication of anticoagulation, forcing it to be discontinued

Chronic PE with associated pulmonary hypertension and cor pulmonale

Immediately post-pulmonary embolectomy

Patients undergoing surgery at high risk of VTE and contraindications to
   anticoagulation

Relative indications for IVC filter placement

>50% occlusion of pulmonary vascular bed in a patient who will not tolerate
   further embolization

Patients with a propagating iliofemoral thrombus despite anticoagulation

High-risk patient with a free-floating iliofemoral thrombus on venogram

---

significant bleeding in these patients. Current guidelines calling for surgical prophylaxis are dependent on the type of surgery being performed. For vascular surgery cases, recommendations for preoperative anticoagulation are different than in either general or orthopedic cases.

The majority of vascular procedures require high doses of anticoagulation prior to vessel clamping or device delivery that obviates the need to give preoperative anticoagulation in the majority of cases. Therefore, in vascular surgery patients with no additional risk factors for VTE, early ambulation is the only recommendation. In those patients who do have additional risk factors, prophylaxis should be given in the form of heparin 5000 SC within two hours of surgery and then two to three times per day after surgery until ambulation or LMWH (*e.g.* enoxaparin 40 mg SC within two hours of surgery and once daily after until ambulation). All trauma, orthopedic, and general surgery patients should receive thromboprophylaxis with either heparin or LMWH prior to surgery unless there is a documented contraindication.

2.6 *Pulmonary embolism*

Pulmonary embolism remains a dreaded complication of DVT and in its most severe form can present as hypotension with circulatory collapse. PE can often be confused with other conditions such as myocardial infarction, pneumothorax, sepsis, or pneumonia, so accurate diagnosis is imperative. Diagnosis classically has involved angiography which today is done in conjunction with computed tomography as well as magnetic resonance imaging. Ventilation perfusion scanning is an older test that is still useful as a screening tool to exclude the diagnosis of PE in patients with a low clinical suspicion, but due to its low specificity, its use has been supplanted by spiral CT and MRA.

Thrombolysis for PE should be done in cases of hemodynamic instability including hypotension, systemic hypoperfusion, right ventricular dysfunction, and pulmonary hypertension. The greatest benefit to thrombolysis is seen in the first 24–48 hours as it induces faster clot lysis and more quickly improves pulmonary arterial perfusion. However, the long-term results of thrombolysis show no differences versus heparin, with equivalent mortality, PE resolution, and recurrent PE. Thrombolytic agents used include tPA (100 mg infusion over two hours), streptokinase (250,000 U over 30 minutes, maintenance 100,000 U/hr for 24 hours), and urokinase (4400 U/kg over 10 minutes, 4400 U/kg/hr for 12–24 hours). Catheter-based approaches to embolectomy have seen increasing use both as sole therapy as well as in conjunction with systemic thrombolysis. A myriad of devices have been constructed to fragment, macerate, and aspirate clot, but there is no consensus as to the best device, if any, to achieve lysis.

Open pulmonary embolectomy can be performed in patients with chronic PE and elevated pulmonary pressures and in those with a contraindication to lytic or catheter-based therapies. These patients are often extremely unstable and open embolectomy requires that patients be placed on full or partial cardiopulmonary bypass with mortality rates of approximately 30% and 10%, respectively.

As in DVT, anticoagulation is the mainstay of treatment for PE. However, due to the risks of hypoxemia and hemodynamic instability associated with PE, close monitoring and supportive therapy are necessary. For mild and hemodynamically stable PE, anticoagulation is the same as for DVT with IVC filter placement in selected circumstances as described in the previous section.

2.7 Long-term sequelae

A significant number of patients who have DVT later develop post-thrombotic or post-phlebitic syndrome. This complication develops because of damage to the venous valvular system that produces the symptoms of chronic venous insufficiency described in the previous section. However, unlike with GVS disease, the post-phlebitic syndrome is difficult to treat and can be a lifelong problem for these patients.

References

Albers GW, Amarenco P, Easton JD, Sacco RL, Teal P. Antithrombotic and thrombolytic therapy for ischemic stroke: the Seventh ACCP Conference on Antithrombotic and Thrombolytic Therapy. *Chest.* 2004; **126**(3 Suppl):483S–512S. Review.

Comerota AJ. Randomized trial evidence supporting a strategy of thrombus removal for acute DVT. *Semin Vasc Surg*. 2010; **23**(3):192–8.

Gale SS, Lee JN, Walsh ME, Wojnarowski DL, Comerota AJ. A randomized, controlled trial of endovenous thermal ablation using the 810-nm wavelength laser and the ClosurePLUS radiofrequency ablation methods for superficial venous insufficiency of the great saphenous vein. *J Vasc Surg*. 2010; **52**(3):645–50. Epub 2010 Jul 17.

Geerts WH, Pineo GF, Heit JA, Bergqvist D, Lassen MR, Colwell CW, Ray JG. Prevention of venous thromboembolism: the Seventh ACCP Conference on Antithrombotic and Thrombolytic Therapy. *Chest*. 2004; **126**(3 Suppl):338S–400S. Review.

Gillespie DL; Writing Group III of the Pacific Vascular Symposium 6, Kistner B, Glass C, Bailey B, Chopra A, Ennis B, Marston B, Masuda E, Moneta G, Nelzen O, Raffetto J, Raju S, Vedantham S, Wright D, Falanga V. Venous ulcer diagnosis, treatment, and prevention of recurrences. *J Vasc Surg*. 2010; **52**(5 Suppl):8S–14S. Epub 2010 Aug 3. Review. No abstract available.

Goldhaber SZ. Risk factors for venous thromboembolism. *J Am Coll Cardiol*. 2010; **56**(1):1–7. Review.

Guex JJ, Schliephake DE, Otto J, Mako S, Allaert FA. The French polidocanol study on long-term side effects: a survey covering 3,357 patient years. *Dermatol Surg*. 2010; **36**(Suppl 2):993–1003.

Henke P; Writing Group I of the Pacific Vascular Symposium 6, Vandy F, Comerota A, Kahn SR, Lal BK, Lohr J, Meissner M, Caprini J, McLafferty R, Bender D, Jarvis G, Meyer P, Wu D, Wakefield T. Prevention and treatment of the postthrombotic syndrome. *J Vasc Surg*. 2010; **52** (5 Suppl):21S–28S. Epub 2010 Aug 1.

Houman Fekrazad M, Lopes RD, Stashenko GJ, Alexander JH, Garcia D. Treatment of venous thromboembolism: guidelines translated for the clinician. *J Thromb Thrombolysis*. 2009; **28**(3):270–5.

Knipp BS, Blackburn SA, Bloom JR, Fellows E, Laforge W, Pfeifer JR, Williams DM, Wakefield TW; Michigan Venous Study Group. Endovenous laser ablation: venous outcomes and thrombotic complications are independent of the presence of deep venous insufficiency. *J Vasc Surg*. 2008; **48**(6):1538–45. Epub 2008 Oct 1.

Mandalà M, Falanga A, Roila F; ESMO Guidelines Working Group. Venous thromboembolism in cancer patients: ESMO Clinical Practice Guidelines for the management. *Ann Oncol*. 2010; **21**(Suppl 5):v274–6. No abstract available.

Marston W. Summary of evidence of effectiveness of primary chronic venous disease treatment. *J Vasc Surg*. 2010; **52**(5 Suppl):54S–58S. No abstract available.

Marrocco CJ, Atkins MD, Bohannon WT, Warren TR, Buckley CJ, Bush RL. Endovenous ablation for the treatment of chronic venous insufficiency and venous ulcerations. *World J Surg*. 2010; **34**(10):2299–304.

Meissner MH. The effectiveness of deep vein thrombosis prevention. *J Vasc Surg*. 2010; **52**(5 Suppl):65S–67S.

O'Connell JB, Chandra A, Russell MM, Davis G, Sanchez I, Lawrence PF, Derubertis BG. Thrombolysis for acute lower extremity deep venous thrombosis in a tertiary care setting. *Ann Vasc Surg*. 2010; **24**(4):511–7.

Puggioni A, Kalra M, Carmo M, Mozes G, Gloviczki P. Endovenous laser therapy and radiofrequency ablation of the great saphenous vein: analysis of early efficacy and complications. *J Vasc Surg*. 2005; **42**(3):488–93.

Raju S, Neglén P. Clinical practice. Chronic venous insufficiency and varicose veins. *N Engl J Med*. 2009; **360**(22):2319–27. Review. No abstract available.

Stevens SM, Douketis JD. Deep vein thrombosis prophylaxis in hospitalized medical patients: current recommendations, general rates of implementation, and initiatives for improvement. *Clin Chest Med*. 2010; **31**(4):675–89.

Subramonia S, Lees T. Randomized clinical trial of radiofrequency ablation or conventional high ligation and stripping for great saphenous varicose veins. *Br J Surg*. 2010; **97**(3):328–36.

Tapson VF, Decousus H, Pini M, Chong BH, Froehlich JB, Monreal M, Spyropoulos AC, Merli GJ, Zotz RB, Bergmann JF, Pavanello R, Turpie AG, Nakamura M, Piovella F, Kakkar AK, Spencer FA, Fitzgerald G, Anderson FA Jr; IMPROVE Investigators. Venous thromboembolism prophylaxis in acutely ill hospitalized medical patients: findings from the International Medical Prevention Registry on Venous Thromboembolism. *Chest.* 2007; **132**(3):936–45. Epub 2007 Jun 15.

Welch HJ. Endovenous ablation of the great saphenous vein may avert phlebectomy for branch varicose veins. *J Vasc Surg.* 2006; **44**(3):601–5.

Yamaki T, Hamahata A, Soejima K, Kono T, Nozaki M, Sakurai H. Factors Predicting Development of Post-thrombotic Syndrome in Patients with a First Episode of Deep Vein Thrombosis: Preliminary Report. *Eur J Vasc Endovasc Surg.* 2010. [Epub ahead of print]

Chapter 12
Vascular Access

Hugh A. Gelabert

Learning Objectives

- Understand the principles of central venous catheter access, its indications, benefits, and limitations.
- Understand the principles, benefits, and limitations of peritoneal dialysis.
- Understand the principles, benefits, and limitations of hemodialysis.
- Become familiar with the differences between arteriovenous fistulas and grafts, techniques for placement, and salvage.

1. What Is Vascular Access?

Vascular access refers to a broad set of indications and operations, which are designed to provide reliable, repeated access to circulation in patients whose disease process requires administration of medication, sampling of blood, or treatment of their blood.

There is a spectrum of devices, which has been designed for particular interventions. Each of these devices has particular characteristics which are optimized toward certain functions. This allows the use of devices appropriate to the clinical need.

2. Venous Catheter Access

The applications for venous access are generally related to administration of fluids, nutrients, and medications. A second important use for central venous catheter access is to allow sampling blood. Reasons for sampling blood range from routine blood testing (such as CBC or Chem panels) to treatment of the blood (such as pheresis or dialysis) prior to re-infusion.

The clinical goal of the catheter is the most important consideration in determining which catheter is best suited for the proposed job. For occasional infusions, a smaller device would suffice. For a repeated infusion of blood in the course of hemapheresis or hemodialysis, then a minimal flow rate of 250 cc per minute would require a large diameter catheter.

The frequency of use will also impact the device characteristics. If the goal is a frequent or continuous infusion, then a catheter which allows semi-permanent connection is needed. Such is the case with the external catheters which have a sub-cutaneous tunneled cuff. Examples of these are the Hickman or Groshong catheters. These are ideal for administration of TPN or daily administration of antibiotics or chemotherapy. They are durable, effective, and simple to use. They have the disadvantage of being external catheters, which exposes the catheters to potential damage.

An additional distinction which needs to be considered is the requirement for anticoagulation. Open-tip catheters such as the Hickman catheter require periodic flushing with heparin in order to prevent clotting of the catheter. The Groshong catheter is designed with a closed tip and a valve which eliminates the need for heparin flushes. This may be a significant element in choosing a catheter when issues of thrombocytopenia and possible HIT are factored into the patient's care plan.

If the purpose of the catheter is periodic but not frequent administration of medication, then a catheter with a subcutaneously implanted reservoir may be a better choice. Examples of these include the Port-a-cath and similar devices. These have the advantage of being totally implanted and thus not subject to trauma and infection. They also have the advantage of being simpler to care for, not requiring special care in bathing and dressing. Finally, for patients the absence of an external catheter offers a psychological benefit with regard to body image. They have the disadvantage of requiring a needle to traverse the skin and access the subcutaneous port. Applications for such catheters include monthly administration of chemotherapy. It should be noted that earlier generations of these catheters did not allow for infusion of contrast from power injectors. This limited their utility in that patients who required frequent CT scans could not use their port-a-cath as the access site for contrast injection. A newer generation of these devices has been developed which is capable of withstanding very high injection pressures.

3. Advantages and Disadvantages of Cuffed Catheters and Ports

The main advantage of cuffed catheters and implanted ports is their durability (Table 1). These devices are designed to resist infection and thrombosis. Their positioning within the central venous system makes them durable to the point where they may last for years. The principal disadvantages are that these devices are more expensive than temporary access and expose patients to increased risk at the time of

Table 1. Catheter distinctions and uses.

	Example	Indication
Non-cuffed catheter	Percutaneous catheter	Short-term access
Tunneled cuffed catheter	Hickman catheter	Long-term infusion
Valve tip catheter	Groshong catheter	Long-term infusion where heparin may be problem
Implanted reservoir catheters	Port-a-cath	Intermittent long-term infusion
Large bore tunneled cuffed	Permacath	Hemodialysis or hemapheresis

their implantation. For this reason, general guidelines as to the utility of the cuffed catheters and ports suggest that these be reserved for instances where treatment is likely to be ongoing over a period of time of at least two to three months. For shorter periods of time, access may often be adequately provided for by use of less permanent catheters and PICC lines.

4. Risk of Catheter Access

Risks associated with venous access are grouped into immediate risks and long-term risks. Immediate risks are those potentially encountered at the time of implantation. The most common immediate risks associated with tunneled cuffed catheters and port include infection, central bleeding, and hemo- or pneumothorax. The long-term risks are those which may occur after implantation and extend as long as the catheter is in place. These include infection and deep-vein thrombosis (Table 2).

Table 2. Risks of catheter placement.

Perforation of central vessels
Hemothorax
Pneumothorax
Infection
Long- term risks of catheters
Infection
Deep-vein thrombosis

5. Implantation Guidelines

5.1 *Antibiotic prophylaxis*

Current antibiotic prophylactic guidelines indicate that a single dose of antibiotics should be administered within 30 minutes of commencing the procedure. No further antibiotics are required. The choice of antibiotics should be directed toward anticipated skin organisms. In most instances, a first-generation cephalosporin is the antibiotic of choice. A reserve drug such as Vancomycin may be indicated in circumstances where the risk of MRSA is considered to be increased. Examples of such instances include known colonization of the patient with resistant bacteria, or in an institution which has an elevated incidence of resistant organisms.

5.1.1 *Sterile environment*

A sterile operating environment is essential to catheter placement as the risk of bacterial infection is elevated in patients requiring catheters.

5.1.2 *Ultrasound-guided puncture of vessels*

Central venous puncture based on skin topography is a well-recognized clinical skill. Still this method is inexact and subject to anatomical variations which may not be detectable to the naked eye. Portable ultrasound devices have made a significant improvement for placement of central venous access, as these machines allow easy bedside identification of the major vessels. They further allow determination of vessel patency and diameter. These two characteristics are vital in selecting the best vessel for central puncture. Finally, ultrasound allows for direct visualization of the vessels as they are punctured, affording a visual guide to assist with cannulation of the vessels.

5.1.3 *Intra-operative fluoroscopy*

The use of fluoroscopy in the course of passage of the catheter is vitally important. From passage of guide wires and introducers to the positioning of the tip of the catheter, fluoroscopy allows increased margin of safety and prompt identification of problems. Identifying specific normal and abnormal radiographic patterns of guide wire positioning will allow the operator to recognize and avoid potential problems. Similarly once the catheter is near its final position, fluoroscopy allows evaluation of the optimal site.

5.1.4 *Postoperative radiograph*

The post-op x-ray is obtained for several purposes. First it allows evaluation of potential problems such as pneumothorax, hemothorax, and malpositioning of the catheter. Second it affords documentation of the successful completion of the case. Lastly it allows comparison at later date should a concern arise about the catheter function or position.

6. Complications of Venous Access

The most common risks associated with placing tunneled cuffed catheters and ports include infection, central bleeding, and hemo- or pneumothorax. The most common long-term risks include infection and deep-vein thrombosis.

Infection is a concern with any implanted prosthetic device. To reduce this risk, the devices should be implanted in a sterile environment such as an operating room. Antibiotic prophylaxis should be administered at the time of implantation. Specifically antibiotics should be provided to reduce the risk of infection by skin flora, primarily *Staphylococcus* bacteria. Current antibiotic prophylactic protocols suggest that one dose of antibiotic should be administered about 30 minutes before the device is implanted.

Long-term infection risks are present throughout the period that the catheter is implanted. The only way to reduce this risk is to remove the catheter entirely once its use is at end.

Pneumothorax occurs following puncture of the lung with leakage of air into the chest. The result of air leaking from the lung into the chest is collapse of the lung. If not treated, the ongoing air leak may eventually result in the development of a tension pneumothorax with compression against the mediastinum and displacement of the mediastinum toward the contralateral hemithorax. Treatment is chest tube thoracostomy with evacuation of the air. The lung puncture will often seal by itself. If the air leak from the lung persists, then VATS (video-assisted thoracoscopic surgery) may be required to close the leak from the lung. Pneumothorax is a potentially life-threatening condition which requires prompt identification and treatment. Fortunately these events are uncommon. In experienced hands and with use of intra-operative ultrasonography the incidence of pneumothorax is under 1%. When discovered and managed in a timely manner, it is controllable and is usually remedied with little difficulty.

Central vessel bleeding at the time of insertion may occur as a consequence of central venous perforation, or inadvertent cannulation of an adjacent artery. These events are rare and occur at a rate far below 1%. Central venous perforation occurs when the catheter insertion sheath fails to follow the centrally placed guidewire. In these instances the perforation may occur in any of the vessels starting from the point of insertion through the right atrium or right ventricle. Potentially fatal hemorrhage may ensue. Rapid recognition of the perforation is the most certain way to successfully remedy the problem. Steps to correction of the problem include positioning the patient in a full upright position to reduce central venous pressure, and possible surgical repair of the perforation.

Hemothorax occurs as a consequence of central venous perforation with bleeding into the chest. The blood flow into the chest displaces the lung and results in gradual loss of circulating blood volume. This is a potentially life-threatening condition where the bleeding is occult to the operating surgeons. A high index of suspicion may be triggered by observing an abnormal course of the catheter or introducer under fluoroscopic guidance. Treatment includes chest tube drainage of the blood and correcting the source of bleeding. A hemothorax may be identified by upright chest radiography. The same condition may not be identified by a supine fluoroscopic examination of the chest.

Deep-vein thrombosis (DVT) is not a frequent complication, yet remains a significant risk. The rate of DVT associated with central venous catheters may range from 1% to 10%, depending on the patient's coagulation status. These DVTs most often present with aching and swelling of an arm (in the case of subclavian catheters) or the side of the neck (in the case of jugular catheters). The diagnosis is usually established with duplex ultrasound scanning. The treatment is to anticoagulate the patient for at least three months. In many instances where the catheter is placed for treatment of malignancy the anticoagulation may be lifelong.

7. Outcome of Venous Access

Overall, the success of central venous access is remarkably high. In most instances, these devices are effective and present a low risk to patients. Complication rates are relatively low in experienced hands. For this reason they have become commonplace, and clinicians may underestimate the risk considerations involved in placing these devices.

8. Dialysis Access

8.1 *Overview*

Dialysis refers to the exchange of solutes across semi-permeable membranes to accomplish a clinically significant task. In common understanding, dialysis is taken to refer to hemodialysis, although the term is also used in reference to peritoneal dialysis.

Hemodialysis is a technique where a patient's blood is extracted and passed through a machine which allows the removal of substances from the blood. Most commonly, it is used as a form of replacement of renal function. Hemodialysis may be used to correct physiological abnormalities in the blood such as hyperkalemia and acidosis. Hemodialysis may also be used to remove some toxic substances and drugs from circulation. Dialysis may be very effective in removing excess fluid volume in instances of congestive failure with fluid overload.

Peritoneal dialysis is a technique where the selective permeability of the peritoneum is used to filter solutes from the circulation. The technique is based on instillation of a fluid into the peritoneal cavity which will drive osmotic gradients, yet is not absorbed. This fluid will then draw substances from the circulating blood into the peritoneal cavity. The fluid is then drained and along with it, the dialyzed substances are removed. The principal advantages of PD are its simplicity and reliability. It is most often done at home, by the patient or a caregiver. It thus allows for independence and the convenience of being able to establish a dialysis schedule according to individual convenience.

The PD access is by means of a surgically placed subcutaneously tunneled cuffed catheter which is placed in the abdomen. The PD fluid is instilled by a gravity feed. The fluid is drained passively by siphoning into a collection sac. In order for this siphoning mechanism to work properly, the catheter tip should rest in the pelvis in a dependent location.

8.2 *Advantages of PD*

The most significant advantage of PD is physiologic: since the dialysis is done on a daily basis the process is more homeostatic, with narrower shifts in fluid and electrolyte balance between dialysis sessions. This may avoid dramatic shifts in blood pressure. It avoids the ill feeling some patients may experience with hemodialysis as it is commonly administered three times per week. At the same time PD allows patients a significant element of control over their treatment. The convenience of dialysis at home and the relatively simple mechanism of dialysis make this an accessible technique.

8.3 *Disadvantages of PD*

The most significant disadvantage of PD is the need for daily connection to the dialysis machine. The need to physically lift and connect the bags of dialysis solution may be a physical challenge to some patients. The need to understand and implement sterile dialysis technique may be beyond the capability of some individuals.

8.4 *Patient selection*

The ideal candidates for PD are individuals who have sufficient strength and capacity to care for themselves, to manage the bags of PD fluid (two to four liters per bag), and who are capable of learning and implementing sterile technique. Most individuals who opt for PD are fairly healthy and highly functional. They find the independence afforded by PD to be a major advantage. In addition, the ideal candidate should not have had many prior abdominal operations — as scar tissue and adhesions from prior operations may present a significant impediment to successful PD. Body mass may be a consideration in electing against PD. Persons who are very obese may not be able to undergo effective PD as the efficiency of the PD may not allow effective dialysis in very large individuals.

8.5 *PD catheter access technique*

PD catheters should be placed surgically in a sterile operating room environment. Currently the most common technique is the laparoscopic placement method where laparoscopy is performed to assess the abdominal cavity and to observe and direct the positioning of the catheter tip within the peritoneal cavity. Laparoscopic placement requires general anesthesia and the creation of a pneumoperitoneum. The need for general anesthesia may be a significant limitation in certain individuals. Alternatively the catheters may be placed under local anesthesia by using an open technique.

Open surgical approach to catheter placement is an older technique which allows placement of the catheter into the peritoneum under direct visualization. This may be done under general or local anesthesia. The open technique suffers the disadvantages of requiring a larger incision, and not being able to clearly assess the condition of the peritoneal cavity or the final position of the catheter tip. Open technique may be required under certain circumstances. The most common of these is where there have been multiple prior abdominal operations and trocar entry is impeded. Another indication is when the patient may not tolerate general anesthesia. Open techniques are frequently used in very small children who are not ideal candidates for laparoscopy due to their size.

8.6 *Complications of PD access*

The PD catheter, as with any prosthetic material, is subject to infection. Infection is the most common complication of PD. Infections may affect the catheter, the peritoneal cavity, or both. An infection isolated to the catheter itself is rare. Most often this involves one of the subcutaneous cuffs along the abdominal wall. On occasion it may present as an exit site infection. In these instances, the infection is not only the catheter but also involves the adjacent tissue of the abdominal wall.

If a catheter becomes infected the peritoneal cavity may become infected as well. This presents as peritonitis with abdominal tenderness, fever, and leukocytosis. The severity of the infection may range from mild to life-threatening. In mild infections, intravenous antibiotic directed toward the infectious organism may allow clearing of the infection.

If a catheter infection does not respond to intravenous antibiotics, then the catheter must be removed in order to resolve the infection. Recurrent peritoneal infections may reduce the efficacy of the peritoneum to act as a dialysis membrane. Additionally, recurrent peritoneal infections may result in intra-abdominal adhesions. Both the loss of permeability and the development of adhesions can result in the inability to continue with peritoneal dialysis.

The catheters may occlude or clot. Fibrin from within the peritoneal cavity may occlude the catheter tip and stop its normal function. The most important means of preventing occlusion of the catheter is correct catheter care — specifically flushing the catheter periodically if it is not being used. The most significant cause of intra-peritoneal fibrin accumulation is peritoneal infections. For this reason, avoidance of infection and flushing of the catheters is important in preventing this problem. In the event that a catheter becomes occluded, a pressure flush may be attempted. If this fails it is likely that the catheter would need replacement.

Catheter migration is another less common complication of PD catheter access. When placed, the catheter is not secured within the peritoneal cavity. Intestinal peristalsis may move the catheter within the peritoneal cavity. On occasion the catheter tip may come to be lodged over the spleen or the liver. If it remains in that position it will frequently not work properly. Occasionally, the catheter may be returned to a dependent position by spontaneous action of the intestine, or by exercising (*i.e.* jumping jacks) with the intention of jarring the catheter back to its normal position. If the catheter fails to return to correct position then it need to be surgically repositioned.

Less common complications of PD catheters include erosion of the catheter into a viscous, erosion into a blood vessel, involvement of the catheter in a bowel obstruction, and entrapment of the catheter tip within an inflammatory cavity.

8.7 *Outcomes of PD access*

Overall PD access is effective and has a high success rate. The most common limitation is the patient's ability to manage the catheters and avoid infection.

9. Hemodialysis

As noted, hemodialysis refers to the process where blood is removed from the patient's body, waste products and fluid are extracted, and the blood is then returned to the patient.

The means by which hemodialysis is accomplished are commonly referred to as dialysis access. Historically several techniques have been employed to accomplish this goal. Currently there are three fundamental techniques: catheter dialysis access, arteriovenous fistulas (AVF), and arteriovenous grafts (AVG).

9.1 *Modalities of HD access*

Catheter access, as described in the previous section, relies upon large-diameter catheters placed in the central venous circulation. Through these, blood may be withdrawn and returned to the patient. Dialysis access catheters may be temporary or permanently placed. The temporary catheters are intended for short-term use. They are not cuffed and not tunneled and so are at a significant risk of infection. They are used as a means of temporary dialysis access while other more permanent access is placed.

9.2 *HD catheter access*

The permanently placed dialysis catheters are tunneled cuffed catheters which are placed in a sterile environment. Their use is intended to be temporary — they are designed to last for months at a time. In current use, they are intended to temporize dialysis access until permanent access such as an AVF may be created and placed into use. These catheters are not commonly used for permanent access because they are at significant risk of infection. The infections which may accompany these catheters, as with all other catheters, may be life-threatening. Other significant complications of catheter access include DVT and central vein stenosis. These may ultimately result in loss of central venous patency with the consequence of inability to provide dialysis. The ultimate consequence may be the patient's death.

10. AV Fistula and AV Graft

Arteriovenous fistulas (AVF) and arteriovenous grafts (AVG) are access conduits whereby an artificial connection is established between arterial and venous circulation. An AV Fistula (AVF) is a dialysis access construct where a donor artery is directly joined to a recipient vein. The vein will then be used as the dialysis access conduit. An AV Graft (AVG) is a dialysis access construct where a prosthetic conduit is used to bridge the donor artery and the recipient vein. Typically these access conduits are established in the arms. Occasionally they may be constructed in the thigh. The central vessels of the chest and abdomen are not used as the risk of infection in these vessels is prohibitive.

Unlike catheter access, AV access requires cannulation of the AV conduit with large bore (14 or 16 gauge needles). The portion of the conduit nearest the arterial source is called the arterial limb. A needle in the arterial limb of the conduit connects to tubing which leads to the dialysis machine. Inside the dialysis machine, a filter consisting of semi-permeable material is bathed in dialysis fluid to allow exchange of fluid and solutes from the blood. The blood is then returned through a second tube and a second needle in the venous limb of the access. Parameters of dialysis include the flow rates and the flow pressures in the arterial and venous limbs. Flows and pressures are maintained within a specified range. Elevated venous pressures and reduced flows may indicate a blockage in the venous limb of the access (outflow stenosis). Reduced arterial pressures and flow may suggest an inflow stenosis.

10.1 *Nomenclature*

The naming of AV access follows a specific protocol: the name reflects the inflow artery and then the outflow vein. If the access is a graft or a transposed vein then the name will reflect the configuration of the graft or vein. Grafts are termed loop or bridge grafts depending on their construction. A loop graft describes a loop on the arm whereas a bridge graft describes a gentle curve between the donor artery and recipient vein. Accordingly, a graft may be termed a radio-antecubital bridge graft, or an axillary-axillary loop graft. The one prominent exception to the rules of nomenclature is the Brescia-Cimino fistula. This is a radial-cephalic AV fistula constructed at the wrist (Fig. 1). This fistula is unique in its history and efficacy and is popularly known by the names of two of the authors who described its construction.

10.2 *Materials*

AV grafts may be constructed from a number of materials. The most common material is PTFE (polytetrafluoroethylene). This is commonly marketed by the Gore (Gore Medical, Flagstaff, AZ, USA) company as Gore-tex and by the Bard (Tempe, AZ, USA) company as Impra grafts. PTFE is a pliable synthetic material which is able to tolerate repeated puncture and allows incorporation of the graft into the limb. The process of incorporation refers to the growth of fibrous tissue into the graft interstices, as the graft remains implanted. This process is vital in providing AV grafts resistance to infection. Incorporation is also important in preventing bleeding from

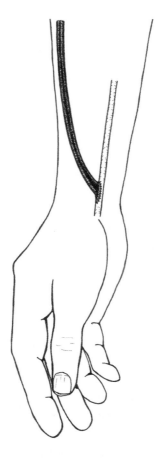

Fig. 1.

puncture points along the AV graft. Other materials, which have been used, include dacron and polyurethane. Bio-prostheses have been made from bovine and porcine vessels. These benefit from supple handling characteristics. Variations in the construction of the prosthetic grafts have been devised to allow immediate cannulation. An example of this is the Bard Vectra graft which has multiple layers that are capable of self-sealing and that allow the graft to be used immediately.

10.3 *Anatomic considerations*

In order to establish an AV access, several anatomic requirements need to be present. There must be adequate arterial supply of blood, and there must be adequate venous drainage. Adequate arterial supply requires that the inflow arteries to the limb be free of stenosis or occlusion. Blood pressure in the limb must be sufficient to maintain blood flow across the fistula or graft. If the blood pressure falls below a critical level then the fistula or graft may clot and cease to work. The distal arterial supply to the

Table 3.   Causes of AV access failure.

Stenosis
Hypotension
Hypercoagulability

limb must be free of occlusions or preferential blood flow in the graft may result in diminished flow in the distal extremity. The consequence of this would be ischemia with pain and ulceration and possible limb loss. If the venous drainage of the AV access is restricted, then the flow across the fistula will be insufficient to prevent clotting and the access will fail (Table 3).

10.4 *Pre-op evaluation*

Factors to consider include the patient's hand dominance, perioperative vein exam, vein mapping, arterial pulse exam, Allen test, and arterial duplex scan.

In determining who is a candidate for hemodialysis access, several elements should be taken into account. If the access is to be established in an arm, the arm dominance should be considered. The non-dominant arm is preferred in most cases. This allows the patient use of the dominant arm while connected to the dialysis machine. In the unlikely event of a problem complicating the access then the dominant arm is spared.

Anatomical elements prevail in determining the success of AV access. Accordingly pre-operative evaluation of the arterial pulses is very important. Part of this evaluation is palpation of the pulse at the axillary, brachial, and radial locations. Allen testing is routinely performed to assess the contribution of radial and ulnar arteries to the circulation of the hand and to assess the competence of the palmar arterial arches. If questions arise as a consequence of physical examination, noninvasive testing is used to assess arterial patency.

Evaluation of the venous anatomy is first done by assessing limb size (swelling may be an indicator of central venous occlusion), the presence of venous congestion, and collateral venous patterns across the shoulder and upper chest. The veins of the forearm and antecubital fossa should be examined and they are assessed for size and patency. If the veins are not clearly seen to be of adequate size, then noninvasive examination may be performed. The venous exam should include the evaluation of patency of the deep venous system. An additional test is vein mapping where the patency and size of the cephalic and basilic veins are measured using a duplex ultrasound scanner. The minimal acceptable diameter for a cephalic vein to be used in construction of an AV fistula is 2.5 mm. In the event of no superficial veins of adequate size, then an AV graft may be required. The AV graft may be joined with the deep veins to the arm to form an access. Accordingly if the deep venous system is not patent, then the access cannot be established.

10.5 *Sequencing of access sites*

In order to maximize the longevity of a patient, access sites are usually approached in sequence leading from distal to proximal. This is done because the establishment of a proximal site may later prevent the use of a distal site. In addition, current recommendations are to use veins before resorting to the use of synthetic graft material. This is due to improved durability and lower infection rates of the vein conduits. Dialysis outcomes quality initiative (DOQI) is an effort to improve dialysis outcomes by encouraging best practices in dialysis. With reference to dialysis access, DOQI guidelines indicate preferential use of cephalic vein conduits before basilic veins, and synthetic grafts as a last choice. This sequence has been described as the "fistula first" approach.

10.5.1 *Femoral access*

When the upper extremities are no longer usable for dialysis access, then femoral vessels may be considered. As with upper extremities, arterial inflow must be free of stenosis and the arterial tree of the lower extremity must be patent. Atherosclerosis is more common in the lower extremities than the upper extremities and so careful evaluation is necessary. Pulse examination should be accompanied by noninvasive testing. Specifically arterial pressures and duplex scanning will allow the assessment of the arterial tree plaque and patency. Similarly the venous drainage of the limb needs to be patent or the access will fail. Of particular importance is any history of deep-vein thrombosis as this may indicate the presence of compromised venous outflow. In the event of any uncertainty, evaluation of the venous drainage is most effectively done by means of venography. Femoral access is usually considered a last alternative because of concerns regarding patency and infection. Infection is thought to be more common in the femoral region. Some fear that patency may be compromised by repeated flexion of the leg.

10.6 *Surgical techniques*

10.6.1 *AV fistula*

An AV fistula is constructed by joining a superficial vein to the side of an artery. The anatomical construct may be one of several variations (side to side, end to end, or end to side). Of these, the most common is the end of vein to side of artery construct. The most successful grouping is the cephalic vein anastomosed to the radial artery at the wrist. This particular fistula is called the Brescia–Cimino fistula. When successful it is the most durable fistula. Most other fistulas are referred to by their anatomic names (brachio-cephalic or brachio-basilic).

Before they may be used, AV fistulas need to proceed through a period of fistula maturation. Maturation involves the dilatation of the vein and growth of the vein wall thickness. Maturation requires about six to eight weeks to proceed to the point where the fistula may be usable. Initial use of the fistula may require a further four weeks to achieve reliable access with large bore needles.

Depending on the location and depth of the vein, the fistula conduit may need to be superficialized or translocated. If the vein is more than 4 mm deep it may be difficult to use. In these instances the vein will require "superficialization," which refers to moving the vein from its normal location to a more superficial location in the arm. The skin overlying the vein is opened and the vein is transferred to a more superficial location.

If the basilic vein is used, then translocation will be necessary. This is because the course of the basilic vein is in a relatively inaccessible portion of the arm. Additionally the basilic vein is frequently too deep to allow successful puncture. Translocation of the vein requires removing the vein from its normal location and tunneling it in a different location which is more readily accessible.

10.6.2 *AV graft*

An AV graft is constructed by anastomosing a synthetic conduit to an artery on one end and to a vein on its other end. The conduit is tunneled just beneath the skin. As blood flows through the conduit, puncture with needles allows removal and return of blood in the dialysis process. Grafts allow establishment of dialysis access in the absence of adequate superficial veins. The placement of the graft results in pain and swelling of the limb which typically lasts 10–14 days. The AV graft may be used once the initial pain and swelling have resolved. While grafts are convenient means of providing for dialysis access, they suffer several disadvantages — the prosthetic material is susceptible to infection; it will not tolerate low systemic blood pressure with consequent low blood flow and will tend to clot and will require periodic de-clotting. Finally, the junction of the prosthetic material to the venous system frequently generates an exaggerated scar response called intimal hyperplasia which over time may block the venous outflow of the graft.

10.7 *Complications of HD access*

The most common complications of HD access include infection and clotting (Table 4). Infection is a potential problem more common with prosthetic access

Table 4.   Complications of HD access.

Infection
Clotting
Stenosis
Ischemic steal
Neuropathy

---

grafts. While the incidence of infection of these grafts may vary between clinical settings, overall it is estimated to be about 10%. In most instances these infections represent cellulitis of the skin overlying the graft. In a minority of instances, the graft itself may become infected. Once the graft is infected, it must be removed in order to resolve the infection. If the graft infection occurs soon after implantation, then removal of the graft may be as simple as disconnecting it from the vessels and tugging it out. On the other hand, most serious graft infections occur long after the graft is implanted and removal requires sharp dissection to excise the graft and the surrounding soft tissue. Disconnecting the graft from the artery may be a complex operation where the artery is repaired with a small portion of vein. The physiological impact of a graft infection varies greatly. It may be of minor importance, or may lead to systemic sepsis with hemodynamic collapse. Thus an AV graft infection is a dangerous costly event. For this reason the DOQI guidelines indicate grafts are a second choice for dialysis access.

Clotting is the most common complication of hemodialysis access. Clotting may occur for any one of several reasons. While removing the clot and restoring blood flow through the AV access is usually a straightforward task, understanding and correcting the cause of the clotting is vital to long-term success of the access. The common causes of clotting of an AV access include loss of venous outflow due to intimal hyperplasia and venous stricture and poor arterial inflow due to arterial stenosis. Both of these may be addressed with either endovascular (balloon angioplasty and stenting) or open surgical technique. Clotting may occur because of hemodynamic causes — hypotension while on dialysis or after dialysis, hypovolemia, and cardiac insufficiency. Correcting the fluid volume at the end of dialysis may reduce this risk. Clotting may be precipitated by a primary coagulation abnormality. Anticoagulation with Coumadin may help correct these events.

A significant subset of failed AV access is the early occlusion of AV fistulas. The rate of initial failure of AV fistulas is between 10 and 25%. In most instances the fistula is not retrievable. The reasons for these early failures are a combination of venous stenosis, coagulation, poor blood flow, and inability of vessels to accommodate and compensate (Table 5). The incidence of early fistula failure is

Table 5.   Modalities of failure of central venous catheters.

Failure to withdraw blood	Catheter infection
Failure to allow infusion	Erosion through skin (reservoir port)
Insufficient catheter flow volume	Kinking in subcutaneous tunnel
Intermittent function (ball valve effect)	Fragmentation of catheter
Thrombosis of catheter	
Thrombosis of central venous structures	
Fracture of catheter	
Embolization of catheter fragments	
Erosion of central venous structures	
Withdrawal of catheter (pulled out)	

related to initial vein diameters. Fistulas based on smaller veins are more prone to fail. Other elements include the age of the patient population, and the incidence of comorbidities such as heart disease and diabetes.

Determining which of these causes is responsible for a given thrombotic event requires analysis of the patient's dialysis records: recorded blood pressures during and after dialysis as well as the recorded pressures of the dialysis machine. Removal of the clot may allow evaluation for the presence of intimal hyperplasia at the arterial or venous anastomosis. Hypercoagulable conditions may be detected by specific blood test. In many instances the cause of clotting may not be evident. At times these may respond to empiric anticoagulation for a non-specified coagulation abnormality.

10.8 *Management of AV access thrombosis*

The management of a patient with acute thrombosis of their AV access requires several specific steps. First, the patient needs to be evaluated to assess volume and electrolyte status. Next a decision must be made as to whether declotting is an option. Recently created AV fistulas tend to present a problem for declotting procedures — they tend to re-clot on short order. The reasons for this are several: the initial cause of clotting is often not remediable (if a marginal vein was used then this will not be improved by the declotting procedure). Endothelium of the veins tends to be injured by the presence of thrombus and by the passage of a thrombectomy balloon. This injury then predisposes to further clotting. For reasons such as these, under certain circumstances, it may be prudent to abandon a marginal access site and plan for a new access operation.

If the patient is stable for declotting then the next question is which declot technique to employ: open surgical declotting or endovascular procedures. Open surgical technique tends to be more successful and allows longer period of use before access fails again. On the other hand, it is a more invasive approach.

10.9 *Open surgical declotting*

With open surgical approach, the patient must be able to proceed to the operating room, undergo anesthesia, and undergo an operation. The operation may be a simple removal of the clot (thrombectomy) or an exploration of the AV access, with possible revision such as patch angioplasty or reconstruction of an anastomosis or replacement of the graft. The fundamental problem with open surgery for declotting an AV access is the unpredictable nature of the operation. The operation is undertaken without exact knowledge of the cause of clotting. Accordingly the operation requires astute observation and experience in order to succeed. The surgeon must be able to recognize clues as to why the access failed. Based on these observations revisions may be then be undertaken to correct the access function. It is this ability to fundamentally revise and correct the access malfunction that gives open surgical declotting an advantage over endovascular techniques.

10.10 *Endovascular thrombectomy*

Endovascular procedures provide an important alternative to open surgical thrombectomy. They enjoy the benefit of being less invasive and capable of being performed with local anesthesia. They are usually performed with radiographic imaging and allow for immediate assessment of the AV access structure and patency. The presence of stenosis may be readily identified and treatment implemented at the same sitting.

The principal endovascular techniques include thrombolysis and mechanical thrombectomy. Thrombolysis refers to the infusion of thrombolytic agents such as tPA in order to dissolve the clot in the graft. Mechanical thrombectomy refers to the disruption of the clot by means of direct mechanical action. Some approaches combine both techniques: thrombolysis is enhanced by mechanical agitation or ultrasound vibration.

A significant benefit of thrombolysis over open thrombectomy is the ability to image the AV graft or fistula at the time of intervention. This allows one to assess the presence of stenosis or occlusion of the access. Stenoses are most commonly found at the venous anastomosis of an AV graft. They may also occur at the arterial anastomosis or at any point along the length of the conduit (graft or fistula). The presence of a significant stenosis (greater than 50% lumen reduction) in the context of a clotted AV access is taken as an evident cause of the thrombotic event. While this may not always be the cause of thrombosis, in most instances, a stenosis presents a significant risk of causing further clotting and will be treated with angioplasty and possibly with stenting. Balloon angioplasty and stenting may be employed to correct any stenosis. Unfortunately the long-term success of these techniques is limited, and re-thrombosis is not uncommon.

10.11 *Ischemic steal*

On occasion an AV access may work so well that it impairs the blood flow to the distal limb. When the blood flow in the AV access is so great that it reduces the blood to the distal limb, resulting in ischemic symptoms, the condition is called an ischemic steal. In essence, the AV access is thought to be stealing blood from the distal limb. Hemodynamic loss of perfusion pressure to some degree is a common event following establishment of HD access. In most instances, the degree of reduction in perfusion is low and is well tolerated. Compensatory mechanisms may come into play — the arterial tree may hypertrophy and enlarge to increase the amount of blood supplied to the limb. In some patients the ability to compensate is inadequate, and the amount of blood removed by the AV access is so great that symptoms of ischemia are encountered.

The most common symptoms are coolness and mild tingling of fingertips. More severe symptoms include numbness and tingling (paresthesias), pain, and weakness of the fingers and hands. These are urgent symptoms and require urgent intervention to correct them. The longer these symptoms are allowed to persist, the more likely they may become permanent. Some patients may have underlying neuropathy with sensitization of their nerves. These patients may be particularly sensitive to changes in circulation. And a relatively minor reduction of blood flow may result in the development of symptoms. Diabetics are prone to this eventuality. For this reason ischemic steal is noted to occur in up to 5% of diabetic patients.

The diagnosis of ischemic steal may be accomplished with noninvasive testing. Pulse volume recording of finger tips may show a significant change when the AV access is temporarily occluded. Arteriography may show preferential blood flow through the AV access.

Correction of ischemic steal may be performed by reducing the blood flow through the AV access. Most commonly this is done by reducing the diameter of the access conduit near the arterial anastomosis with either sutures or bands applied around the conduit ("banding operation"). An alternative procedure is to change the inflow to a more proximal artery. Finally a specific re-orienting of the blood flow may be accomplished with a DRIL (distal revascularization, interval ligation) operation. The banding operation carries an increased risk of clotting of the AV access as it will reduce the flow in the conduit. The DRIL operation is not associated with such increased clotting of the conduit, but it is a more complex operation and presents the risk if limb ischemia inherent to ligation of the arterial tree.

10.12 *Outcomes of HD access*

The results of HD access are far from ideal. A general opinion holds that results of AV fistulas are significantly different from those of AV grafts. When comparing AV grafts to Brescia–Cimino AV fistulas there are significant differences over the long range period of time. Fistulas tend to last longer and have fewer thrombotic events.

Fistulas are considered to be the optimal dialysis access as they tend to be durable, resist clotting, and are less susceptible to infection. The construction of AV fistulas comes at a price however. Between 10 and 25% of AV fistulas will fail within the first two months of creation. Only about 45–60% will reach functional maturity within a year. The long-term patency of a Cimino AV fistula was thought to be about 80%. More recent publication have indicated a much lower primary patency of 35% and assisted primary patency of 50% after 12 months.

Graft access is far from ideal. On the average an AV graft will clot once in every six to nine months. The average 18-month patency of an AV graft is between 30% and 50%. The risk of infection is as high as 10%.

11. Conclusions

Dialysis access is a broad field where knowledge of the limitations and benefits of the various techniques allows optimal care for individual patients. It is difficult to understate the importance of these techniques. They are life-saving and life-sustaining for patients who suffer from renal failure. Loss of access is a critical event which may result in the demise of these patients.

Unlike some other areas of surgery, the incidence of failure and the need for revision are significant. Patients and physicians need to be aware of the limitations of the techniques. Careful planning and pre-operative preparation will yield optimal results.

References

Brescia MJ, Cimino JE, Appel K, Hurwich BJ. Chronic hemodialysis using venipuncture and a surgically created arteriovenous fistula, *N Engl J Med* 1966; **275**(20):1089–1092.
Bakken AM, Protack CD, Saad WE, *et al.* Long-term outcomes of primary angioplasty and primary stenting of central venous stenosis in hemodialysis patients, *J Vasc Surg* 2007; **45**(4):776–783.

Biuckians A, Scott EC, Meier GH, Panneton JM, Glickman MH. The natural history of autologous fistulas as first-time dialysis access in the KDOQI era, *J Vasc Surg* 2008; **47**(2):415–421; discussion 420–421.

Eastridge BM, Lefor A. Complications of indwelling venous access devices in cancer patients, *J Clin Oncol* 1995; **13**:233–238.

Glazer S, Diesto J, Crooks P, Yeoh H, Pascual N, Selevan D, Derose S, Farooq M. Going beyond the kidney disease outcomes quality initiative: hemodialysis access experience at Kaiser Permanente Southern California, *Ann Vasc Surg* 2006; **20**(1):75–82.

Knox RC, Berman SS, Hughes JD, Gentile AT, Mills JL. Distal revascularization-interval ligation: a durable and effective treatment for ischemic steal syndrome after hemodialysis access, *J Vasc Surg* 2002; **36**(2):250–255; discussion 256.

Lumsden AB, MacDonald MJ, Isiklar H, *et al.* Central venous stenosis in the hemodialysis patient: incidence and efficacy of endovascular treatment, *Cardiovasc Surg* 1997; **5**:504–509.

NKF-DOQI clinical practice guidelines for vascular access. National Kidney Foundation-Dialysis Outcomes Quality Initiative, *Am J Kidney Dis* 1997; **30**(4 Suppl 3):S150–S191.

Puel V, Caudry M, Le Métayer P, *et al.* Superior vena cava thrombosis related to catheter malposition in cancer chemotherapy given through implanted ports, *Cancer* 1993; **72**(7):2248–2252.

Schutz JC, Patel AA, Clark TW, *et al.* Relationship between chest port catheter tip position and port malfunction after interventional radiologic placement, *J Vasc Interv Radiol* 2004; **15**(6):581–587.

Yaghoubian A, Lewis RJ, de Virgilio C. Can the National Kidney Foundation guidelines for first-time arteriovenous fistula creation be met in underserved end-stage renal disease patients? *Ann Vasc Surg* 2008; **22**(1):5–10.

Yaghoubian A, de Virgilio C. Plication as primary treatment of steal syndrome in arteriovenous fistulas, *Ann Vasc Surg* 2009; **23**(1):103–107. Epub September 21, 2008.

Chapter 13
Thoracic Outlet Syndrome

Hugh A. Gelabert

————————

Learning Objectives

- Learn and understand the relevant anatomy of the thoracic outlet and its relationship to TOS syndromes.
- Identify key elements of the history and physical examination which aid in the diagnosis of TOS.
- Differentiate between neurogenic, venous, and arterial presentations of TOS.
- Familiarize yourself with the important diagnostic tests relevant to TOS.
- Learn and understand medical and surgical treatment options for patients with TOS.
- Familiarize yourself with potential complications of surgery for TOS.

1. Definition of TOS

Thoracic outlet syndrome (TOS) is the constellation of symptoms that arises from the compression of the neurovascular structures as they cross the anatomic outlet of the thorax. The symptoms are derived from compression of the brachial plexus trunks, the axillo-subclavin artery, or the axillo-subclavian vein. The genesis of the compression is varied and depends on a combination of congenital and developmental variables, which will result in compression. Compression of these structures then results in the symptoms that account for the clinical syndrome.

2. Anatomical Considerations

The anatomy of the thoracic outlet is a complex three-dimensional anatomy which includes bony elements, muscles and ligaments, and the neurovascular structures (the brachial plexus trunks, the axillo-subclavian artery, or the axillo-subclavian vein). These elements interact in both a scissoring motion (the movement of clavicle with relation to the first rib) and a choke-collar-like constriction (the elevation of the rib and tendinous bands against the neurovascular structures) (Fig. 1).

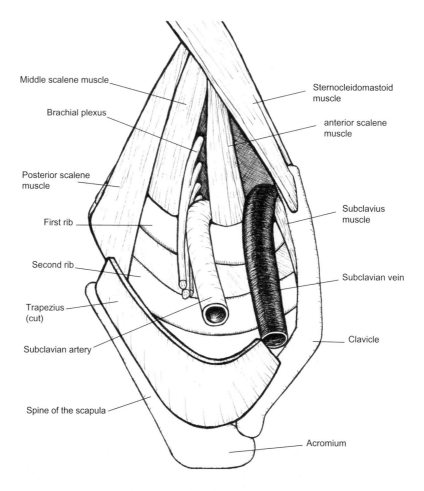

Fig. 1.

The anatomical definition of the thoracic outlet is that space bounded by the first rib, vertebral body, and sternum. Thus the first ribs describe a circular structure at the top of the thoracic cage — this is both the inlet and outlet to the thorax. The neurovascular structures exit the chest and drape over the first rib.

The brachial plexus is a confluence of nerves arising from the C4–T1 nerve roots. These branch and reform to generate the roots, trunks, cords, and branches of the brachial plexus. Eventually these form the median nerve, the radial nerve, and the ulnar nerve as the principal innervation of the upper extremity. In addition, several important nerves derive from the brachial plexus. The long thoracic nerve innervates the subscapularis and anterior serratus muscles and is important in maintaining the stability of the scapula.

The thoracodorsal nerve innervates the latussimus dorsi muscle of the chest wall. The subclavian arteries arise in different manner on the right and left sides.

The right subclavian artery arises as a branch of the innominate (or brachio-cephalic) artery.

The left subclavian artery arises directly from the aortic arch. Both of these arteries are typically described as having a first, second, and third segment. The boundary is the anterior scalene muscle. The first segment is between the origin of the artery and the anterior scalene muscle. The second segment is behind the muscle. The third segment is the portion between the lateral border of the anterior scalene and the lateral margin of the first rib. Beyond the first rib, the artery is called the axillary artery. The veins are named in a similar manner. For this reason the vessels coursing the thoracic outlet are often referred to as the axillo-subclavian artery or veins.

The first rib forms the bony floor of the thoracic outlet. In addition, Sibson's fascia, the thickened condensation of pleura at the apex of the chest, forms a soft-tissue extension of the thoracic outlet floor.

Above the neurovascular structures course the clavicles. On the underside of the clavicles runs the subclavius muscle. Normally a small muscle, it lines the lower aspect of the clavicle and attaches onto the dorsal aspect of the first rib by means of a dense ligament. This ligament is located medially, at the junction of the clavicle and the first rib with the sternum. The effect of the subclavius muscle is to elevate the rib toward the clavicle.

The scalene muscles are central elements of the thoracic outlet structure. The anterior and middle scalene muscles originate on the cervical spine and insert on the dorsal aspect of the first rib. The two muscles are separated by the trunks of the brachial plexus and the subclavian artery. As indicated by its name, the anterior scalene muscle is the first one encountered in frontal view. It is a unique muscle because it inserts between the subclavian artery and subclavian vein. The thoracic outlet is the only place in the body where a muscle inserts between an artery and a vein.

The action of the scalene muscles is to elevate the first rib, and in doing so, elevate the thoracic cage. These are accessory muscles of respiration. Innervation is somatic and under voluntary control. Taking a deep breath activates the muscles in a coordinated effort to assist respiration by elevating the first rib and pulling up the thoracic cage.

Several anomalies of the anatomical development of the throracic outlet are well described. Dr. Roos, of Colorado, described several patterns of musculo-tendinous insertions which he identified in the course of surgical dissection. Of these anomalies, by far the most common is the scalenius minimis muscle.

The scalenius minimis muscle is a vestigial muscle, the remnant of developmental involution. It is located between the brachial plexus and the subclavian artery. It may insert on the first rib or onto Sibson's fascia. It may have fibers which join with

H. A. Gelabert

the lower fibers of the anterior or middle scalene muscles to complete a musculo-
tendinous sling beneath these structures.

The second most common anomaly in the thoracic outlet anatomy is the cervical
rib. Cervical ribs are the result of failure of involution of an early developmental
structure. The cervical ribs normally involute during early embryonic development.
When the involution fails to occur there may be a complete cervical rib with articu-
lation to the sternum. When the involution is near complete there may be a residual
elongated transverse process of C7 vertebral body and a dense fibrous band from
this transverse process extending to the first rib. The most common patterns include
a fully developed cervical rib with complete articular attachment to the first rib, a
fully developed cervical rib with a fibrous attachment to the first rib, and a partially
formed cervical rib with a fibrous band reaching to the first rib. The Gruber classification of the cervical rib is a simple means of organizing these according to length
and the nature of the junction with the first rib (Fig. 1).

3. Pathology of TOS

Two fundamental injuries are thought to account for the onset of most TOS: acute
distraction of the thoracic outlet musculature or a chronic repetitive compression of
the neurovascular structures. In many instances these two mechanisms are related.
The acute injury is most readily comprehended as a traumatic force resulting in rapid,
abrupt, and uncompensated distraction of the structures of the thoracic outlet. Thus
both pulling of the upper extremity away from the torso or pulling the head away
from the shoulder both would be expected to result in acute injury. The magnitude of
the force may result in varying degrees of injury. The muscles, nerves, or vessels may
be partially or completely torn. Adjunctive injury may be identified in the muscles
and ligaments of the shoulder or upper extremity. In those instances with a small
tear, healing processes may result in scarring and contraction of the structures and
in sensitization to further stress.

The chronic repetitive compression injury is the result of repeated use of the
extremities for purposeful activity. This may result in overdevelopment of muscles
associated with these activities. Thus hypertrophy of the anterior scalene and middle
scalene muscles as well as the subclavius muscle may result. Repeated stressful exer-
tion may also lead to forceful contraction of these muscles which, when repeated,
may result in traction on the periosteum of the first rib resulting in bony growth
(exostosis) at the point of insertion of the muscle. Depending on which muscles
hypertrophy, compression may result in narrowing of the subclavian vein, the subclavian artery, or the brachial plexus.

Repetitive use of the muscles of the thoracic outlet or chronic pain, resulting in
sustained muscle spasm and contraction, has been demonstrated to result in a change

254

of muscle fiber type. The change results in replacement of the rapid contraction fibers with fibers capable of sustained contraction. Thus both acute and repetitive injury may result in contraction and spasm of the scalene muscles. This in turn may result in compression of the neurovascular structures and the development of resultant symptoms. Compression of the brachial plexus nerves results in pain and paresthesia (numbness and tingling), weakness, and muscular atrophy. Occasionally compression of the sympathetic nerve fibers results in Raynaud's-like vasomotor instability with color changes. Other repeated symptoms may include sweating or burning pain.

Compression of the axillo-subclavian artery may result in arm fatigue, pallor, heaviness, and weakness. The artery may develop post-stenotic aneurismal dilatation. Within this aneurysm or at the point of compression the artery may form thrombi which then embolize down the arm. Thrombosis of the subclavian artery with retrograde extension has been reported as a cause of vertebral embolization and stroke.

Compression of the axillo-subclavian vein may result in symptoms of arm swelling, congestion, heaviness, or discoloration. After reaching a critical stage, the compression will result in reduced venous flow within the vein and subsequent thombosis of the subclavian vein. This will often present as an abrupt onset of arm swelling. The thrombus may propagate and dislodge centrally, becoming a pulmonary embolus.

4. Diagnosis of TOS

The diagnosis of TOS is, in essence, a clinical one. It is based on recognition of symptoms, clinical presentations, and elicitation of physical exam findings. The diagnosis is supported by the appropriate testing. It is common that patients presenting with TOS may have coexisting conditions which may overlap in presentation. The injuries which lead to TOS are often the same ones which may result in injury to the cervical spine, shoulder, or extremity. For this reason both exclusionary and inclusive testing is routinely performed.

Exclusionary testing is done to exclude confounding diagnoses such as cervical degenerative disease, rotator cuff injury, ulnar nerve entrapment (cubital tunnel syndrome), and median nerve entrapment (carpal tunnel). Specific testing includes MRI of the cervical spine, physical evaluation of the shoulder, and electromyography (EMG)/nerve conduction velocity (NCV) testing of the arm.

Inclusive testing includes those tests which are diagnostic of TOS. These include MRI of the brachial plexus, somato-sensory-evoked potential (SSEP) evaluation, median antecubital cutaneous (MAC) nerve testing, and anterior scalene muscle block. These tests are designed to confirm the diagnosis of TOS.

4.1 Differential diagnosis

In evaluating patients with TOS, one must consider associated diagnoses which may coexist and may confuse the presentation. Specifically, cervical degenerative disease, rotator cuff injury, ulnar nerve entrapment (cubital tunnel syndrome), median nerve entrapment (carpal tunnel).

4.2 Related musculoskeletal syndromes: Rotator cuff, cervical spine

It is important to recognize that TOS may often present in the company of associated clinical syndromes such as rotator cuff tear or cervical degenerative disease. For this reason history, physical evaluation, and testing must address these conditions. History of pain or injury to the neck or shoulder should be elicited. Examination of the shoulder and neck is required as part of the assessment. MRI scan of the cervical spine should be performed in most patients. Orthopedic evaluation of the shoulder should be required when suspicion of injury is present. It is important to proceed with these assessments prior to reaching a final diagnosis and embarking on surgical intervention as one may take precedence over another. For example, in the presence of a severe cervical disk bulge, TOS surgery would be deferred until the cervical spine is stabilized.

4.3 Cubital tunnel syndrome and carpal tunnel syndrome

Cubital tunnel syndrome and carpal tunnel syndrome are the result of compression of the ulnar and median nerves at the elbow and wrist (respectively). These are common coexisting conditions. The diagnosis of TOS is often obscured by these, and it is not uncommon that patients will undergo decompressive procedures for these conditions prior to coming to the diagnosis of TOS. The coexistence of some of these conditions is so common that a term has been established for the phenomena where TOS is accompanied by carpal tunnel syndrome or cubital tunnel syndrome: the double crush phenomenon.

4.4 True neurogenic TOS and diagnosis disputed TOS

One of the problems with management of patients with TOS is differences in opinion regarding diagnosis of the condition. A wide spectrum of opinions exists within medical communities. At the extreme, some physicians take the posture that there is no such entity as thoracic outlet syndrome. A more stringent group accepts only the most advanced presentations: wasting and atrophy of the musculature of the hand of limb accompanied by MEG evidence of denervation. This presentation is referred to as true neurogenic TOS. A more liberal group of doctors accept the concept

Table 1.   Chronic pain syndromes
often associated with TOS.

Central pain syndrome
Raynaud's
Chronic regional pain
Fibromyalgia
Myofascial pain
Anxiety/Depression

that true neurogenic TOS is a far advanced stage of the condition, and that earlier manifestations are likely. These manifestations would precede the onset of muscle wasting and denervation — thus may not be detectable by such criteria. These are common neurogenic TOS. The term "diagnosis disputed TOS" has been applied to these later cases, since by definition, the diagnosis is not secured by the presence of muscle wasting and EMG documented denervation.

4.5 *Associated conditions*

A number of conditions may be associated with TOS and may result in significant pain and disability. These conditions are important to identify as their presence would strongly suggest that the goals of intervention with TOS would be limited at best. In instances where these conditions coexist with the TOS, patients will be anticipated to have persistent symptoms despite adequate decompression of the thoracic outlet. Intervention in these instances is done with a limited goal of reducing one area which may contribute to the overall pain syndrome (Table 1).

5. Clinical Presentations

Compression of the neurovascular structures at the thoracic outlet will result in symptoms relating to the structure compressed. Accordingly patients may present with arterial, venous, or neurogenic symptoms. In many cases there is compression of more than one structure and thus there is overlap of symptoms (Table 2).

Arterial presentations range from intermittent compression of the axillo-subclavian artery to the development of thrombo-embolic events with obliteration of the arterial tree in the upper extremity. The prototypical presentation is unilateral arm ischemia. Most commonly this is an acute event with pulselessnes, pallor, paretehesia, pain, and paralysis. The presentation is that of acute limb-threatening ischemia and requires emergency intervention.

Table 2.   Common presentations of TOS.

Neurogenic	85–95%
Venous	5–10%
Arterial	0–3%

Unilateral arterial insufficiency (lack of pulse, evidence of ischemia, or emboliza-tion) should trigger a suspicion of arterial TOS. Mild vasomotor abnormalities (dis-coloration, cold sensation, and sensitivity to cold exposure) may be a presentation of chronic repetitive embolization to a hand.

The severity of the presentation may vary: from minor emboli with little or no pain to major thrombosis of the limb with pain, paralysis, pulslessness, paresthesia, and limb threat. A presentation of unilateral upper extremity Raynaud's-like discol-oration should be considered an embolic event until proven otherwise. Arterial TOS should be considered in any differential causes of unilateral embolic events to the upper extremity.

Central symptoms are also seen with vascular presentations. Arterial compres-sion may result in thrombosis of the axillo-subclavian artery. In rare instances, the clot may undertake extension and thus retrograde propagation to the proximal sub-clavian artery. If the retrograde extension reaches the ostia of the vertebral artery then vertebral embolization or occlusion may result in a stroke.

Venous presentations of TOS are mostly related to obstruction of blood flow from the arm. Venous compression and thrombosis result in swelling and discoloration of the arm and hand. Thus the most common presentation is that of abrupt onset of arm swelling and discoloration. This is accompanied by varying degrees of pain or congestion.

Paget Schroetter syndrome refers to the spontaneous development of axillo-subclavian vein thrombosis. Spontaneous in this context signifies no prior history of instrumentation, catheterization, traumatic injury, or surgery. The most common cause of Paget Schroetter syndrome is extrinsic compression of the axillo-subclavian vein at the thoracic outlet. For this reason Paget Schroetter syndrome if often con-sidered almost synonymous with venous TOS.

A less common presentation is intermittent compression with swelling, pain, and discoloration. This presentation carries the name of McCleery's syndrome and is thought to be caused by intermittent compression of the axillo-subclavian vein with changes in the position of the arm.

Chronic venous occlusion from an established axillo-subclavian thrombosis may result in chronic congestive symptoms in an arm. Typically these patients suffered an acute episode where the subclavian vein clotted, often associated with a period of intense arm exercise. Initial partial resolution of symptoms is achieved with resting the extremity or with anticoagulation. Symptoms present with resumption of arm use. In those instances where the thrombosis does not resolve, the arm will experience congestion, discoloration, and aching with use.

Central symptoms are also seen with venous presentations of TOS. Subclavian venous thombosis may result in pulmonary embolization. The incidence is estimated to be between 5% and 15%.

5.1 *Neurogenic presentations*

Neurogenic presentations of TOS are believed to be the result of impingement on the brachial plexus by bony, muscular, and ligamentous structural elements of the thoracic outlet. Pinching of the nerves results in pain, numbness, and tingling. If the compression is severe and lasting then disruption of nerve conduction may result in weakness and denervation. Denervation will later result in atrophy of the target muscles.

The classic neurogenic symptoms include pain and paresthesia. If the compression of neurovascular structures occurs at the thoracic outlet, then it is understandable that symptoms will present in the affected extremity.

The classic pattern is of pain and paresthesia radiating from the base of the neck into the hand. Ulnar distribution along the underside of the arm and into the fourth and fifth fingers is more common than radial distribution. Occasionally the entire hand is involved (both radial and ulnar).

5.2 *Less typical distributions*

A large number of patients will also experience symptoms in regions beyond the extremity. In cases presenting with pain, the pain may be noted in the torso, the shoulder, the neck, the scapula, the head, or the face. Pain along the head and face may be indistinguishable from migraine. At times migraine may be the result of muscle spasm and pain in the neck and shoulder.

5.3 *Mixed presentations*

Most presentations will include a combination of arterial and neurogenic symptoms. These presentations include pain, paresthesia (numbness and tingling), weakness, and atrophy. They may also include cold sensation, color changes, and swelling in the hand and fingers. Distinguishing between transient symptoms from positional arterial compression versus positional exacerbation of compression of a nerve trunk may be difficult as both etiologies may share a similar presentation.

5.4 *Pectoralis minor syndrome*

This is an unusual cause of neurovascular compression in the upper extremity and is frequently considered a subset of TOS. The compression occurs as the neurovascular bundle enters the upper arm. The pectoralis minor tendon crosses over the neurovascular bundle and is able to compress it against the upper humerus. This results in pain and paresthesia down the arm and is typically associated with spasm and tenderness in the pectoralis muscle.

6. Physical Examination for TOS

The physical examination of TOS patients should include not only evaluation for signs of thoracic outlet compression, but should also include a general assessment of the musculoskeletal function of the upper extremity, shoulder, and neck.

General posture and skeletal orientation should be assessed by inspection and range of motion. Posture should be observed. The bearing of the shoulders, the position, and function of the scapula should be recorded. Range of motion of the shoulder and neck is assessed to identify possible shoulder and neck problems. Additionally these areas should be palpated to assess for point tenderness which would be considered a specific indicator of problems in these areas.

Vascular observations include the presence of subungual splinter hemorrhages or Roth spots in the hands and fingers as signs of embolization. The presence of venous collaterals across the shoulders and chest, swelling of the hand and arm, and congestion of the upper extremity are also to be noted.

Hands are inspected to assess the evidence of denervation and muscular atrophy. This is most evident in the thenar and hypothenar eminence of the palm and in the interosseous muscle of the hand.

Motor function is assessed for all major muscle groups. Grip strength and opponens function of the thumb and fifth fingers will reveal function of the median and ulnar nerves respectively. Sensory examination is performed with light touch for all dermatomes (C6 through T1), bilaterally. Deep tendon reflexes are tested for biceps, triceps, and brachioradialis.

Neurovascular evaluation of the extremity should include several specific observations as to the sensitivity of peripheral nerves, the effect of stress maneuvers on symptoms, the presence or absence of pulses with scalene muscle contraction, and arm elevation.

Tests of nerve sensitivity are performed to establish the presence of compression points along the course of the nerves arising from the brachial plexus.

Erbs point palpation is performed over the scalene muscles.

Tinnel testing is performed by percussing over the median nerve at the wrist at the carpal tunnel, the ulnar nerve at the elbow over the cubital tunnel, and the brachial plexus beneath the scalene muscle (at Erb's point). The patient is asked to report pain or paresthesia as a result of the percussion.

Phalen testing is performed with flexion and extension of the wrist. Again the patient is asked to report pain or paresthesia as result of the exam.

The tests of pulse response to scalene muscle contraction and arm elevation include the Adson maneuver and the AER test.

Adson maneuver is performed bilaterally with hands in lap, head turned, and deep breath holding. The deep breathing activates scalene muscle contraction and may result in reduction or loss of the radial pulse.

Abduction external rotation (AER) maneuver is done with deep breath holding, the head is turned away from the arm being examined, and the arm is raised above the head.

The radial pulse is again assessed for reduction or absence. The subclavian artery should be auscultated for the presence of a bruit. The AER maneuver is more sensitive than the Adson test, but is not as well known.

The tests of musculoskeletal compression include the elevated arm stress test, hyper abduction test, clavicular compression, and pectoralis palpation.

The roos elevated arm stress test (EAST) is performed by having the patient elevate arms and open and close hands repeatedly. The test is often graded by duration (one, three, or five minutes). Patients are asked to report pain, paresthesia, arm heaviness, and fatigue. The hands are evaluated for pallor. The test commonly detects both neurogenic and arterial symptoms. Patients with venous compression may complain of arm swelling or tightness and blue discoloration.

Wright hyperabduction testing is performed by bringing the arms backward from a neutral position. The test places stress on the brachial plexus and elicits symptoms of pain or paresthesia.

Costo-clavicular compression is performed by pressing down on the clavicle or distracting the arm downward toward the feet. This test seeks to elicit pain or paresthesia by compressing the clavicle against the brachial plexus.

Pectoralis and subclavius palpation is performed to elicit tenderness or paresthesia in the extremity which may suggest pectoralis or subclavius muscle impingement relating to the patient's symptoms (Table 3).

7. Diagnostic Testing

Diagnostic testing includes two broad categories of tests. The exclusionary tests and the inclusive tests. The exclusionary tests are required to exclude conditions which

Table 3.   Physical examination tests for TOS.

Erbs point palpation
Tinnel percussion
Adson maneuver
Abduction external rotation (AER)
Elevated arm stress test (EAST. Roos test)
Hyperabduction (Wright test)
Costo-clavicular compression
Pectoralis and subclavius palpation

---

may mimic TOS. These conditions are frequently found to coexist with TOS. They may be severe and require intervention. Their identification allows for informed discussion of expectations with regard to TOS treatments. The inclusive tests are those which are specific to the diagnosis of TOS. A positive result of one of these tests would support the diagnosis of TOS. These tests are performed with the intention of supporting the diagnosis of TOS and often allow prescription of care and prognostication of outcomes.

Exclusionary testing is performed to evaluate the presence of coexisting conditions which may confound the diagnosis of TOS and may require additional intervention in order to alleviate the overall presentation of symptoms. At the very least, an appreciation of the presence of coexisting conditions allows appreciation that treatment of TOS alone may not result in complete relief of symptoms.

The tests included in this group are EMG/NCV, MRI of cervical spine, epidural injection, MRI of shoulder, and shoulder injections. Of these, the MRI of the cervical spine and the EMG/NCV exams are essential due to the observed frequency of cervical and extremity nerve compression in TOS patients.

MRI of the cervical spine is used to assess the presence of disk disease, foraminal stenosis, cord compression, and degenerative disease of the spine. A significant finding of any of these should lead to evaluation by a spine surgeon prior to proceeding with treatment of TOS.

EMG/NCV testing is done in the upper extremity to identify compression of the median, ulnar, and radial nerves in the arm. Most commonly, these are seen at the carpal tunnel and cubital tunnel. A positive test would be the reason for evaluation and treatment. In many instances decompression of the thoracic outlet would precede decompression of the more peripheral lesions. A preoperative appreciation of the presence of these lesions is important in advising a patient about the possibility of postoperative symptoms following TOS surgery.

These tests do not often provide evidence to support the diagnosis of TOS. The test may provide indirect evidence suggesting possible TOS. Most often this is in the form of prolonged f-waves. It is also important to note that a normal EMG/NCV test result does not exclude the diagnosis of TOS.

7.1 *Testing specific to the diagnosis of TOS (inclusive testing)*

Cervical x-rays are a simple yet significant test which leads toward the diagnosis of TOS. The goal of the x-rays is to identify the presence of a cervical rib. The presence of a cervical rib in the setting of appropriate symptoms is highly significant in establishing the diagnosis of TOS. A 15-degree apical-lordotic view of the chest will offset the ribs sufficiently to effectively demonstrate the seventh cervical vertebrae and a cervical rib.

Magnetic resonance imaging (MRI) of the brachial plexus is a specific test to confirm the diagnosis of compression at the thoracic outlet. The brachial plexus MRI evaluates the presence of extraneous mass resulting in compression at the thoracic outlet. Additionally MRI may identify deviation of the normal course of the brachial plexus or edema within the nerves of the brachial plexus. Additionally unusual structural elements such as scalene hypertrophy of scalene muscles may be identified. A more exacting diagnostic MRI is the TOS evaluation MRI which includes the standard MRI of the brachial plexus, but supplements this with MR angiogram of the axillo-subclavian artery and MR venogram of the subclavian vein. These exams are usually done with views of the extremities in both neutral (arms by the side of the torso) and stress (arms elevated overhead) positions. The inclusion of these vascular elements results in increased sensitivity to the exam and offers insight to the frequently observed clinical overlap of vascular and neurogenic symptoms.

Somato-sensory-evoked potentials (SSEP) are a type of nerve conduction evaluation which assess the time a nerve signal takes to travel from the extremity to the cerebral cortex. The nerve signal is stimulated at the hand and recordings are made along the nerve tract (median and ulnar). Recordings are taken at Erb's point (at the base of the neck) and over the spine. The recordings are made with the extremity in both neutral and stress positions. The nerve signal is evaluated for latency (how long it takes to travel) and amplitude (how strong the signal is). In positive examinations, a decrease in amplitude and increase in latency may be seen at Erb's point. This may be accentuated by placing the limb in the stress position.

MAC (medial antebrachial cutaneous) nerve testing is a more recent addition to the diagnostic evaluation. It is highly specific and sensitive for the diagnosis of TOS. In this electrophysiologic exam, electrodes are placed on the forearm and signals are evaluated for amplitude.

7.2 Anterior scalene block

The anterior scalene muscle block is a very specific and sensitive test for TOS. It is the only test which relates anatomical structure with symptoms. In this test a local anesthetic (lidicaine or marcaine) is injected directly into the anterior scalene muscle. The injection is done with some form of guidance (ultrasound, CT, MRI, fluoroscopy, or EMG) to assure that the injection is correctly placed into the muscle. The test requires the patient to report changes in symptoms following injection. The anterior scalene muscle block serves several purposes at once: The block may provide pain relief. A positive block confirms that thoracic outlet syndrome is present. The block serves to illuminate the mechanism of TOS-related pain. A positive result indicates that scalene muscle spasm is central to the pain syndrome and that relief of this spasm will result in relief of symptoms. A positive block also allows prescription of treatments. Based on the result of the block a patient may be a candidate for either BOTOX (botulinum toxin) injection to the anterior scalene muscle or surgical decompression. The BOTOX would be used with the intention of affording her an opportunity to then use physical therapy exercises to stretch the scalene muscle. This may be sufficient to resolve the thoracic outlet syndrome. A positive block also indicates that the patient would be a very good candidate for surgical decompression. Thoracic outlet decompression surgery would be expected to be very effective in relieving symptoms and bringing an end to the TOS. The last goal of the block is to prognosticate outcome with treatment. Based on past experience we would anticipate that a positive block would have a 66% chance of improvement with BOTOX, although the BOTOX effect is expected to last only three to four months. The positive scalene block also predicts a 93% chance of improvement with surgery. This is typically a long-lasting benefit.

Pectoralis minor block is a test similar to the anterior scalene block, but directed at discovery of the impact of pectoralis minor muscle compression in the genesis of upper extremity symptoms. Positive blocks resulting in significant relief of pain or paresthesia would be an indication to proceed with either BOTOX injections or possible surgical intervention.

7.3 Vascular testing

Vascular testing is performed when symptoms suggest possible compression of the axillo-subclavian artery or vein. These have included noninvasive laboratory exams and vascular imaging studies.

7.4 Noninvasive testing

The noninvasive laboratory is often called to perform testing of the upper extremities.

Noninvasive arterial testing includes segmental pressures, digit-brachial index, digit PPG, and upper extremity arterial duplex scan.

Segmental pressure testing refers to use of blood pressure measurements along the length of the upper extremity to assess possible occlusions within the arterial tree.

Digit brachial index is a ratio of blood pressures between an affected digit and the best (between right and left) brachial artery pressure. In normal instances the ratio should be 1.0. In instances when there is occlusion of the arterial tree either in the digit or in the extremity, then the ratio will be reduced.

Digit PPG is a test where pressure cuffs are placed on the finger tips and changes in finger volume with pulse cycle are recorded. It is a sensitive test for acute and chronic occlusion and is frequently used in instances where vasomotor instability such as Raynaud's syndrome is suspected.

Upper extremity arterial duplex scan uses the combination of B-mode imaging and pulse-Doppler scan to assess the arterial blood flow in the upper extremity. These scans are particularly sensitive in their ability to assess the axillary, brachial, radial, and ulnar arteries. The area of the subclavian artery may be difficult at times due to body habitus and the presence of the clavicle and ribs which may limit scanning of certain segments.

7.5 *Stress positioning*

These tests may be performed in a neutral position or in a stress position according to clinical indication. In instances where a static occlusion is suspected (embolus to the hand or thrombosis of the brachial artery) a neutral position exam is adequate. In instances where symptoms are related limb position, then testing in the stress position is indicated.

7.6 *Vascular imaging*

Arteriography is indicated for both diagnostic and therapeutic purposes. Arteriographic imaging modalities include CT angiograms, MR angiograms, and conventional angiograms. While conventional arteriograms are more invasive than the other modalities, they afford the opportunity to treat thrombotic lesion with intra-arterial thrombolysis or angioplasty.

Venography is the most accurate means of assessing axillo-subclavian vein compression or occlusion. The venogram (contrast venogrpahy) may be performed by direct injection of contrast into the veins of the upper extremity. Alternate methods of venography include CT venograms and MR venograms. Of these three, contrast venography is the most cost-effective and is the one which most readily allows assessment of venous flow patterns (direction and velocity). Additionally contrast venography allows the implementation of catheter-directed intervention (thombolsysis or angioplasty) where there may be indicated.

7.7 *Contralateral venography in Paget–Schroetter patients*

Given a very high incidence of significant compression of the vein in the contralateral arm, it is advisable to assess the contralateral axillo-subclavian veins before evaluation is completed. Failure to assess may expose a patient to recurrent DVT in the un-evaluated arm. Studies have indicated that the contralateral vein is compressed in up to 75% of cases. In about 5% of these cases, the compression is considered pre-occlusive and may warrant surgical decompression.

8. Non-Surgical Treatment of TOS

The first step to management of TOS is to identify the extent and severity of symptoms. There is a wide spectrum of severity in the presentations of TOS. Many people have mild symptoms and are able to manage well without seeking medical attention. Most patients who do seek attention have moderate symptoms. These are symptoms that present significant impairment to their ability to function productively. A minority of TOS patients present with severe or advanced symptoms and will require urgent intervention.

A review of inciting events, activities, or actions, or uses of the affected limb which may serve as triggers will help establish both the degree limitation and severity of the presentation. Additionally it may serve to identify interventions which may alleviate the symptoms.

8.1 *Ergonomic assessment of work space*

Workspace ergonomic optimization includes correct lighting, adjustment of desk, chair and computer monitor height relative to the individual size, and the use of hands-free headsets for telephones all help alleviate common workplace problems. More detailed assessment of repetitive movement and mechanical stress may be required, particularly in industrial locations.

Initial care of patients with moderate symptomatic TOS presentations includes consideration of physical therapy, chiropractic care, acupuncture, and massage. Medical attention to associated conditions is particularly important. Patients who have significant comorbid conditions such as auto-immune disorders such as Lupus or rheumatoid disease should be assessed by their physicians to optimize care of these conditions.

8.2 *Physical therapy, pharmacological, pain management*

Alternate therapies for skeletal balancing and muscular tone — chiropractic, yoga, pilates — are available. Alternate therapies for pain relief include acupuncture, massage, and TENs. Pharmacological management often involves non-steroidal anti-inflammatory (SAID), muscle relaxants, narcotics, and neuralgesics. Pain management plays a vital role in relief of symptoms. Pain management physicians have at their disposal a number of interventions including medications, injections, and blocks. Additional modalities include the use of radiofrequency and electrostimulation of involved nerves. Physical therapy may help up to 85% of patients with TOS improve.

9. Surgery for TOS

Surgery is indicated for relief of severe neurogenic symptoms, prevention of recurrent thrombosis, or limb threat. Patients should have attempted and failed physical therapy, and an attempt at pain management. Testing should support the diagnosis, and comorbid conditions should have been assessed prior to proceeding with TOS decompression.

The fundamental goal of surgical intervention is to relieve compression at the thoracic outlet. The compressive elements which constitute the scalene triangle include the anterior and middle scalene muscles and the first rib. Surgery is designed to disrupt this triangle by removing one or all of the elements.

Resection of the anterior scalene muscle is one of the first successful operations devised for relieving thoracic outlet compression. This is performed via a cervical incision. The goal of this operation is to excise as much of the anterior scalene as possible. Particular care is taken to preserve the phrenic nerve which typically runs on the anterior border of the muscle. The advantage of this operation is that it is relatively simple. It allows inspection of the anterior aspect of the brachial plexus. It allows division of anterior and middle scalene muscle fibers which may occasionally interdigitate between the trunks of the brachial plexus. The principal disadvantage is that it allows only limited decompression of the thoracic outlet. Even in the event of a successful operation, the middle scalene and the first rib remain in place. Additionally it does not allow for resection of common ligamentous bands which may course beneath the lower trunks of the brachial plexus. For this reason some patients may find residual symptoms from incomplete decompression.

Resection of the first rib is the alternative to anterior scalenectomy. The first rib serves as the point of attachment for the scalene muscles. Resection of the first rib will effectively release the scalene muscle attachments. In the course of first rib resection, partial scalene muscle resection is commonly performed in order to facilitate removal of the rib. The first rib resection may be approached by way of a supraclavicular (cervical) incision or through a trans-axillary approach. Supraclavicular rib resection has the advantage of being a familiar approach to many surgeons. Like the anterior scalene resection it allows inspection of the anterior aspect of the brachial plexus and attention to interdigitation of scalene fibers. The cervical approach allows for removal of most but not all of the first rib. Many thoracic outlet surgeons advocate this approach for resection of cervical ribs. It suffers the disadvantage of difficult exposure of the most anterior and most posterior elements of the first rib. In cases of subclavian vein compression, an additional infraclavicular incision is required to remove the anterior aspect of the first rib, which may be compressing the vein. Exposure of the posterior portion of the rib requires anterior retraction of the brachial plexus and may account for reports of nerve paresthesias and palsy which may attend this operation.

The trans-axillary first rib resection approaches the rib from its lateral aspect. The operation requires special instrumentation and training. The approach is analogous to laparoscopic surgery in that the operative field is somewhat remote from the incision. The advantages of this approach are that the entire first rib is easily removed with no need to retract the brachial plexus. A more complete assessment and resection of the insertion of the muscles, extraneous muscle, and ligamentous bands is possible. Cervical rib resection may be successfully performed via the trans-axillary approach. Cases of venous compression are readily managed through the trans-axillary approach. The principal disadvantage is the inability to approach the upper portions of the scalene muscle or the brachial plexus. The trans-axillary approach would not allow reconstruction of the subclavian vessels. In this instance the rib resection is followed by re-positioning and then a separate cervical or para-costal incision.

Pectoralis minor tenotomy involves the division of the pectoralis minor muscle tendon before its insertion onto the humerus. The objective of this operation is to relieve compression by the pectoralis minor tendon against the neurovascular bundle as this enters the arm. Its advantage is that it results in minor disability and little postoperative discomfort. Surgical complications are low. The operation has not gained widespread appeal and as such the efficacy has not been widely corroborated.

Vascular reconstruction is frequently required in arterial TOS cases, it is less often required in venous cases. Arterial reconstruction may require graft replacement of an aneurysm or bypass of an occluded arterial segment. More recently hybrid operations have been fashioned where open surgery for rib resection is accompanied by endovascular interventions for repair of aneurysms.

Venous reconstructions are not as common. The indication for venous reconstruction is demonstrated occlusion without recanalization and poor collateralization. In selected cases, the subclavian vein may be repaired with open angioplasty, patch angioplasty, or segmental replacement with a vein graft.

9.1 Surgical complications

Common surgical concerns such as bleeding and wound infection are rare. The most common surgical effects relate to nerve injuries — bruising or transection of the sensory nerve in the region of the surgical incision and approach. Most common of these are numbness of the neck and axilla following surgery. Axillary anesthesia or paresthesia is seen in as many as 30–50% of cases. Most of these are transient and fully recover with time. A few of these nerve injuries are long-lasting.

The second most common surgical injury is to branches off the brachial plexus — the long thoracic nerve and the thoracodorsal nerve. Overall the incidence of these injuries is between 0 and 5% of cases. Phrenic nerve injuries are a concern with cervical rib resection and scalenectomy. The incidence of these injuries is also very low.

9.2 Vascular injuries

Injuries to the major vessels are a rare complication. The subclavian artery and subclavian vein are at risk due to their direct involvement: they are compressed by the scalene muscles and the rib. Vascular surgical technique allows working with these vessels without undue risk of injury.

Pneumothorax and pleural effusions are potential complications to thoracic outlet decompression surgery. Removing the first rib offers the opportunity for pleural disruption, and chest tube evacuation of the thorax may be performed in as many as 25% of cases. Since a pulmonary parenchymal injury is rarely encountered the chest tube is required only for evacuation of the air from the chest and is not a long-lasting item. Pleural effusion may result from rib resection. Drainage may be required in a small number of cases (less than 1%) for relief of dyspnea or pleuritic discomfort.

Complex regional pain syndrome may result from decompression of the brachial plexus. Paradoxically, some patients may respond to the relief of long-standing nerve compression by developing intense burning sensation, hyperalgic pain, and paresthesia. The DRP syndrome may overwhelm the presenting neuralgia, and the onset of this condition may nullify the benefit of relief from thoracic outlet compression. Fortunately this is a rare event. Management consists of pain medication and stellate ganglion blockade.

9.3 *Failure of relief*

Failure to relieve symptoms may be seen in a small number of patients following thoracic outlet decompression. This may be the result of incomplete decompression. It is thought to be slightly more common in patients undergoing anterior scalene resection, but may attend first rib resection. The resolution in these instances is to proceed with further decompression. If the first operation was a scalenectomy, then a first rib resection should be considered. If the first operation was a first rib resection then a scalene muscle resection should be considered. Another consideration which must be taken into account is whether a second cause of pain may be present and unattended. Concomitant compression at the carpal tunnel or cubital tunnel (double crush syndrome) is not an uncommon event. Similarly, neuralgia from cervical spine disease should also be considered. Treatment of the second source of pain should be undertaken where appropriate. Finally, a small number of patients may have chronic centralized pain or one of the associated pain syndromes. In these instances complete resolution of symptoms despite thoracic outlet decompression is unlikely and pain management may be more appropriate.

9.4 *Postoperative care*

Following decompression for TOS, most patients will require a few days hospital stay for pain control. Support with intravenous medication and IV fluids may be necessary for 24 to 48 hours. Provision should be made for anti-emetics as many patients will respond to intravenous analgesics with nausea. A chest x-ray should be routinely reviewed to assess for possible pneumothorax.

On discharge, patients should be sufficiently independent as to be able to attend most self-care functions. Pain medication is anticipated to be necessary on a scheduled basis for the first week or two. Many patients feel sufficiently recovered as to drive after two weeks.

Arm exercises are started within the first three to four days post-op. The initial goal is to preserve range of motion at the shoulder with pendulum and circle exercises. Physical therapy is usually started after the first or second post-op week. The goals of PT are the gradual return to normal range of motion and improvement in strength and posture.

9.5 *Post-intervention assessment*

Following decompression for vascular presentations, noninvasive testing or imaging to assess the outcome is routinely performed. Instances where arterial or venous stenosis resulted in thrombotic or embolic events should be assessed to be certain the stenosis is relieved. Angioplasty is indicated where a significant ($>50\%$) residual stenosis is identified. Past experience indicates that this is necessary in up to 40–50% of cases.

Interval thrombosis may be seen in as many as 10% of venous cases. In these instances the thrombosis responds well to intravenous catheter-directed thrombolytic therapy. Due to the risk of bleeding, imaging and intervention are delayed until after 14 days post-op.

During the post-op evaluation, the contralateral limb should be assessed as well (if it has not already been examined) since as many as 70% of patients will have some degree of compression in their contralateral extremity.

10. Postoperative Outcomes

Results are usually evaluated according to presentation: arterial, venous, and neurogenic.

Neurogenic TOS responds well to surgical decompression. Most results are stratified according to preoperative testing and operation. Patients undergoing transaxillary rib resection and subtotal scalenectomy generally do better than those undergoing anterior scalene resection alone. The difference is between 5 and 15 percentage points and varies amongst reports.

Those whose diagnosis is based on exam and history alone will anticipate between 50 and 70% improvement following surgery. Those whose diagnosis was supported with abnormal electrophysiologic testing will anticipate 75–90% chance of improvement. Those whose response to a scalene muscle block was positive anticipate as much as 94% chance of improvement when undergoing first rib resection.

The vascular indications for surgery are generally considered to have good outcomes. Most patients will resume normal activity with no limitations. When considered from the perspective of preoperative vessel status (patent, chronically occluded, and stenosed) those patients whose vessels were occluded and underwent successful thrombolysis will almost uniformly have restoration of normal vessel patency and function after decompression. Many of those who do not have patent vessels prior to surgery may experience relief of the occlusion with decompression; however some may not. Even in the instance of an occluded vessel, symptomatic improvement is the rule.

10.1 *Re-operation for TOS*

10.1.1 *Complementary decompression: anterior scalenectomy,*
       first rib resection

Both rib resection and scalenectomy present limitations to the efficacy of decompression. Both operations will have an element of overlap — one will supplement the other. A number of patients undergoing first rib resection will ultimately require scalenectomy. A number of patients undergoing scalenectomy will later require first rib resection. The specific numbers vary according to the criteria employed in selecting patients for surgery. In cases where patients are selected based on less stringent criteria, the number with persistent or recurrent symptoms and the number of subsequent complementary surgeries will be greater. Thus secondary operation rates for first rib resection following scalenectomy range from 30% to 15%. Similarly in cases managed with rib resection, about 5–20% may require later scalenectomy.

10.2 *Prognosis of TOS*

Of these patients who improve with surgical decompression, about 30% are cured and have no residual symptoms and about 60% are improved but still may have significant symptoms. For this later group then long-term provision should be made for pain management and physical therapy.

Finally it is important to note that following an initially successful operation there is about a 10–20% risk of recurrent TOS symptoms arising again following an initial thoracic outlet operation. This may require a second operation. Following this we would anticipate similar outcomes as following a first operation.

Ultimately there will be a small number of patients who will not benefit from surgical decompression and will require lifelong pain management and physical therapy. This number is small yet it is difficult to predict who will fall within this category.

Finally it should be evident that patients who present with untreated coexisting conditions will continue to experience symptoms related to these. Some conditions may benefit from intervention (*e.g.*, peripheral nerve compression syndromes), while others may require chronic medical management (*e.g.*, fibromyalgia).

11. Conclusion

Thoracic outlet syndrome is an unusually complex medical condition where disability and pain intersect with anatomy and physiology. The magnitude of disability confronted by surgical care is more severe than that commonly seen in vascular surgery. The patients present with complex problems. The stakes are high — preservation of limb use, alleviation of suffering, restitution of employability, and financial viability. The purely medical issues of diagnosis and treatment are compounded by issues of contiguous pathology and synchronous injury. The result of correct diagnosis and decision is restoration of the patient to healthful life.

References

Axelrod DA, Proctor MC, Geisser ME, Roth RS, Greenfield LJ. Outcomes after surgery for thoracic outlet syndrome, *J Vasc Surg* 2001; **33**(6):1220–1225.

Chang DC, Rotellini-Coltvet LA, Mukherjee D, De Leon R, Freischlag JA. Surgical intervention for thoracic outlet syndrome improves patient's quality of life, *J Vasc Surg* 2009; **49**(3):630–635; discussion 635–637. Epub January 14, 2009.

Gelabert HA, Machleder HI. Diagnosis and management of arterial compression at the thoracic outlet, *Ann Vasc Surg* 1997; **11**(4):359–366.

Hagspiel KD, Spinosa DJ, Angle JF, Matsumoto AH. Diagnosis of vascular compression at the thoracic outlet using gadolinium-enhanced high-resolution ultrafast MR angiography in abduction and adduction, *Cardiovasc Intervent Radiol* 2000; **23**(2):152–154.

Jordan SE, Machleder HI. Diagnosis of thoracic outlet syndrome using electrophysiologically guided anterior scalene blocks, *Ann Vasc Surg* 1998; **12**(3):260–264.

Machanic BI, Sanders RJ. Medial antebrachial cutaneous nerve measurements to diagnose neurogenic thoracic outlet syndrome, *Ann Vasc Surg* 2008; **22**(2):248–254.

Machleder HI. Evaluation of a new treatment strategy for Paget-Schroetter syndrome: spontaneous thrombosis of the axillary-subclavian vein, *J Vasc Surg* 1993; **17**(2):305–315; discussion 316–317.

Makhoul RG, Machleder HI. Developmental anomalies at the thoracic outlet: an analysis of 200 consecutive cases, *J Vasc Surg* 1992; **16**(4):534–542; discussion 542–545. Review.

Roos DB. Transaxillary approach for first rib resection to relieve thoracic outlet syndrome, *Ann Surg* 1966; **163**(3):354–358.

Sanders RJ, Hammond SL, Rao NM. Diagnosis of thoracic outlet syndrome, *J Vasc Surg* 2007; **46**(3):601–604. Review.

Sharp WJ, Nowak LR, Zamani T, Kresowik TF, Hoballah JJ, Ballinger BA, Corson JD. Long-term follow-up and patient satisfaction after surgery for thoracic outlet syndrome, *Ann Vasc Surg* 2001; **15**(1):32–36.

Chapter 14
Complications and their Management Following Vascular Surgery and Intervention

Carolyn Glass and Ankur Chandra

Learning Objectives

- Recognize and understand the common medical perioperative complications associated with patients undergoing vascular surgery and their ideal management strategies.
- Recognize and understand the complications associated with open vascular surgery and their ideal management strategies.
- Recognize and understand the common complications associated with endovascular therapy and their ideal management strategies.

1. Introduction

Medical and surgical complications are an inescapable part of the modern practice of vascular surgery. While continuous efforts are made to prevent or avoid these complications, it is early recognition and management that often differentiates a successful outcome from a fatal result. Although common complications of open vascular surgery have been firmly established, the recognition and management of complications from newer endovascular interventions are evolving. The purpose of this chapter is to provide an overview of complications and their management following vascular surgery and intervention. The chapter is divided into medical perioperative complications, complications of open vascular surgery, and complications of endovascular interventions.

2. Medical Perioperative Complications

Patients undergoing vascular surgical procedures have associated systemic disorders such as atherosclerosis, diabetes, chronic renal insufficiency, and various cardiopulmonary diseases which place them at high preoperative baseline risk. Attention to comorbid factors not only guides intraoperative and perioperative management but also dictates which type of vascular intervention is most safe and optimal for the patient.

2.1 *Cardiac*

The most common cause of perioperative mortality in vascular surgery patients is cardiac related. The risk of a major cardiac complication, including nonfatal or fatal myocardial infarction, unstable angina, congestive heart failure, and arrhythmia, can be calculated using the revised Lee's index risk factor scale. Patients are stratified into low-, intermediate-, or high-risk categories based on the number of risk factors present. Factors leading to increased morbidity include high-risk surgery (open aortic, extra-anatomic bypass, or infrainguinal revascularization), ischemic heart disease, congestive heart disease, cerebrovascular disease, insulin-dependent diabetes mellitus, renal failure (defined by creatinine $>2.0\,\text{mg/dL}$), hypertension, and age >75 years. Vascular patients are considered low risk for a major cardiac complication with no risk factors (0.4%), intermediate with 1–2 risk factors (1–7%), and high with ≥ 3 risk factors (11%).

2.1.1 *Ischemia*

Myocardial infarction (nonfatal and fatal MI) is the most important perioperative outcome measure in determining cardiac morbidity and mortality after vascular surgery. Coronary plaque stability rather than degree of stenosis predicts the occurrence of most acute coronary events. The Cleveland Clinic study reported significant coronary artery disease (CAD) in 36% patients with abdominal aortic aneurysms (AAA), 32% with extracranial carotid disease, and 28% with lower extremity ischemia. Meta-analysis studies show the highest incidence of nonfatal and fatal MI in elective vascular surgeries occurs with infrainguinal revascularization and open AAA surgery.

The American College of Cardiology and American Heart Association (AHA) 2007 guidelines for the perioperative management of patients undergoing vascular surgery is evidence based (Class I — benefit of treatment, Class II — conflicting opinions on treatment, Class III — treatment ineffective or potentially harmful). Results from the Coronary Artery Revascularization Prophylaxis (CARP) trial showed no significant difference in MI-related mortality between patients with stable CAD randomized to preoperative coronary revascularization and observation at 30 days and six years. Class I evidence supports that only patients with active cardiac conditions (defined as unstable angina, decompensated heart failure, significant arrhythmia, or severe valvular disease) undergo preoperative noninvasive cardiac stress testing (treadmill test, dobutamine stress echocardiography, and perfusion scintigraphy). Preoperative angiography or coronary revascularization in vascular surgery patients is indicated for a positive stress test, unstable angina, MI <30 days prior to procedure, left ventricular systolic dysfunction, or a need for valve replacement.

Strict blood pressure and glycemic control along with use of beta-blockers, statins, and antiplatelet agents are imperative in patients with perioperative MI. Prior to 2007, routine beta-blocker therapy (Bisoprolol) was recommended in all patients undergoing vascular surgery at least one week prior through 30 days post-op. The current AHA class I recommendation is to continue beta-blockade if the patient is already on the medication or to start a beta-blocker before vascular surgery only in patients with a positive stress test. Class IIa recommendations support starting a beta-blocker in only high-risk vascular surgery patients. Two recent prospective trials (Metoprolol after Vascular Surgery Study, and Perioperative Ischemic Evaluation Trial) showed minimal or no difference in the incidence of perioperative MI in patients treated with Metoprolol at 30 days and six months. They also showed a concurrent increase in the rate of intraoperative bradycardia and hypotension resulting in a significant increase in death and stroke rates with beta-blockade. The Scandinavian Simvastatin Survival study showed a reduction in MI, stroke, and death with extended release statin therapy initiated at least 30 days prior to the procedure in all patients undergoing vascular surgery. In addition to statin therapy, the American College of Surgeons recommends antiplatelet therapy with 81 mg aspirin given just before and continued after certain vascular procedures for MI risk reduction, embolic protection in carotid interventions, and prothrombotic protection in lower extremity revascularization. The Clopidogrel versus Aspirin in Patients at Risk of Ischemic Events (CAPRIE) study showed superiority of dual antiplatelet therapy over aspirin for the prevention of cardiac events. The current AHA guideline recommends uninterrupted dual antiplatelet therapy with aspirin and a thienopyridine, such as clopidogrel, for a minimum of 30–45 days following percutaneous coronary intervention (PCI) in patients with a bare metal stent and six months to one year following PCI with drug eluting stents.

2.1.2 *Arrhythmia*

The etiology of perioperative arrhythmias is multifactorial. Pre-existing cardiac disease, drug toxicity, hypoxia, intravascular hypervolemia, metabolic derangements, and sepsis may all contribute. Frequently, pre-existing arrhythmias are exacerbated by the stress response of surgery resulting in a surge of catecholamines and inotropic stimulus on cardiac muscle. Supraventricular tachycardias such as atrial fibrillation are most common, but patients may also develop brady- and ventricular tachyarrhythmias. Patients undergoing carotid intervention may experience bradycardia and hypotension due to operative manipulation near the carotid bulb.

Pre-existing or perioperative arrhythmias should be closely monitored with telemetry for a minimum of 24–48 hours postoperatively. All suspected arrhythmias must be confirmed by a 12-lead EKG. Underlying electrolyte abnormalities and anemia should be corrected and accurate home medication dosages restarted. Close attention to anticoagulant dosages in patients with atrial fibrillation and diuretics in patients with pre-existing heart failure are important. Atrial fibrillation causes up to two-thirds of peripheral emboli in the general population. Postoperative patients with persistent atrial fibrillation warrant vigilant postoperative monitoring for symptomatic embolization. Rate control with a beta or calcium channel blockers should be started immediately with new onset of perioperative atrial fibrillation with adjunctive use of intravenous amiodarone for suboptimal control. Prompt treatment of other tachyarrhythmias is necessary to prevent an increase in oxygen demand that exceeds the capability of the coronary artery supply. Unstable supraventricular tachycardia can be treated with several intravenous boluses of adenosine (6 and 12 mg) with or without a continuous intravenous beta-blocker infusion. Patients with persistent bradycardia may require fluid resuscitation, atropine to block parasympathetic effects, or in extreme cases vasopressors with intensive care unit monitoring. Severe bradycardia due to beta-blocker overdose can be treated with an initial bolus followed by continuous infusion of intravenous glucagon.

2.2 Pulmonary

Postoperative pulmonary complications include atelectasis, pneumonia, pulmonary edema, acute respiratory distress syndrome (ARDS), and respiratory failure. The morbidity and mortality of vascular surgery patients is significantly greater in the setting of chronic tobacco use and pre-existing pulmonary disease. Specific procedure-related factors such as incision site, duration of surgery, and type of anesthesia may also contribute to the risk or pulmonary complications.

2.2.1 Nosocomial pneumonia

Pneumonia is the most common cause of death due to hospital-acquired infections. Vogel showed a 3.7% incidence of postoperative pulmonary infectious complications after elective vascular surgery. The highest rate of infection occurred with open abdominal aortic surgery, followed by open thoracic procedures and aortic-iliac-femoral bypass. Pneumonia was also the most common infectious complication after open aortic surgery. Mechanical ventilation was the greatest single risk factor for developing pneumonia (1% risk per day) with colonization frequently occurring within 48 hours of intubation. Nosocomial pathogens identified include *Enterobacter, E. coli, Klebsiella, Proteus, Serratia, Pseudomonas, Acinetobacter*, antibiotic sensitive and resistant *S. aureus*, and *S. pneumoniae*. Other known risk factors include age >70 years, chronic lung disease, large volume aspiration, incision site near chest wall or diaphragm, nasogastric tube, tube feeds, reintubation, antacid therapy resulting in increased gastric pH, and supine positioning.

Patients on mechanical ventilation should be assessed daily using a spontaneous breathing trial for possible weaning or extubation. Initiating appropriate empiric antibiotic therapy increases survival if pneumonia is suspected. Untreated pneumonia increases the risk of developing acute respiratory failure, sepsis, and acute respiratory distress syndrome.

2.2.2 *Reduced mechanical or chemical diaphragm function*

A reduction in lung volume demonstrated by a decrease in functional residual capacity occurs as a result of surgery. The type of anesthesia influences risk for this pulmonary complication. Patients receiving spinal or epidural anesthesia have a 40% decreased incidence of pneumonia and 60% reduction in respiratory depression compared to those receiving general anesthesia. Those patients who do undergo general anesthesia have a three-fold decrease in pulmonary complications with shorter acting neuromuscular agents such as vecuronium. Certain procedures occurring near the phrenic nerve, such as carotid-subclavian bypasses, can result in temporary or permanent hemidiaphragm paralysis from nerve traction or injury (Fig. 1). A reflexive increase in the intercostal and abdominal muscle tone after surgical incision can also reduce diaphragmatic function. The incidence of pulmonary complications is greatest with incisions closest to the diaphragm (thoracic or upper abdominal operations). Other mechanical causes of respiratory failure may include pneumothorax, hemothorax, mucous plug, ascites, or abdominal compartment syndrome.

The positive end expiratory pressure (PEEP) and tidal volumes should be adjusted to prevent alveolar collapse and subsequent ventilation-perfusion mismatch in intubated patients. For those patients not on mechanical ventilation, adequate pain control and use of an incentive spirometer to allow sufficient tidal volume inflow are essential to prevent atelectasis and pneumonia. Conversely, administration of excessive narcotics may depress respiratory function. A symptomatic pneumo- or hemothorax should be drained *via* tube thoracostomy to prevent respiratory compromise and loculation, respectively. Peak airway pressures and bladder scans should be used to closely monitor patients with suspected increased abdominal pressures.

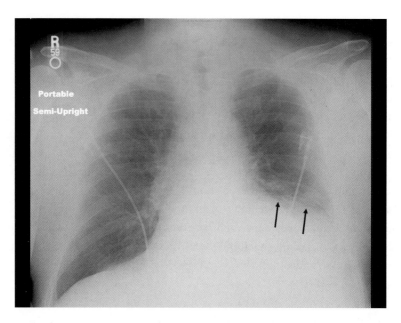

Fig. 1. Anterior–posterior chest radiograph from a patient recently having undergone a left carotid-subclavian artery bypass shows elevation of the left hemidiaphragm (black arrows). This is a result of traction injury to the phrenic nerve and most will regain full left hemidiaphragm function in three to six months.

2.3 *Renal*

Postoperative vascular surgery patients in acute renal failure (ARF) commonly present with sudden oliguria and an elevated creatinine level and are at significant risk for higher morbidity and mortality. Perioperative ARF in vascular surgery patients is most commonly a result of prerenal or renal (parenchymal) causes.

2.3.1 *Prerenal acute renal failure*

Prerenal ARF is due to inadequate perfusion of the kidney and prominent during the perioperative or early post-op period. Intravascular fluid losses, inadequate fluid replacement, and third space sequestration are potential contributors. Vascular patients may also present with prerenal ARF secondary to cardiogenic causes such as left heart failure. Occlusive renal disease (also termed ischemic nephropathy) from chronic atherosclerosis or emboli from vessel manipulation has also been classified as a cause of prerenal failure in vascular surgery patients.

Urinalysis, urine sodium, creatinine concentrations, urine osmolality, and fractional excretion of sodium (FeNa) can be used to diagnose prerenal ARF. A FeNa $<1\%$, urine sodium $<30\,\text{mmol/L}$, and urine osmolarity $>400\,\text{mOsm/L}$ are common. Treatment of hypovolemic prerenal azotemia requires administration of isotonic intravenous fluid. Patients reabsorb extravascular fluid back into the intravascular space by approximately postoperative days 2–3. Fluid administration should be reassessed and adjusted accordingly to prevent fluid overload. Renal dysfunction of cardiogenic origin is treated with afterload reduction, inotropic agents (dobutamine) and diuretic therapy. Fluids should be administered while monitoring cardiac output, central venous, and pulmonary artery wedge pressure. Renal duplex sonography may be used to detect hemodynamically significant renal artery stenosis (renal artery to aortic velocity ratio (RAR) >3.5) or occlusion.

2.3.2 *Parenchymal (renal) dysfunction/contrast nephropathy*

Acute tubular necrosis (ATN) is a dysfunction of the renal parenchyma causing ARF. ATN can be self-limited or result in permanent renal failure. In vascular surgery, ATN is commonly caused by ischemic injury (suprarenal clamp, shock, acute renal artery occlusion, and atheroembolic injury) or toxic insult (contrast dye, medications, and myoglobinemia). The shedding of the cells lining the tubules results in obstruction, interstitial swelling, and disruption of glomerular filtration. An abrupt rise in the serum creatinine, tubular cells in the urinary sediment, and an increase in resistance index are pathopneumonic.

Contrast-induced nephrotoxicity is caused by agents with iodine designed to absorb x-ray photons. The incidence is 1–2% in patients with preoperative normal renal function, but can reach up to 12% in all patients. The risk of nephropathy is directly related to the amount and duration of contrast exposure and pre-existing kidney disease. It is a common practice to limit contrast agents to <50–75 mL per case in patients with a GFR of <20–30 mL/min. Alternatives to contrast exposure include carbon dioxide gas angiography, gadolinium-based angiography, or duplex ultrasound. Patients with GFR <30 mL/min are no longer candidates for gadolinium-based studies due to an increased rate of nephrogenic systemic fibrosis (NSF). The damage occurs at the level of the renal tubules, and patients with pre-existing renal insufficiency or diabetes (specifically type 1) are less likely to recover from contrast injury, requiring permanent dialysis. Preoperative intravenous hydration, with 0.9% saline or sodium bicarbonate solution (3 amps $NaHCO_3$ per liter sterile water), at a rate of 3–5 mL/kg for 1 hour before angiography and continued at 1 mL/kg/hr for six hours after the study is recommended. N-acetylcysteine is also commonly used prophylactically in at-risk patients for its reactive oxygen species scavenger properties (600 mg orally before and after angiography). One study showed a significant reduction in serum creatinine with oral acetylcysteine and hydration compared with placebo and hydration. Current management of parenchymal ARF is largely supportive with dialysis as needed. If long-term hemodialysis is required, attempts should be made to avoid prolonged central venous catheterization and plan for early autologous fistula options.

3. Open Surgical Complications

3.1 *Carotid endarterectomy*

3.1.1 *Stroke*

The goal of carotid endarterectomy (CEA) is to prevent stroke. However, perioperative stroke is itself a major complication of CEA, occurring with an incidence of ~1–3%. The majority of perioperative strokes occur within six hours of procedure and are usually associated with technical problems such as internal carotid artery (ICA) thrombosis or embolism from the endarterectomy site. An intimal flap caused by dissection or residual plaque may result in acute thrombosis of the endarterectomy site (Fig. 2). The risk of developing cerebral ischemia after CEA drops significantly after 24 hours. Some studies report an increased risk of perioperative stroke associated with a distal intimal flap with eversion CEA which employs a transverse arteriotomy and reimplantation of the carotid artery in contrast to a longitudinal arteriotomy for conventional CEA. However, a recent Cochrane review showed no significant differences in the rate of perioperative stroke or death between eversion and conventional CEA (1.7% vs. 2.6%, respectively).

Surgical manipulation, the use of carotid shunts, and atrial fibrillation have all been associated with perioperative stroke due to embolization. Carotid shunts, in particular, have been associated with debris embolization as well as with distal ICA

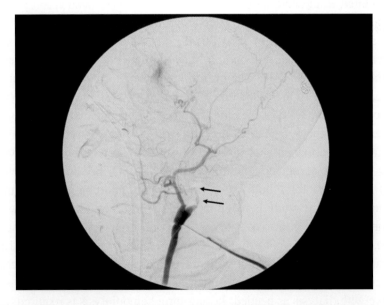

Fig. 2.   Completion angiogram after a carotid endarterectomy shows an absence of flow (black arrows) through the internal carotid artery. This patient underwent immediate thrombectomy and reconstruction of the patch over the carotid bifurcation with good results and no residual neurological deficits.

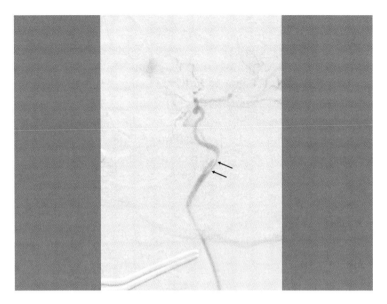

Fig. 3. Cerebral angiogram after carotid endarterectomy reveals a dissection flap (black arrows) in the distal internal carotid artery just below the skull base. This can occur as a result of trauma to the vessel, operative manipulation, or secondary to shunt insertion.

dissection and thrombosis (Fig. 3). A recent prospective randomized trial, however, comparing the results of routine versus selective shunting based on stump pressure measurement showed no differences in the combined perioperative transient ischemic attack and stroke rates between the two groups (2% and 2.9% in the routine and selective shunt groups, respectively). The study concluded the method in which the surgeon is most experienced and comfortable with should be employed. Although rare, other causes of carotid thrombosis may include sticky platelet syndrome, an autosomal dominant platelet disorder characterized by hyperaggregability of platelets in platelet-rich plasma with adenosine diphosphate and heparin-induced thrombocytopenia.

Patients with neurological changes immediately following CEA require immediate operative exploration with or without adjunctive color duplex scanning to detect intimal flaps and/or thrombosis. Patients with early symptomatic thrombosis after CEA at the Cleveland Clinic benefited from immediate surgical management (thrombectomy, thrombectomy and vein patch angioplasty, and thrombectomy of the external carotid artery) with return of neurologic function. If an intimal flap or thrombosis defects are absent on exploration or ultrasound, further acute imaging with a diffusion-weighted brain MRI or emergent intracranial angiography may confirm an embolic ischemia while a noncontrast head CT may confirm intracranial hemorrhage. Emergent intra-arterial clot retrieval with or without thrombolytic therapy is considered for patients with intracranial embolism on cerebral angiography.

3.1.2 Cranial nerve injury

Cranial nerve injuries occur in 2–15% in patients undergoing CEA, with higher incidences reported (up to 30%) when formal pharyngeal studies are performed. Nerve injury was reported to occur in 8.6% of patients in the NASCET trial and 4.9% of patients in the ACAS trial. The majority of cranial nerve injuries are transient with complete recovery in >90% of patients. The vagus or hypoglossal is most commonly injured, followed by the marginal mandibular branch of the facial nerve. The most serious vagal injury results in recurrent laryngeal nerve dysfunction and ipsilateral vocal cord paralysis. Hoarseness and an ineffective cough may be signs of early recurrent nerve injury. Bilateral recurrent laryngeal nerve injury may result in airway obstruction and inability to protect the airway. Because of this concern, simultaneous bilateral CEA is avoided and documentation of normal vocal cord function by laryngoscopy is recommended for those patients undergoing staged CEA. The hypoglossal nerve descends medially and loops over the external carotid anteriorly to innervate the tongue muscles. Injury to this cranial nerve results in ipsilateral tongue palsy. Mobilization of the hypoglossal often requires division of the descending branches of the ansa cervicalis arising from the cervical plexus. Division of the ansa however does not result in any clinically significant neurologic deficit. The marginal mandibular nerve, a branch of the facial nerve, courses along the inferior ramus of the mandible and may drop to the lower neck. Retractor compression against the mandible or direct injury to this nerve results in drooping at the corner of the mouth. Injury to other nerves and adjacent structures may result in dysfunction (Table 1). Fortunately the majority of cranial nerve injuries are transient. Patients

Table 1. CEA CN injury.

Structure	Deficit
CN X (vagus — recurrent laryngeal)	Ipsilateral vocal cord paralysis
CN XII (hypoglossal)	Ipsilateral tongue palsy
CN VII (facial — marginal mandibular)	Ipsilateral facial droop
CN IX (glossopharyngeal)	Swallowing impairment, recurrent aspiration
CN XII (spinal accessory)	Ipsilateral shoulder droop/weakness, winging of scapula
Superior laryngeal	Voice fatigue, high-pitch problems
Greater auricular	Ipsilateral paresthesia or hypesthesia
Sympathetic chain	Horner's syndrome

with glossopharyngeal injury will require aspiration precautions and a permanent feeding tube in severe cases.

3.1.3 *Hyperperfusion syndrome*

Cerebral hyperperfusion syndrome is a rare (<1%) but serious complication after carotid revascularization. The normal brain maintains constant intracranial pressure by cerebrovascular reactivity; the cerebral arterioles constrict or dilate in response to the alterations of blood flow. Patients with extracranial carotid stenosis maximally vasodilate their cerebral arterioles in order to maintain sufficient cerebral blood supply and exhaust the cerebrovascular reactivity regulatory response. Correction of the stenosis restores blood flow resulting in increased perfusion. This absence of cerebral autoregulation coupled with increases in blood flow after CEA causes hyperperfusion of the cerebral arterial circulation. This hyperperfusion is further exacerbated by postoperative systemic hypertension. The cause of postoperative hypertension after CEA is multifactorial but may include pre-existing essential hypertension, elevated cranial norepinephrine levels from perioperative stress, and the use of specific anesthetic agents. Symptoms range from mild, including confusion and unilateral migranous headaches, to severe involving aphasia, epileptic focal seizures, or generalized seizures. Ataxia and visual disturbances may also occur within 24–48 hours of surgery. Symptoms may present several days after revascularization. Noncontrast head CT should be performed in all patients suspected of having hyperperfusion syndrome to evaluate for intracranial hemorrhage and/or cerebral edema. Severe brain edema, intracranial hemorrhage, or death can occur if left untreated.

Treatment strategies are directed toward regulation of blood pressure and limiting rises in cerebral perfusion pressure. A recent review of cerebral hyperperfusion syndrome showed there are few randomized trials comparing optimal perioperative management protocols due to the rarity of the complication. A high index of suspicion is imperative. Intensive care hemodynamic monitoring, control of systemic blood pressure, use of anticonvulsants with onset of seizures, and alleviation of cerebral edema with administration of mannitol are routine. Avoidance of cerebral vasodilating medications such as dihydralazin, nitrate, or calcium channel antagonists is prudent.

3.1.4 *Postoperative bleeding/neck hematoma*

Perioperative and long-term postoperative antiplatelet therapy reduces the risk of perioperative thromboembolic events (stroke or death) by 27% and outweighs any risk of bleeding complications. Current evidence shows aspirin doses of 80–325 mg/day are most appropriate for CEA patients. A recent study showed patients concurrently on clopidogrel can safely undergo CEA without increased risk of hematoma or neurological complications. Intraoperative anticoagulation with heparin reduces the risk of stroke or mortality from thromboembolic events. Recent data from the VSGNNE database showed a decrease in postoperative hematomas when protamine was used to reverse the effects of heparin at the conclusion of CEA. There is no evidence supporting anticoagulation beyond the intraoperative period due to increased bleeding complications unless there are other indications such as a documented hypercoagulable state.

Significant bleeding requiring hematoma evacuation occurs in 1–3% of cases after CEA. A neck hematoma causing tracheal deviation or respiratory compromise warrants immediate evacuation at the bedside or in the OR to prevent airway compromise. Jackson–Pratt drains are placed prophylactically by some to prevent neck hematomas. Youseff *et al.* evaluated the utility of neck wound drains after CEA in a prospective randomized trial and found no benefit in volume reduction in those patients who developed hematoma. A selective policy of drain use after CEA was therefore recommended.

3.2 *Aortic reconstruction*

3.2.1 *Aortic cross-clamping*

Cardiac complications account for the highest cause of mortality after open aortic repair. Proximal aortic clamping causes an abrupt increase in cardiac afterload resulting in hypertension and precipitating ischemia. Administration of vasodilators is required to minimize this complication. Conversely, sudden declamping is associated with hypotension requiring adequate fluid and blood resuscitation. Intraoperative monitoring with arterial pressure measurements, pulmonary capillary wedge pressure, and transesophageal echocardiography is performed by a specialized anesthesia team to assess accurate volume status and optimize cardiac function. Proximal aortic clamping, particularly supraceliac clamping, may also cause distal ischemia and embolization of pre-existing proximal thrombus. Heparin is therefore administered just prior to clamping. To prevent morbid ischemic complications such as renal failure or mesenteric ischemic, the duration of aortic clamping should be limited to under 30 minutes. A supraceliac clamp is moved to the infrarenal aorta as soon as proximal control is gained. Studies show using a long beveled anastomosis during aortic aneurysm repair which obviates the need for reimplantation reduces clamp time and fewer complications.

3.2.2 *Hemorrhage*

Bleeding complications from elective abdominal aortic aneurysm repair occur in 3–5% of cases, and increase with ruptures and thoracoabdominal aortic surgery. Suture line bleeding, commonly from the posterior aspect of the proximal anastomosis, must be identified intraoperatively, preferably prior to removal of the proximal clamp. Calcified or friable vessels with poor wall integrity often require pledgeted sutures to prevent bleeding from adventitial tears. Iatrogenic injury to iliac or left renal veins during difficult exposures may also occur. Venous anomalies such as a retroaortic left renal vein or large lumbar veins are susceptible to aortic clamp injuries and can result in uncontrolled bleeding. If venous anomalies are suspected, meticulous dissection is necessary to prevent inadvertent injury from aortic clamp placement. Endovascular aortic balloon occlusion may also be used for proximal control. In a small percentage of cases, a left renal vein may be circumferential, always demanding clinical suspicion for a retroaortic component. For many iliac vein injuries, division and subsequent repair of the overlying iliac artery may be necessary to control bleeding. With both elective and emergent aortic operations, blood loss may be exacerbated by hypothermia, thrombocytopenia, and dilutional coagulopathy from excessive isotonic fluid resuscitation. Massive transfusion protocols (replacement with a set ratio of platelets, fresh frozen plasma, and packed red blood cells with or without factor VII concentrate) have shown to improve survival.

3.2.3 *Embolization*

Distal embolization occurs with repair of both aneurysmal and occlusive aortic disease. Manipulation of mural thrombus or clamping of heavily calcified arterial segments showers debris, occasionally resulting in symptomatic end-organ ischemia. Visceral emboli commonly lodge in proximal SMA and its branches due to its anatomic caudal angulation. The incidence of mesenteric ischemia after elective aortic aneurysm repair is low (1–2%), but increases to ~3–30% after ruptured AAA repair. The associated mortality of postoperative bowel infarction ranges from 40% to 100% warranting a high index of suspicion. Signs may include abdominal pain and distention, diarrhea, fever, and leukocytosis. Bloody diarrhea occurs in one-third of patients with proven ischemic colitis and mandates prompt flexible sigmoidoscopy if present within 24–48 hours of aortic surgery. Flexible sigmoidoscopy is highly sensitive for detecting ischemic colitis as ischemia occurs within the rectosigmoid colon the majority of the time after aortic surgery. Ischemia involving the mucosal and muscularis layers may be treated with antibiotics and bowel rest. Transmural ischemia (pseudomembranes) requires immediate bowel resection to prevent perforation and sepsis. Fortunately, infarction is infrequent due to the rich collateral networks of the bowel. The meandering mesenteric artery and marginal artery of Drummond both connect the SMA and the IMA. The sigmoid colon also receives collateral circulation from the internal iliac artery *via* the superior rectal artery and from the profunda femoris artery *via* the circumflex femoral if the internal iliac artery is occluded. Celiac or SMA flow integrity should be recognized prior to aortic surgery with CT angiogram or ultrasound. However, the decision to reimplant the IMA is commonly an intraoperative one. An abnormally large IMA and meandering mesenteric artery collateral suggests poor SMA circulation. The IMA is temporarily clamped and backbleeding is assessed after restoring aortic flow. Pulsatile backbleeding through the IMA orifice indicates the IMA can be safely ligated close to its aortic origin. At present, there is no level I evidence recommending routine IMA reimplantation.

Lower extremity ischemia occurs in 1–7% after open aortic surgery. Most of these embolic complications can be divided into large and small vessel involvement. The clinical presentation of small vessel emboli, commonly referred to as "trash foot", results from pre-existing atheromatous debris from occlusive disease or thrombus from the aortic aneurysm sac embolizing distally after aortic mobilization or clamping. These patients frequently have palpable dorsalis pedis or posterior tibial pulses when the forefoot is affected and demarcated. Patchy areas of dusky or "blue toes" mark the areas of microembolization. These patients may experience ischemic toe pain and tissue loss requiring amputation. One review of 1601 aortic reconstructions showed distal embolization occurred in 23 cases followed by aortic aneurysm repair, 13.6% resulting in early amputation and 20.5% delayed amputation. The lower extremities should be routinely inspected intraoperatively (prior to incision closure) for changes in the baseline pulse exam. Systemic anticoagulation should be instigated if embolization is suspected. Large vessel emboli should be treated with operative embolectomy. Contrast angiography may be performed for diagnosis and treatment of persistent ischemia after operative embolectomy. Unfortunately, in small vessel emboli, operative intervention may not be useful due to the small size and distal nature of the obstruction.

3.2.4 *Spinal cord ischemia*

Paraplegia from spinal cord ischemia is one of the most devastating complications of aortic aneurysm surgery, occurring in ∼5–20% of patients undergoing thoracoabdominal aneurysm repair based on extent. Spinal cord ischemia can be precipitated by prolonged aortic clamp with disruption of the collateral blood supply to the spinal cord after graft reconstruction. Blood flow to the spinal cord is received from the anterior spinal artery and two posterior spinal arteries, which are supplied by segmental radicular arteries. The largest of the radicular arteries, the artery of Adamkiewicz, supplies the anterior spinal artery *via* a left intercostal or lumbar artery most commonly arising between T8 and L2. There is minimal collateralization between the anterior and posterior spinal networks so that sufficient anterior spinal artery disruption alone can cause anterior horn ischemia and paralysis. For this reason, paraplegia is observed predominantly during descending thoracic aortic repair where the artery of Adamkiewicz is compromised. Although rare after infrarenal AAA repair, paraplegia due to anatomic anomalies (lower anatomic origin) of the anterior radicular artery or disruption of anterior spinal artery collateral flow *via* the hypogastric arteries has been reported.

Many adjunct strategies have been shown to reduce the risk of spinal cord ischemia. An earlier study showed the incidence of paraplegia was 27% with an aortic cross clamp time of >60 minutes and 8% if <30 minutes. Coselli demonstrated a lower rate of paraplegia in a group of patients who underwent thoracoabdominal aneurysm repair utilizing left heart bypass, but other studies showed no difference. Revascularization of the spinal cord with reimplantation of intercostal arteries is also widely practiced among vascular surgeons. Studies show that re-implantation of significant patent arteries at the T11–T12 level is associated with lower paraplegia rates. Effort should also be made to maintain flow in at least one internal iliac artery to preserve spinal artery collateral vessels.

Spinal cord perfusion pressure is the mean arterial pressure (MAP) minus the cerebrospinal fluid pressure (CSF). CSF pressure rises with ischemia during aortic clamping or reduced MAP. A randomized controlled trial of CSF drainage in patients who underwent type I or II thoracoabdominal aneurysm repair showed a significant reduction in paraplegia rates (13% vs. 2.6%) in the CSF drainage group. The CSF pressure was maintained at 10 mmHg and continued 48 hours after surgery. Both groups had left heart bypass and reattachment of critical intercostal arteries. In patients who develop delayed signs of neurological compromise postoperatively, a CSF drain may be inserted. Cambria demonstrated that epidural cooling reduces the risk of neurological injury in patients who have type I–III thoracoabdominal aneurysm repair. Rises in CSF temperature (reaching 25–28°) during aortic cross clamping were associated with higher rates of cord injury. Unfortunately spinal cord ischemia may still occur in 10–15% of patients after these adjunct strategies have been employed and remains a highly morbid vascular complication.

3.2.5 *Graft infection*

Graft infection after aortic repair occurs in <1% of patients. A recent study of over 12,000 open repairs showed a two-year aortic graft infection rate of 0.19%. The highest risk occurred within the first postoperative year and in patients with septicemia and surgical site infection during the periprocedural hospitalization. Patients with femoral anastomosis are also at higher risk. The standard treatment for an infected aortic graft is extra-anatomic bypass followed by graft excision and local debridement to healthy tissue. A recent meta-analysis, however, comparing extra-anatomic bypass, rifampin bonded prostheses, cryopreserved allografts, and autogenous veins favored *in situ* options over extra-anatomic bypass based on amputation and reinfection rates. Although rare, an aortoenteric fistula can also present as or cause a graft infection. The fistula commonly involves the duodenum and presents in an estimated 5% of patients approximately 10 years after AAA repair. Patients present with fever, GI bleed, and diarrhea. A high index of suspicion is required, and upper endoscopy is the test of choice for accurate diagnosis.

3.2.6 *Impotence*

The para-aortic autonomic nerves course along the left side of the infrarenal aorta near the IMA, and across the proximal left common iliac artery. Impotence or retrograde ejaculation after open aortic surgery may result from injury to these autonomic nerves. This complication has been reported in up to 25% of patients. A recent study reported that the baseline incidence of sexual dysfunction prior to aortic surgery is approximately 30% and doubles over seven years. Postoperative impotence may also be associated with reduced pelvic blood flow due to internal iliac occlusion or embolization. Management is supportive, and therapy with phosphodiesterase inhibitors is frequently ineffective for neurogenic impotence.

3.3 *Peripheral revascularization*

3.3.1 *Graft thrombosis*

Surgical bypass from the femoral artery to the popliteal or tibial arteries is a common revascularization procedure performed to treat complications of peripheral occlusive disease. Compared to aortoiliac disease, infrainguinal vessels are smaller and require longer bypass conduits. Bypass graft thrombosis is the most frequent complication after infrainguinal reconstruction and can be classified into three different time points. Early thrombosis occurring within 30 days of surgery is associated with technical problems involving untreated inflow disease, outflow obstruction, or the conduit itself. Inflow problems may include undiagnosed stenoses, injury from vascular clamping, dissection, narrowing of the proximal anastomosis, sizing mismatch from the proximal (smaller diameter) end of a reversed saphenous vein graft, or unlysed valves from *in situ* vein grafts. Severe tibial disease, clamp injury, dissection, narrowing of the distal anastomosis, and unlysed valves from *in situ* vein bypass grafts are common causes of outflow obstruction. Folding or twisting of the conduit during tunneling and suboptimal vein quality (reversed saphenous vein diameter <3.5 mm, excessive instrumentation for *in situ* saphenous vein, thick phlebitic vein) are other predisposing factors for early postoperative thrombosis.

Thrombosis which occurs one month to one year after surgery may be attributed to cellular changes of the bypass graft or anastomotic sites secondary to intimal hyperplasia. Intimal hyperplasia is triggered by injury followed by vascular smooth muscle proliferation and migration from the media to the intima. This process is mediated by growth factors and cytokines. Injury is multifactorial and may include increased turbulent flow, compliance mismatch, and instrumentation of the conduit. Fibrotic changes of the venous valves in reversed saphenous vein grafts may also cause stenosis, turbulence, and eventual thrombosis. Thrombosis occurring after one year is attributed to the progression of atherosclerotic disease and is increased with the use of prosthetic grafts due to the absence of a true intima with its antithrombotic properties.

Postoperative surveillance of infrainguinal vein grafts with noninvasive duplex scanning is recommended and should be completed every three to six months within the first year to detect stenosis or early signs of graft thrombosis. Percutaneous angioplasty of hemodynamically significant stenoses in the graft body or the anastomotic sites is commonly performed to prevent graft failure. Patch angioplasty may also be completed at the site of stenosis. If thrombosis occurs, percutaneous pharmacomechanical thrombolytic therapy has been used with good results. Surgical thromboembolectomy is also very effective. For chronic thrombosis, a second open revascularization is usually required, with vein as the preferred conduit. Curi *et al.* showed that patients with serologically proven congenital or acquired hypercoagulable states (heparin-induced platelet aggregation, anticardiolipin antibodies, lupus anticoagulant, protein C or S deficiency, antithrombin III deficiency, and factor V Leiden mutation) have inferior long-term patency and limb salvage rates after infrainguinal bypass. Patients with hypercoagulability were younger (63 ± 2 years vs. 69 ± 1 years, p = .007), had more prior revascularization attempts (38% vs. 21%, p = .003), and had chronic anticoagulation therapy after previous surgeries (46% vs. 25%, p = .001). Prosthetic conduit choice was an independent predictor of graft failure (p = .0001) in hypercoagulable patients. Serological screening should be completed in all patients where a high degree of suspicion for hypercoagulability exists.

3.3.2 *Wound infection*

The Szilagyi clinical classification for infection is frequently used to describe postoperative vascular wound infections. Surgical site infection can be confined to the dermis (Grade I), penetrate the subcutaneous tissue without involving the graft material (Grade II), or involve the graft material (Grade III). Wound complications after infrainguinal bypass are frequent (10–40%), and deep wound infections may be limb-threatening and cause sepsis. Multivariate analysis in patients who underwent infrainguinal bypass at the Minneapolis Department of Veterans Affairs Medical Center showed that obesity and the development of a postoperative incisional hematoma were two main independent predictors of wound infection. Surprisingly diabetes mellitus, duration of operation, length of preoperative hospital stay, prosthetic graft placement, and steroid use were not significant. Longitudinal groin incisions have been shown to have a higher associated rate of infection than transverse incisions. Surgical dissection of the profunda femoris artery has been associated with an increase in the risk of lymph leaks. Illig showed a reduced incidence of serious wound complications and shortened postoperative hospital stay in selected patients who underwent lower extremity bypass using endoscopic vein harvest. However in an extension of this study, Julliard *et al.* recently showed no differences in wound complication rates in a larger group of patients with endo harvest compared to conventional means.

The treatment for early deep groin infections is antibiotics and surgical debridement down to healthy tissue. If the graft is involved or exposed, graft excision and extra-anatomic or *in situ* bypass with autologous vein, rifampin soaked or silver impregnated prosthetics, and cryopreserved allografts have been used. If the graft is only partially infected, the patient is not septic, and *Pseudomonas aeruginosa* is not the infecting organism, preservation of the graft may be attempted with debridement, intravenous antibiotics, and muscle flap coverage. Dosluolglu recently reported an alternative treatment method for early deep groin infections (12 grafts Szilagyi III) with the use of vacuum-assisted closure (VAC) therapy without muscle flap coverage. Twenty-two patients with deep groin infections from various procedures including infrainguinal bypass with PTFE and autologous vein, endarterectomy/patch, and extra-anatomic bypass were studied. VAC therapy was started one to six days after operative debridement along with culture-directed antibiotic therapy. All except for two wounds healed (mean, 49 ± 21 days). One patient had bleeding from the anastomotic heel eight days after debridement with subsequent graft removal and *in situ* replacement. The other presented with reinfection on day 117 and underwent extra-anatomic bypass. There was no perioperative mortality or limb loss.

3.3.3 *Graft infection*

The incidence of peripheral graft infections is much lower than wound infection, occurring in 1–10% depending on the location and type of conduit (fem-pop 1–10%, fem-fem 1–4%, fem-tib 2–3%, ax-fem 5–8%). Prosthetic grafts have a higher risk for infection compared to autogenous conduits. Graft infection may occur from perioperative contamination through the surgical wound, seeding from bacteremia, leakage from lymphatic sources, direct contact from an adjacent infectious process, or through fistulization (Fig. 4). Any microorganism can potentially cause graft infection (bacteria, yeast, and fungi). *Staphlococcal species* is the most prevalent pathogen, with methicillin-resistant *S. aureus* (MRSA) accounting for 25% of

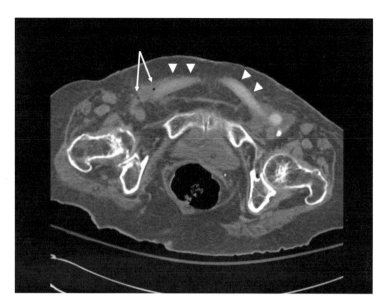

Fig. 4. CT angiogram of the pelvis of a patient having undergone a femoral-femoral bypass (white arrowheads) shows both fluid and air bubbles (white arrows) surrounding the graft. These findings are highly suspicious of a graft infection. This diagnosis must be aggressively pursued with either further imaging and laboratory studies or operative exploration.

early prosthetic graft infections. *S. epidermidis* (coagulase negative staphylococci) is present on normal skin flora and has a strong affinity for biofilm on prosthetic surfaces. Infection with this organism is common, isolated on 50–70% of thrombosed grafts and 80% with anastomotic aneurysms associated with infection. *S. epidermidis* graft infections are indolent and late appearing. The diagnosis of a *S. epi* graft infection is difficult as the gram stain is routinely negative. Identification of *S. epi* requires sonication of the biofilm for organism isolation. Infection from Gram-negative bacteria such as *E. coli*, *Pseudomonas*, *Klebsiella*, *Enterobacter*, and *Proteus* species occur earlier (within three to four months) and are highly virulent. These infections are likely hospital acquired, and patients present with sepsis, bacteremia, and serious wound infections (Szilagyi grade III).

Stewart *et al.* examined the effectiveness of specific perioperative strategies to prevent graft infection in patients undergoing peripheral arterial reconstruction. Meta-analysis of 34 randomized trials (prophylactic systemic antibiotics, rifampicin bonded grafts, preoperative skin antisepsis, and suction wound drainage) showed that prophylactic systemic antibiotics reduced the risk of wound infection and early graft infection, and antibiotic prophylaxis for >24 hours appeared to be of no added benefit. There was no evidence of decreased wound and graft infection rates with prophylactic rifampin bonded Dacron grafts, suction groin wound drainage, or preoperative bathing with antiseptic agents.

Appropriate treatment for an infected graft is dependent on a combination of factors including organism virulence, extent of graft infection, and patient's clinical status (sepsis and bleeding). Patients with sepsis or anastomotic disruption require urgent intervention with aggressive debridement of infected tissue, removal of the entire graft, and revascularization with extra-anatomic bypass or *in situ* graft replacement. Delay in removing the infected graft in critically ill patients is not recommended. If the initial indication for the bypass graft was disabling claudication, revascularization may be delayed until the patient is more stable.

Local treatment of partial graft infections with aggressive perigraft tissue debridement without graft excision, antibiotic use, and muscle flap coverage is reasonable. Multiple small series have shown healing occurs in approximately 70% of cases with local treatment and does not harm the patient given he or she does not exhibit signs of sepsis or anastomotic disruption.

3.4 *Hemodialysis access*

3.4.1 *Ischemic steal syndrome*

Distal ischemic steal syndrome refers to hypoperfusion to the hand after dialysis access placement. Excessive arterial flow to the venous segment of the fistula "steals" perfusion from the hand resulting in palor, pain, paresthesia, paralysis, or tissue loss. This occurs more commonly when the venous anastomosis is located more proximally on arteries with larger diameters, such as the brachial artery. Undiagnosed inflow disease to the hand from arterial occlusive disease either proximal to the fistula anastomosis may also cause steal symptoms. Pain or paresthesia occurs in 10–20% of cases, and more serious symptoms such as tissue loss and motor dysfunction requiring immediate intervention occur in 3–5%. Patients with diabetes, multiple access procedures, constructions based on proximal arteries, and female gender are more prone to ischemia.

Doppler ultrasound evaluation of the inflow artery with finger pressures and waveform analysis can be performed before creation of a fistula as a preventative measure. If steal occurs however, balloon angioplasty may be used for inflow artery stenosis in mild cases. Other operative techniques include banding or ligation of venous collaterals, distal revascularization, and interval ligation (DRIL) or as a last resort, ligation of the fistula. In the DRIL procedure, the greater saphenous vein is commonly used as a bypass conduit to make a proximal anastomosis at the proximal brachial artery and a distal anastomosis immediately distal to the fistula anastomosis. The brachial artery immediately proximal to the distal bypass anastomosis is then ligated. A recent study of 64 DRIL procedures reported relief of ischemic symptoms in 78% of cases. Residual symptoms included paresthesia in 13%, pain in 5%, tissue loss in 4%, and motor deficit in 2%. The secondary DRIL patency rates were 81%, 76%, and 76% at one year, three years, and five years, respectively.

3.4.2 *Bleeding*

Bleeding from the access site after renal replacement therapy (RRT) is one of the most common complications dialysis patients will present with in the urgent care or emergency room. This is a potentially life-threatening complication and requires urgent diagnosis and management. With profuse arterial bleeding, rupture of a pseudoaneurysm should be suspected. Repeated punctures at the same site of a dialysis graft or vein during RRT can result in a pseudoaneurysm (Fig. 5). If not evident on clinical exam, duplex ultrasound can be used to identify a pseudoaneurysm. Because fistulas are a high-flow, low-pressure system direct pinpoint pressure of the bleeding site using a finger, rather than large sandbags or IV bags, is much more efficient to control the initial bleeding. Primary repair or replacement with an interposition graft is necessary for bleeding pseudoaneurysms.

3.4.3 *Central venous stenosis*

Central venous obstruction, frequently of the innominate and subclavian veins, results from repeated catheterization by central lines (40–50% of patients with subclavian lines develop central stenosis) or chronic intimal changes from high-flow turbulence. Outflow venous obstruction results in venous hypertension, edema and pain

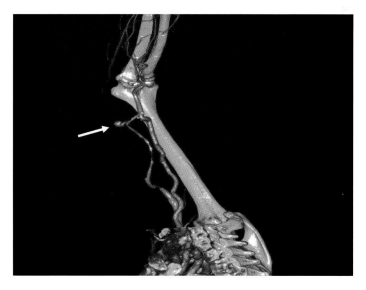

Fig. 5. This three-dimensional reconstruction of a CT angiogram of the upper extremity shows a patent brachiobasilic arteriovenous fistula with a distal pseudoaneurysm (white arrow). These commonly form secondary to multiple punctures and inadequate hemostasis after removal of dialysis cannulas.

of the upper extremity, and eventual dysfunction of the distal fistula. Endovascular intervention with balloon angioplasty with or without stent placement, subclavian vein to right atrial bypass, and superior vena cava or innominate reconstruction using a spiral saphenous vein graft have all been reported as treatment options for central venous stenosis. In a small percentage of patients, dialysis patients may have extrinsic compression of the thoracic outlet requiring first rib or claviculectomy decompression to alleviate the central obstruction.

4. Endovascular Complications

4.1 *Carotid stenting*

Similar to carotid endarterectomy, carotid angioplasty and stenting (CAS) is performed to prevent a stroke from occurring but has the potential to cause inadvertent strokes as a result of the procedure itself. The peri-procedural life-threatening stroke rate associated with CAS has been shown in multiple trials to be similar to that of carotid endarterectomy. Recent evidence, however, shows that CAS has a higher rate of minor strokes. Further studies attribute this higher rate of minor strokes to microemboli which are released during the angioplasty and stent placement. MRI studies from patients, especially elderly patients >80 years old, who have undergone CAS, show multiple small areas of infarcts which have been linked to a more rapid decline in cognitive function as they age. If CAS results in intraprocedural internal carotid artery or middle cerebral artery thrombosis/occlusion, immediate interventional neurorescue therapy is mandatory. This may include mechanical clot retrieval and/or thrombolysis as is standard in the setting of acute strokes. Often patients may experience clinical cerebral ischemia, including slurred speech, loss of consciousness, or hemiparesis, during the procedure at times such as balloon inflation and stent placement. Treatment usually involves rapidly completing the procedure and removal of any embolic-protection device in place, followed by a diagnostic angiogram to look at the results. On completion of angiography, defects such as carotid dissections from catheter and wire manipulation, spasm of the internal carotid artery from embolic-protection devices, or evidence of distal emboli causing regional filling defects must be dealt with on a case-by-case basis but have the potential for catastrophic outcomes.

4.2 *Aortic aneurysm repair*

4.2.1 *Access site complications*

Femoral access for endovascular aortic aneurysm repair is obtained through a cutdown or percutaneous approach. A recent meta-analysis of 22 studies using the percutaneous approach reported an arterial closure success rate of 92%, access related complication rate in 4.4%, and reduced operative time. Whether to use the cutdown or percutaneous approach is surgeon dependent. Access site issues are the most common complications with endovascular procedures, most frequently occurring at the common femoral artery and its bifurcation. These complications include groin hematoma, pseudoaneurysm, arteriovenous fistula, and less commonly acute arterial occlusions. Groin hematomas cause severe pain, progressive edema, and occasionally necrosis of the overlying skin, all which are indications for evacuation. Groin puncture may also result in a retroperitoneal hematoma when bleeding enters the fascia of the iliopsoas muscle commonly due to a posterior arterial wall puncture. The hematoma compresses the psoas muscle which contains the lumbar plexus and may cause compression neuropathy. Thigh pain, numbness, or quadriceps weakness results from femoral nerve compression requiring urgent hematoma evacuation and repair of the arterial puncture site.

Hematomas may be associated with a pseudoaneurysm in 1% of cases and should be further studied with duplex ultrasound. A pseudoaneurysm represents bleeding contained by the surrounding soft tissue due to failure of hemostasis at the arterial puncture site. A duplex examination of the pseudoaneurysm can detect the source, size, and neck type (wide or long). Small pseudoaneurysms spontaneously thrombose either with time (2–4 weeks) or with direct compression (~20 minutes duration) of the pseudoaneurysm neck with the ultrasound transducer. However, direct compression using the ultrasound probe causes patient discomfort and is considered labor intensive. If pseudoaneurysms have sufficiently long necks, duplex-guided thrombin injection is commonly used to thrombose the pseudoaneurysm sac.

Although rare, an inadvertant puncture of the profunda femoral artery and the profunda vein may result in an arteriovenous fistula. The incidence is <1% with cardiac catheterizations and the majority are asymptomatic not requiring treatment due to small shunt volumes. Duplex ultrasound confirms the presence of a fistula with a characteristic systolic–diastolic flow pattern in the venous system. However with endovascular aortic repair, the catheter and sheath sizes are much larger, and interventionalists should be aware of this possible complication. Fistula ligation is necessary in high-flow states causing enlargement, limb ischemia, and high-output cardiac failure. The role of covered stents in traumatic fistulae is not clearly defined but has been used successfully as a treatment option.

4.2.2 *Endoleaks*

An endoleak is defined as persistent blood flow into the aneurysm sac after the deployment of an endovascular aortic stent graft, resulting in persistent blood flow in the sac. A type I endoleak results from incomplete sealing of either the proximal (Ia)

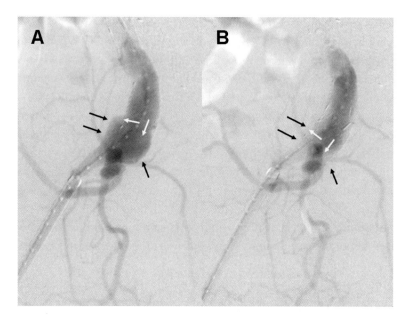

Fig. 6. This patient had undergone endovascular repair of an aortoiliac aneurysm. He was noted to have developed a distal Type I (Ib) endoleak. The operative angiogram (A) shows a leak at the distal iliac attachment site with flow (black arrows) outside of the graft body (white arrows). An aortic extension cuff was placed and the post-implantation angiogram (B) shows no further flow (black arrows) outside of the newly placed cuff (white arrows).

or distal end (Ib) of the stent causing perigraft leakage of blood into the aneurysm sac (Fig. 6). A type II endoleak results from retrograde flow into the AAA sac from patent lumbar, inferior mesenteric, or hypogastric arteries. A type III endoleak occurs with component separation of the stent graft modules, and a type IV endoleak occurs from porosity of the stent graft. A type V endoleak describes a persistently enlarging sac presumed to be caused by persistent flow but without a source that can be confirmed with radiological imaging.

Types I and III endoleaks are usually evident on an intraoperative completion angiogram and are fixed immediately due to the continued risk of aneurysm rupture if left untreated. Balloon angioplasty is attempted to improve apposition of the distal or proximal stent sites to the aortic wall. If needed, extension modules, cuffs, or additional stents are used to cover the leaking areas. Aburhama recently correlated aortic neck length with endoleaks in 238 patients. Aortic neck length was classified into ≥ 15 mm, 10–14 mm, and <10 mm and early type Ia endoleaks occurred in 12%, 42%, and 53%, respectively ($p < .001$). Endovascular aneurysm repair is still plausible with a short aortic neck but is associated with a significantly higher need for proximal aortic cuffs.

Type II endoleaks are the most common and are treated either conservatively with imaging surveillance or intervention. If the type II endoleak persists with concurrent increase in aneurysm sac size, intervention is favored. Coil embolization of backbleeding vessels is attempted through the translumbar, transcaval, or transarterial approach. Laparoscopic ligation has also been used to treat type II endoleaks, but usually after unsuccessful attempts with embolization techniques. Patients with endovascular aortic aneurysm repair require lifelong surveillance with CT angiography or duplex ultrasound. One recent study showed patients with an intraoperative type I or II endoleak were more likely to have an endoleak at 1.5 years (31.4% vs. 21.6%, p = .02) and required more frequent reintervention. The authors concluded there should be a high degree of suspicion during follow-up in this subset of patients.

4.2.3 *Distal embolization*

Manipulation of endovascular devices such as wires and catheters within the sac during aneurysm repair can result in end-organ damage from embolization to any first-order aortic branches. Embolic debris can lodge in the renal, visceral, or lower extremity arteries. Unnecessary proximal manipulation of endovascular grafts can cause an embolic stroke. Renal failure and bowel infarction due to embolization significantly increase morbidity and mortality. Vigilant monitoring of urine output, creatinine levels, and electrolytes are imperative with injured kidneys to assess the need for dialysis. Serial abdominal exams and lactate levels are important in patients with suspected visceral embolization to detect ischemic bowel and prevent sepsis. As discussed in the open aortic surgery section, flexible sigmoidoscopy is highly sensitive for detecting ischemic colitis within the rectosigmoid colon the majority of the time after aortic surgery. Presence of transmural bowel ischemia mandates resection.

Lower extremity embolization and ischemia have been associated with patients with large mural thrombus at the time of aortic stent deployment. Thompson compared the incidence of distal lower extremity embolization in patients who underwent conventional open versus endovascular aortic aneurysm repair and showed a significantly greater number of gaseous, particulate, and total emboli in the endovascular group compared with the conventional group (p < 0.05) based on sample volume length (emboli velocity × duration = sample volume length). Distal lower extremity embolization requires immediate initiation of anticoagulation, with surgical embolectomy being the gold standard to prevent major amputation.

4.2.4 *Coverage of aortic branches*

End-organ ischemia occurs with inadvertent stent graft coverage of the renals or mesenteric arteries. Proximal stent graft migration, inaccurate stent deployment, and unfavorable aortic neck morphology may lead to this complication. Due to the low incidence, most reports of treatment options are anecdotal. Endovascular techniques can initially be attempted to reposition the stent graft. These include pulling down the graft with kissing balloons, the cross-over wire pull-down technique, and renal stenting using selective catheterization from the upper extremity. Open hepatorenal, splenorenal, iliorenal, or mesenteric bypasses are necessary if revascularization is unsuccessful with endovascular techniques.

4.2.5 *Iatrogenic aortic dissection/rupture*

Although uncommon, guide wires can cause iatrogenic aortic dissection and full thickness tears (rupture) during endovascular repair. Dissection occurs when an intimal tear directs blood flow between the intimal and medial layers resulting in a pressurized false lumen and compressed true lumen. Stanford type A dissections originate in the ascending aorta while Stanford type B originate distal to the left subclavian artery and are confined to the descending thoracic and abdominal aorta. Type A dissections are more common during and following endovascular repair of thoracic aortic aneurysms. Based on the data from the International Registry of Acute Aortic Dissection (IRAD) study, mortality is greatest with cardio-aortic complications such as aortic rupture into the pericardium and acute aortic regurgitation (41.6%). False lumen obstruction of the visceral vessels from a Type B dissection resulting in mesenteric ischemia is also associated with high mortality (13.9%). Iatrogenic Stanford type A dissections may be treated with endovascular or open surgery, depending on the location of the intimal tear entry site. Involvement of the ascending aorta and aortic valve will require open surgery. If the intimal tear is distal to the left carotid artery, endovascular repair with a covered and uncovered stents may be sufficient to prevent further dissection and induce thrombosis of the false lumen.

Iatrogenic aortic ruptures are rare but have been cited in the interventional cardiac catheterization and vascular literature. Traumatic aortic tear is highly lethal in the polytrauma population, and 80–90% of patients die before reaching the hospital. The Parmley Classification for Thoracic Aortic Tears is commonly used to predict mortality; Grades 1 (intimal hemorrhage) and 2 (intimal laceration with intimal hemorrhage) tend to heal spontaneously. Grades 3 (laceration in the media layer), 4 (complete transection), 5 (false aneurysm formation), and 6 (complete transection with periaortic hemorrhage) aortic tears warrant immediate open or endovascular repair. Outcomes for iatrogenic injury are less dismal due to quick accessibility (e.g. patient is already on the table) and lack of comorbid head and visceral trauma. A few randomized clinical trials comparing open versus endovascular repair of traumatic thoracic aortic ruptures have shown clear benefit of the latter approach due to avoidance of thoracotomy, one-lung ventilation, cardiopulmonary bypass with heparin use, and aortic cross clamping. Open repair mortality is >20% compared to 0–6% with the endovascular approach.

4.2.6 *Iatrogenic iliac artery dissection/rupture*

Successful passage of large-sized endovascular sheaths for aortic repair requires adequate femoral and iliac artery vessel diameters, anatomy, and caliber. Young, healthy trauma patients requiring aortic stents grafts usually have nondiseased vessels but may present with hemorrhagic shock and arterial vasospasm. Elderly patients undergoing aneurysmal repair have adequate vessel diameter size but tortuous, heavily calcified arteries increasing the risk of embolization, dissection, and in extreme cases iliac rupture. The caliber of the access vessels can be determined by CT angiogram prior to elective cases and should be reviewed to ensure adequate device-appropriate size ($\geq$7 mm). A retroperitoneal conduit can be placed to prevent iliac dissection and rupture in the majority of cases. Recognition of iliac artery rupture may be delayed due to the tamponade effect of the sheath. When rupture is suspected, maintaining guide wire access is crucial to gain control of bleeding with balloon occlusion so the rupture can be treated.

4.3 *Peripheral intervention*

4.3.1 *Distal vessel embolization/thrombosis*

Occlusive peripheral arterial disease occurs most frequently in the lower extremity at the level of the superficial femoral artery near the adductor hiatus. A variety of endovascular devices have been employed to attempt restoration of flow in severe claudicants and patients with critical limb ischemia. Atherectomy catheters, standard percutaneous balloon angioplasty (PTA), cutting balloons, and a variety of stents have all been widely used. The potential for distal vessel embolization exists with all of these interventions. The AHA Task Force on PTA Guidelines published complications among 3700 patients and reported access site bleeding (3.4%), PTA site thrombosis (3.2%), and distal vessel embolization (2.3%) as most common. Limb loss occurred in only 0.2% after PTA in this review.

Anticoagulation with percutaneous or open embolectomy should be attempted to treat acute limb-threatening ischemia in patients with intra- or post-procedural embolization. A recent study showed patients who underwent thromboembolectomy of the dorsalis pedis and perimalleolar posterior tibial arteries in less than four hours of their original operation had 100% patency and limb salvage at a mean follow-up of 3.0 years. Treatment delay of seven to ten days resulted in progressive foot ischemia requiring bypass to preserve the limb. Percutaneous thromboembolectomy with clot retrieval catheters with or without adjunctive thrombolysis has been successful in treating acute embolization or thrombosis without conversion to open surgery. Rarely, embolization or arterial thrombosis results in severe ischemia requiring distal amputation.

4.3.2 *Access site complications*

Femoral puncture site complications are similar to those discussed in the aortic endovascular repair section. Upper extremity access complications can include the brachial and radial arteries. Hematomas involving the brachial and axillary sheaths can be particularly dangerous. Patients who have axillary or brachial sheath hematomas with concurrent paresthesias in the ipsilateral hand must undergo emergent operative decompression and hematoma drainage. Failure to recognize this complication can result in permanent damage to the nerves innervating the distal arm and hand causing permanent paresthesias or paralysis. Brachial artery thrombosis can be treated with cutdown and immediate thrombectomy. Radial artery thrombosis is acceptable if the dominant ulnar artery is patent.

4.3.3 *Stent mechanics*

The use of intraarterial stents as a primary treatment or adjunctive to balloon angioplasty is accompanied by complications related to both the stent and its delivery to the site of disease. Frequent flexion/extension of the treated arterial segment can lead to stent fracture resulting from metal fatigue. This occurs primarily in locations of bending and twisting of the extremity such as superficial femoral artery, popliteal artery, and axillo-subclavian artery. Metal fatigue and subsequent failure can occur in stents of both nitinol and stainless steel composition. Fracture often leads to restenosis and/or occlusion (Fig. 7). Treatment of such stents commonly requires repeat angioplasty and stenting to regain patency or open bypass if patency of the arterial segment cannot be achieved with percutaneous methods. Another common complication of stent use is misdeployment or delivery device failure. This occurs more with self-expanding stents and less commonly with balloon-expandable stents due to the pre-mounted, precise delivery available with the balloon-expandable variety. Failure to properly deploy a self-expanding stent is most commonly due to failure to properly prepare and flush the stent deployment system with saline. If a stent is not able to be deployed or is in an incorrect location, all attempts should be made to remove it from the artery. In situations where it cannot be removed, it should be deployed in the safest area in proximity. This may require repeat angioplasty or placement of a new stent within the misdeployed stent if concern over stent structure exists.

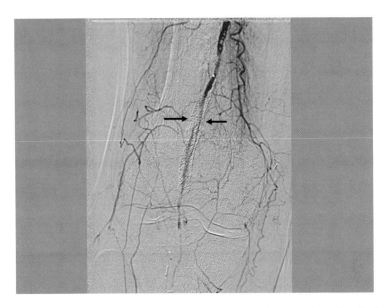

Fig. 7. This patient with rest pain of her lower extremity underwent angioplasty and stenting of a distal femoral and popliteal artery occlusion. On follow-up angiogram done for recurrent pain, the previously placed stent in her popliteal artery is fractured (black arrows) with subsequent thrombosis and repeat occlusion of her popliteal artery. She underwent repeat angioplasty and stenting of this segment to regain patency.

References

Abbott WM, Maloney RD, McCabe CC. Arterial embolism: A 44-year perspective, *Am J Surg* 1982; **143**:460–464.

Aburahma AF, Campbell J, Stone PA, Nanjundappa A, Scott Dean L, Keiffer T, Emmett M. Early and late clinical outcomes of endovascular aneurysm repair in patients with an angulated neck, *Vascular* 2010; **18**(2):93–101.

Aburahma AF, Stone PA, Hass SM, Dean LS, Habib J, Keiffer T, Emmett M. Prospective randomized trial of routine versus selective shunting in carotid endarterectomy based on stump pressure, *J Vasc Surg* 2010; **51**(5):1133–1138.

Ahn S, Marcus D, Moore W. Post-carotid endarterectomy hypertension: Association with elevated cranial norepinephrine, *J Vasc Surg* 1989; **9**:351–360.

Alkon JD, Smith A, Losee JE, Illig KA, Green RM, Serletti JM. Management of complex groin wounds: preferred use of the rectus femoris muscle flap, *Plast Reconstr Surg* 2005; **115**(3):776–783.

Amabile P, Collart F, Gariboldi V, Rollet G, Bartoli JM, Piquet P. Surgical versus endovascular treatment of traumatic thoracic aortic rupture, *J Vasc Surg* 2004; **40**(5):873–879.

Andersen J. Sticky platelet syndrome, *Clin Adv Hematol Oncol* 2006; **4**(6):432–434.

Assadian A, Senekowitsch C, Hagmüller GW, Lax J, Hübl W. Effects of enoxaparin and unfractionated heparin on platelet activity and reactivity during carotid endarterectomy, *Vascular* 2008; **16**(3):161–166.

Bakken AM, Protack CD, Saad WE, Lee DE, Waldman DL, Davies MG. Long-term outcomes of primary angioplasty and primary stenting of central venous stenosis in hemodialysis patients, *J Vasc Surg* 2007; **45**(4):776–783.

Bakker-deWekker P, Alfieri O, Vermeulin F, *et al.* Surgical treatment of infected pseudoaneurysms after replacement of the ascending aorta, *J Thorac Cardiovasc Surg* 1984; **88**:447.

Bandyk DF, Bergamini TM, Kinney EV, *et al. In situ* replacement of vascular prostheses infected by bacterial biofilms, *J Vasc Surg* 1991; **13**:575.

Bandyk DF, Berni GA, Thiele BL, *et al.* Aortofemoral graft infection due to *Staphylococcus epidermidis*, *Arch Surg* 1984; **119**:102.

Bandyk DF, Novotney ML, Back MR. Expanded application of *in situ* replacement for prosthetic graft infection, *J Vasc Surg* 2001; **34**:411.

Bandyk DF. Infection of prosthetic vascular grafts. In: Rutherford RB (Ed.), *Vascular Surgery*, 5th edition, St. Louis: CV Mosby, 1995, p. 566.

Bandyk DF. Vascular graft infections: Epidemiology, microbiology, pathogenesis, and prevention. In: Bernhard VM and Towne JB (Eds.), *Complications in Vascular Surgery*, St. Louis: Quality Medical, 1991, pp. 223–234.

Barr JD, Horowitz MB, Mathis JM, *et al.* Intraoperative urokinase infusion for embolic stroke during carotid endarterectomy, *Neurosurgery* 1995; **36**:606–611.

Bauer SM, Cayne NS, Veith FJ. New developments in the preoperative evaluation and perioperative management of coronary artery disease in patients undergoing vascular surgery, *J Vasc Surg* 2010; **51**(1):242–251.

Benzel E, Hoppens K. Factors associated with postoperative hypertension complicating carotid endarterectomy, *Acta Neurochir (Wien)* 1991; **112**:8–12.

Berman SS, Gentile AT, Glickman MH, Mills JL, Hurwitz RL, Westerband A, Marek JM, Hunter GC, McEnroe CS, Fogle MA, Stokes GK. Distal revascularization-interval ligation for limb salvage and maintenance of dialysis access in ischemic steal syndrome, *J Vasc Surg* 1997; **26**(3):393–402.

Bjorck M, Bergqvist D, Troeng T. Incidence and clinical presentation of bowel ischaemia after aortoiliac surgery-2930 operations from a population-based registry in Sweden, *Eur J Vasc Endovasc Surg* 1996; **12**:139.

Bove E, Fry W, Gross W, Stanley J. Hypotension and hypertension as consequences of baroreceptor dysfunction following carotid endarterectomy, *Surgery* 1979; **85**:633–637.

Braunwald E, Califf RM, Cannon CP, *et al.* Redefining medical treatment in the management of unstable angina, *Am J Med* 2000; **108**:41–53.

Brewster DC, Franklin DP, Cambria RP, *et al.* Intestinal ischemia complicating abdominal aortic surgery, *Surgery* 1991; **109**:447.

Browner WS, Li J, Mangano DT. In-hospital and long-term mortality in male veterans following non-cardiac surgery. The Study of Perioperative Ischemia Research Group, *JAMA* 1992; **268**:228–232.

Calligaro KD, Veith FJ, Yuan JG, *et al.* Intra-abdominal aortic graft infection: Complete or partial graft preservation in patients at very high risk, *J Vasc Surg* **38**:1199.

Cambria RP, Davison JK, Zannetti S, L'Italien G, Brewster DC, Gertler JP, Moncure AC, LaMuraglia GM, Abbott WM. Clinical experience with epidural cooling for spinal cord protection during thoracic and thoracoabdominal aneurysm repair, *J Vasc Surg* 1997; **25**(2):234–241.

Cao PG, de Rango P, Zannetti S, Giordano G, Ricci S, Celani MG. Eversion versus conventional carotid endarterectomy for preventing stroke, *Cochrane Database Syst Rev* 2001.

Caro JJ, Migliaccio-Walle K. Generalizing the results of clinical trials to actual practice: the example of clopidogrel therapy for the prevention of vascular events. CAPRA (CAPRIE Actual Practice Rates Analysis) Study Group. Clopidogrel versus Aspirin in Patients at Risk of Ischaemic Events, *Am J Med* 1999; **107**(6):568–572.

Centers for Disease Control and Prevention. Guideline for prevention of nosocomial pneumonia, *Respir Care* 1994; **39**:1191.

Chalela JA, Katzan I, Liebeskind DS, *et al.* Safety of intra-arterial thrombolysis in the postoperative period, *Stroke* 2001; **32**:1365–1369.

Champagne BJ, Lee EC, Valerian B, Mulhotra N, Mehta M. Incidence of colonic ischemia after repair of ruptured abdominal aortic aneurysm with endograft, *J Am Coll Surg* 2007; **204**(4):597–602.

Chang JK, Calligaro KD, Ryan S, Runyan D, Dougherty MJ, Stern JJ. Risk factors associated with infection of lower extremity revascularization: analysis of 365 procedures performed at a teaching hospital. *Ann Vasc Surg* 2003; **17**(1):91–96.

Chuter TA, Faruqi RM, Sawhney R, *et al.* Endoleak after endovascular repair of abdominal aortic aneurysm, *J Vasc Surg* 2001; **34**:98–105.

Conte MS. Technical factors in lower-extremity vein bypass surgery: how can we improve outcomes? *Semin Vasc Surg* 2009; **22**(4):227–233.

Coselli JS, LeMaire SA, Conklin LD, Adams GJ. Left heart bypass during descending thoracic aortic aneurysm repair does not reduce the incidence of paraplegia, *Ann Thorac Surg* 2004; **77**(4):1298–1303.

Coselli JS, LeMaire SA, Köksoy C, Schmittling ZC, Curling PE. Cerebrospinal fluid drainage reduces paraplegia after thoracoabdominal aortic aneurysm repair: results of a randomized clinical trial, *J Vasc Surg* 2002; **35**(4):631–639.

Coselli JS, LeMaire SA. Left heart bypass reduces paraplegia rates after thoracoabdominal aortic aneurysm repair, *Ann Thorac Surg* 1999; **67**(6):1931–1934.

Coutts S, Hill M, Hu W. Hyperperfusion syndrome: Toward a stricter definition, *Neurosurgery* 2003; **53**:1053–1060.

Crawford ES, Crawford JL, Safi HJ, Coselli JS, Hess KR, Brooks B, Norton HJ, Glaeser DH. Thoracoabdominal aortic aneurysms: Preoperative and intraoperative factors determining immediate and long-term results of operations in 605 patients, *J Vasc Surg* 1986; **3**(3):389–404.

Curi MA, Skelly CL, Baldwin ZK, Woo DH, Baron JM, Desai TR, Katz D, McKinsey JF, Bassiouny HS, Gewertz BL, Schwartz LB. Long-term outcome of infrainguinal bypass grafting in patients with serologically proven hypercoagulability, *J Vasc Surg* 2003; **37**(2):301–306.

De Borst GJ, Moll FL, Van de Pavoordt HD, *et al.* Stroke from carotid endarterectomy: When and how to reduce perioperative stroke rate? *Eur J Vasc Endovasc Surg* 2001; **21**:484–489.

Dehn TC, Taylor GW. Cranial and cervical nerve damage associated with carotid endarterectomy, *Br J Surg* 1983; **70**:365–368.

Dente CJ, Shaz BH, Nicholas JM, Harris RS, Wyrzykowski AD, Patel S, Shah A, Vercruysse GA, Feliciano DV, Rozycki GS, Salomone JP, Ingram WL. Improvements in early mortality and coagulopathy are sustained better in patients with blunt trauma after institution of a massive transfusion protocol in a civilian level I trauma center, *J Trauma* 2009; **66**(6):1616–1624.

DePalma RG, Levine SB, Feldman S. Preservation of erectile function after aortoiliac reconstruction, *Arch Surg* 1978; **113**:958

Diehl JT, Cali RF, Hertzer NR, Beven EG. Complications of abdominal aortic reconstruction: An analysis of perioperative risk factors in 557 patients, *Ann Surg* 1983; **197**:49.

Donadio C, Tramonti G, Lucceshi A, *et al.* Tubular toxicity is the main renal effect of contrast media, *Ren Fail* 1996; **18**:647.

Dorman BH, Elliott BM, Spinale FG, *et al.* Protamine use during peripheral vascular surgery: A prospective randomized trial, *J Vasc Surg* 1995; **22**:248–256.

Dosluoglu HH, Loghmanee C, Lall P, Cherr GS, Harris LM, Dryjski ML. Management of early (<30 day) vascular groin infections using vacuum-assisted closure alone without muscle flap coverage in a consecutive patient series, *J Vasc Surg* 2010; **51**(5):1160.

Durham JR, Rubin JR, Malone JM. Management of infected infrainguinal bypass grafts. In: Bergan JJ, Yao JST (Eds.), *Reoperative Arterial Surgery*, Orlando, FL: Grune & Stratton, 1986, pp. 359–373.

El-Sabrout RA, Duncan JM. Right atrial bypass grafting for central venous obstruction associated with dialysis access: another treatment option, *J Vasc Surg* 1999; **29**(3):472–478.

Eldrup-Jorgensen J, Bredenberg CE. Repair of type III and type IV thoracoabdominal aortic aneurysms by using a long beveled anastomosis: A description of technique, *Surgery* 1998; **123**(3):351–355.

Evans WE, Mendelowitz DS, Liapis C, *et al.* Motor speech deficit following carotid endarterectomy, *Ann Surg* 1982; **196**:461–464.

Fagon JY, Chastre J, Hance AJ, *et al.* Nosocomial pneumonia in ventilated patients: A cohort study evaluating attributable mortality and hospital stay, *Am J Med* 1993; **94**:281.

Faries PL, Cadot H, Agarwal G, *et al.* Management of endoleak after endovascular aneurysm repair: Cuffs, coils, and conversion, *J Vasc Surg* 2003; **37**:1155–1161.

Fearn SJ, Parry AD, Picton AJ, *et al.* Should heparin be reversed after carotid endarterectomy? A randomised prospective trial, *Eur J Vasc Endovasc Surg* 1997; **13**:394–397.

Ferguson GG, Eliasziw M, Barr HW, *et al.* The North American Symptomatic Carotid Endarterectomy Trial: Surgical results in 1415 patients, *Stroke* 1999; **30**:1751–1758.

Fernandez-Ortiz A, Badimon JJ, Falk E, *et al.* Characterization of the relative thrombogenicity of atherosclerotic plaque components: Implications for consequences of plaque rupture, *J Am Coll Cardiol* 1994; **23**:1562–1569.

Fischer PE, Fabian TC, deRijk WG, Edwards NM, DeCuypere M, Landis RM, Barnard DL, Magnotti LJ, Croce MA. Prosthetic vascular conduit in contaminated fields: A new technology to decrease ePTFE infections, *Am Surg* 2008; **74**(6):524–528.

Flanigan DP, Schuler JJ, Keifer T, *et al.* Elimination of iatrogenic impotence and improvement of sexual function after aortoiliac revascularization, *Arch Surg* 1982; **117**:544.

Fleming MD, Stone WM, Scott P, Chapital AB, Fowl RJ, Money SR. Safety of carotid endarterectomy in patients concurrently on clopidogrel, *Ann Vasc Surg* 2009; **23**(5):612–615.

Ford GT, Whitelaw WA, Rosenal TW, *et al.* Diaphragm function after upper abdominal surgery, *Am Rev Respir Dis* 1983; **127**:431.

Gabriel M, Pukacki F, Dzieciuchowicz Ł, Oszkinis G, Checiński P. Cryopreserved arterial allografts in the treatment of prosthetic graft infections, *Eur J Vasc Endovasc Surg* 2004; **27**(6): 590–596.

Gargiulo NJ 3rd, Veith FJ, Lipsitz EC, Suggs WD, Privrat AI, Ohki T. Perimalleolar and pedal thromboembolectomy and bypasses to treat distal embolization during aortoiliac aneurysm repairs, *J Vasc Surg* 2008; **48**(1):43–46.

Glass C, Maevsky V, Massey T, Illig K. Subclavian vein to right atrial appendage bypass without sternotomy to maintain arteriovenous access in patients with complete central vein occlusion, a new approach, *Ann Vasc Surg* 2009; **23**(4):465–468.

Gloviczki P, Cross SA, Stanson AW, *et al.* Ischemic injury to the spinal cord or lumbosacral plexus after aorto-iliac reconstruction, *Am J Surg* 1991; **162**:131.

Goodney PP, Tavris D, Lucas FL, Gross T, Fisher ES, Finlayson SR. Causes of late mortality after endovascular and open surgical repair of infrarenal abdominal aortic aneurysms, *J Vasc Surg* 2010.

Gracey DR, Divertie MB, Didier EP. Preoperative pulmonary preparation of patients with chronic obstructive pulmonary disease, *Chest* 1979; **76**:123–129.

Hagan PG, Nienaber CA, Isselbacher EM, Bruckman D, Karavite DJ, Russman PL, Evangelista A, Fattori R, Suzuki T, Oh JK, Moore AG, Malouf JF, Pape LA, Gaca C, Sechtem U, Lenferink S, Deutsch HJ, Diedrichs H, Marcos y Robles J, Llovet A, Gilon D, Das SK, Armstrong WF, Deeb GM, Eagle KA. The International Registry of Acute Aortic Dissection (IRAD): new insights into an old disease, *JAMA* 2000; **283**(7):897–903.

Hallett JW Jr, Marshall DM, Petterson TM, *et al.* Graft-related complications after abdominal aortic aneurysm repair: Reassurance from a 36-year population-based experience, *J Vasc Surg* 1997; **25**:277.

Hamdan AD, Pomposelli FB Jr, Gibbons GW, *et al.* Perioperative strokes after 1001 consecutive carotid endarterectomy procedures without an electroencephalogram: Incidence, mechanism, and recovery, *Arch Surg* 1999; **134**:412–415.

Harkonen S, Kjellstrand CM. Exacerbation of diabetic renal failure following intravenous pyelography, *Am J Med* 1977; **63**:939.

Hertzer NR, Beven EG, Young JR, *et al.* Coronary artery disease in peripheral vascular patients: A classification of 1000 coronary angiograms and results of surgical management, *Ann Surg* 1984; **199**:223–233.

Hertzer NR, Feldman BJ, Beven EG, Tucker HM. A prospective study of the incidence of injury to the cranial nerves during carotid endarterectomy, *Surg Gynecol Obstet* 1980; **151**:781–784.

Hou SH, Burchinsky DA, Wish JB, *et al.* Hospital acquired renal insufficiency: A prospective study, *Am J Med* 1983; **74**:243.

Huber TS, Brown MP, Seeger JM, Lee WA. Midterm outcome after the distal revascularization and interval ligation (DRIL) procedure, *J Vasc Surg* 2008; **48**(4):926–932.

Hughes MJ, McCall JM, Nott DM, Padley SP. Treatment of iatrogenic femoral artery pseudoaneurysms using ultrasound-guided injection of thrombin, *Clin Radiol* 2000; **55**:749–751.

If intraoperative type I or II endoleak at risk down the road.

Illig KA, Rhodes JM, Sternbach Y, Shortell CK, Davies MG, Green RM. Reduction in wound morbidity rates following endoscopic saphenous vein harvest, *Ann Vasc Surg* 2001; **15**(1):104.

Illig KA, Surowiec S, Shortell CK, Davies MG, Rhodes JM, Green RM. Hemodynamics of distal revascularization-interval ligation. *Ann Vasc Surg* 2005; **19**(2):199–207.

Jimenez JC, Smith MM, Wilson SE. Sexual dysfunction in men after open or endovascular repair of abdominal aortic aneurysms, *Vascular* 2004; **12**(3):186–191.

Jonker FH, Aruny J, Muhs BE. Management of type II endoleaks: preoperative versus postoperative versus expectant management, *Semin Vasc Surg* 2009; **22**(3):165.

Khan AM, Jacobs S. Trash feet after coronary angiography, *Heart* 2003; **89**(5):e17.

Kieburtz K, Ricotta JJ, Moxley RT III. Seizures following carotid endarterectomy, *Arch Neurol* 1990; **47**:568–570.

Kiguchi M, O'Rourke HJ, Dasyam A, Makaroun MS, Chaer RA. Endovascular repair of 2 iliac pseudoaneurysms and arteriovenous fistula following spine surgery, *Vasc Endovascular Surg* 2010; **44**(2):126.

Kreienberg P, Cheema M, Chang BB, Paty PS, Roddy SP, Darling RC 3rd. Primary revision of mid-vein stenoses in venous bypass conduits: venous patch versus interposition vein, *J Vasc Surg* 2007; **45**(5):929–934.

Kuhan G, Raptis S. 'Trash foot' following operations involving the abdominal aorta, *Aust N Z J Surg* 1997; **67**(1):21–24.

Kushner FG, Hand M, Smith SC Jr, King SB 3rd, Anderson JL, Antman EM, Bailey SR, Bates ER, Blankenship JC, Casey DE Jr, Green LA, Hochman JS, Jacobs AK, Krumholz HM, Morrison DA, Ornato JP, Pearle DL, Peterson ED, Sloan MA, Whitlow PL, Williams DO. Focused Updates: ACC/AHA Guidelines for the Management of Patients With ST-Elevation Myocardial Infarction (updating the 2004 Guideline and 2007 Focused Update) and ACC/AHA/SCAI Guidelines on Percutaneous Coronary Intervention (updating the 2005 Guideline and 2007 Focused Update): a report of the American College of Cardiology Foundation/American Heart Association Task Force on Practice Guidelines. American College of Cardiology Foundation/American Heart Association Task Force on Practice Guidelines, *Circulation* 2009; **120**(22):2271–2306. Epub November 18, 2009. No abstract available. Erratum in: *Circulation* 2010; **121**(12):e257.

Landesberg G, Einav S, Christopherson R, *et al.* Perioperative ischemia and cardiac complications in major vascular surgery: Importance of preoperative twelve-lead electrocardiogram, *J Vasc Surg* 1997; **26**:570–578.

Landesberg G, Mosseri M, Wolfe Y, *et al.* Perioperative myocardial ischemia and infarction: Identification by continuous 12-lead electrocardiogram with online ST-segment monitoring, *Anesthesiology* 2002; **96**:264–270.

Landesberg G, Mosseri M, Zahger D, *et al.* Myocardial infarction after vascular surgery: The role of prolonged stress-induced ST segment depression-type ischemia, *J Am Coll Cardiol* 2001; **37**:1839–1845.

Larson JS, Hudson K, Mertz ML, *et al.* Renal vasoconstriction responses to contrast medium, *J Lab Clin Med* 1983; **101**:385.

Lee TH, Marcantonio ER, Mangione CM, Thomas EJ, Polanczyk CA, Cook EF, Sugarbaker DJ, Donaldson MC, Poss R, Ho KK, Ludwig LE, Pedan A, Goldman L. Derivation and prospective validation of a simple index for prediction of cardiac risk of major noncardiac surgery, *Circulation* 1999; **100**(10):1043.

Lennox AF, Delis KT, Szendro G, *et al.* Duplex-guided thrombin injection for iatrogenic femoral artery pseudoaneurysm is effective even in anticoagulated patients, *Br J Surg* 2000; **87**:796–801.

Liapis CD, Satiani B, Florance CL, Evans WE: Motor speech malfunction following carotid endarterectomy, *Surgery* 1981; **89**:56–59.

Liu X, Cheng Y, Zhang S, Lin Y, Yang J, Zhang C. A necessary role of miR-221 and miR-222 in vascular smooth muscle cell proliferation and neointimal hyperplasia, *Circ Res* 2009; **104**(4):476–487.

Longo WE, Lee TC, Barnett MG, *et al.* Ischemic colitis complicating abdominal aortic aneurysm surgery in the U.S. veteran, *J Surg Res* 1996; **60**:351.

Loughlin KA, Weingarten CM, Nagelhout J, Stevenson JG. A pharmacoeconomic analysis of neuromuscular blocking agents in the operating room, *Pharmacotherapy* 1996; **16**(5):942–950.

Malkawi AH, Hinchliffe RJ, Holt PJ, Loftus IM, Thompson MM. Percutaneous Access for Endovascular Aneurysm Repair: A Systematic Review, *Eur J Vasc Endovasc Surg* 2010.

Maniglia AJ, Han DP. Cranial nerve injuries following carotid endarterectomy: An analysis of 336 procedures, *Head Neck* 1991; **13**:121–124.

Marin ML, Veith FJ, Cynamon J, *et al.* Initial experience with transluminally placed endovascular grafts for the treatment of complex vascular lesions, *Ann Surg* **222**:449–469.

Maroulis J, Karkanevatos A, Papakostas K, *et al.* Cranial nerve dysfunction following carotid endarterectomy, *Int Angiol* 2000; **19**:237–241.

Marschall J, Doherty J, Warren DK. The epidemiology of recurrent Gram-negative bacteremia in a tertiary-care hospital, *Diagn Microbiol Infect Dis* 2010; **66**(4):456.

Martens JM, Knippenberg B, Vos JA, de Vries JP, Hansen BE, van Overhagen H. PADI Trial Group. Update on PADI trial: percutaneous transluminal angioplasty and drug-eluting stents for infrapopliteal lesions in critical limb ischemia, *J Vasc Surg* 2009; **50**(3):687–689.

Mason J, Joeris B, Welsch J, *et al.* Vascular congestion in ischemic renal failure: The role of cell swelling, *Miner Electrolyte Metab* 1989; **15**:114.

Massey EW, Heyman A, Utley C, *et al.* Cranial nerve paralysis following carotid endarterectomy, *Stroke* 1984; **15**:157–159.

Mattioli AV, Bonetti L, Carletti U, Ambrosio G, Mattioli G. Thrombotic events in patients with antiplatelet factor 4/heparin antibodies, *Heart* 2009; **95**(16):1350–1354.

Mauney MC, Buchanan SA, Lawrence WA, *et al.* Stroke rate is markedly reduced after carotid endarterectomy by avoidance of protamine, *J Vasc Surg* 1995; **22**:264–270.

McFalls EO, Ward HB, Moritz TE, Apple FS, Goldman S, Pierpont G, Larsen GC, Hattler B, Shunk K, Littooy F, Santilli S, Rapp J, Thottapurathu L, Krupski W, Reda DJ, Henderson WG. Predictors and outcomes of a perioperative myocardial infarction following elective vascular surgery in patients with documented coronary artery disease: results of the CARP trial, *Eur Heart J* 2008; **29**(3):394–401.

Millon A, Deelchand A, Feugier P, Chevalier JM, Favre JP. Conversion to open repair after endovascular aneurysm repair: causes and results. A French multicentric study. University Association for Research in Vascular Surgery (AURC), *Eur J Vasc Endovasc Surg* 2009; **38**(4):429.

Molitoris BA. New insights into the cell biology of ischemic acute renal failure, *J Am Soc Nephrol* 1991; **1**:1263.

Moulakakis KG, Mylonas SN, Sfyroeras GS, Andrikopoulos V. Hyperperfusion syndrome after carotid revascularization, *J Vasc Surg* 2009; **49**(4):1060–1068.

Muther RS. Acute renal failure: Acute azotemia in the critically ill. In: Civetta JM, Taylor RW and Kirby RR (Eds.), *Critical Care*, 2nd Edition, Philadelphia: JB Lippincott, 1992, pp. 1583–1598.

O'Connor S, Andrew P, Batt M, Becquemin JP. A systematic review and meta-analysis of treatments for aortic graft infection, *J Vasc Surg* 2006; **44**(1):38–45.

Ott MC, Stewart TC, Lawlor DK, Gray DK, Forbes TL. Management of blunt thoracic aortic injuries: endovascular stents versus open repair, *J Trauma* 2004; **56**(3):565–570.

Ouriel K, Shortell CK, Illig KA, *et al*. Intracerebral hemorrhage after carotid endarterectomy: Incidence, contribution to neurologic morbidity, and predictive factors, *J Vasc Surg* 1999; **29**:82–89.

Pearson S, Hassen T, Spark JI, Cabot J, Cowled P, Fitridge R. Endovascular repair of abdominal aortic aneurysm reduces intraoperative cortisol and perioperative morbidity, *J Vasc Surg* 2005; **41**(6):919–925.

Picone AL, Green RM, Ricotta JR, *et al*. Spinal cord ischemia following operations on the abdominal aorta, *J Vasc Surg* 1986; **3**:94.

Pittaluga P, Batt M, Hassen-Khodja R, *et al*. Revascularization of internal iliac arteries during aortoiliac surgery: A multicenter study, *Ann Vasc Surg* 1998; **12**:537.

Poldermans D, Bax JJ, Schouten O, Neskovic AN, Paelinck B, Rocci G, van Dortmont L, Durazzo AE, van de Ven LL, van Sambeek MR, Kertai MD, Boersma E. Dutch Echocardiographic Cardiac Risk Evaluation Applying Stress Echo Study Group. Should major vascular surgery be delayed because of preoperative cardiac testing in intermediate-risk patients receiving beta-blocker therapy with tight heart rate control? *J Am Coll Cardiol* 2006; **48**(5):964–969.

Poldermans D, Bax JJ, Steyerberg EW, Thomson IR, Banga JD, van De Ven LL, van Urk H, Roelandt JR; DECREASE Study Group (Dutch Echocardiographic Cardiac Risk Evaluation Applying Stress Echocardiogrpahy). Predictors of cardiac events after major vascular surgery: Role of clinical characteristics, dobutamine echocardiography, and beta-blocker therapy, Boersma E, *JAMA* 2001; **285**(14):1865–1873.

Reilly LM, Stoney RJ, Goldstone J, *et al*. Improved management of aortic graft infection: The influence of operation sequence and staging, *J Vasc Surg* 1987; **5**:421.

Riles TS, Imparato AM, Jacobowitz GR, *et al*. The cause of perioperative stroke after carotid endarterectomy, *J Vasc Surg* 1994; **19**:206–216.

Rodgers A, Walker N, Schug S, McKee A, Kehlet H, van Zundert A, Sage D, Futter M, Saville G, Clark T, MacMahon S. Reduction of postoperative mortality and morbidity with epidural or spinal anaesthesia: Results from overview of randomised trials, *BMJ* 2000; **321**(7275):1493.

Rousseau H, Dambrin C, Marcheix B, Richeux L, Mazerolles M, Cron C, Watkinson A, Mugniot A, Soula P, Chabbert V, Canevet G, Roux D, Massabuau P, Meites G, Tran Van T, Otal P. Acute traumatic aortic rupture: a comparison of surgical and stent-graft repair. *J Thorac Cardiovasc Surg* 2005; **129**(5):1050–1055.

Schauber MD, Fontenelle LJ, Solomon JW, Hanson TL. Cranial/cervical nerve dysfunction after carotid endarterectomy, *J Vasc Surg* 1997; **25**:481–487.

Seify H, Moyer HR, Jones GE, Busquets A, Brown K, Salam A, Losken A, Culbertson J, Hester TR. The role of muscle flaps in wound salvage after vascular graft infections: the Emory experience, *Plast Reconstr Surg* 2006; **117**(4):1325–1333.

Shammas NW, Dippel EJ, Shammas G, Gayton L, Coiner D, Jerin M. Dethrombosis of the lower extremity arteries using the power-pulse spray technique in patients with recent onset thrombotic occlusions: results of the DETHROMBOSIS Registry, *J Endovasc Ther* 2008; **15**(5):570–579.

Shieh SD, Hirsch SR, Boshell BR, *et al*. Low risk of contrast media induced acute renal failure in nonazotemic type 2 diabetes mellitus, *Kidney Int* 1982; **21**:739.

Shimada K, Kobayashi M, Ozawa T. The modulation of heparin-like activity of endothelial cells in experimental systems, *Nippon Ketsueki Gakkai Zasshi* 1989; **52**(8):1337–1342.

Skudlarick J, Mooring S. Systolic hypertension and complications of carotid endarterectomy, *South Med J* 1982; **75**:1563–1565.

Skydell J, Machleder H, Baker J, Busuttil R, Moore W. Incidence and mechanism of post-carotid endarterectomy hypertension, *Arch Surg* 1987; **122**:1153–1155.

Sobel M, Verhaeghe R. American College of Chest Physicians; American College of Chest Physicians. Antithrombotic therapy for peripheral artery occlusive disease: American College of Chest Physicians Evidence-Based Clinical Practice Guidelines, 8th Edition, *Chest* 2008; **133**(6 Suppl):815S–843S.

Solomon R, Werner C, Mann D, *et al*. Effects of saline, mannitol and furosemide to prevent acute decreases in renal function induced by radiocontrast agents, *N Engl J Med* 1994; **331**:1416.

Sreeram S, Lumsden AB, Miller JS, *et al*. Retroperitoneal hematoma following femoral arterial catheterization: A serious and often fatal complication, *Am Surg* 1993; **59**:94–98.

Srivastava SD, Eagleton MJ, O'Hara P, Kashyap VS, Sarac T, Clair D. Surgical repair of carotid artery aneurysms: a 10-year, single-center experience, *Ann Vasc Surg* 2010; 24(1):100–105.

Stewart AH, Eyers PS, Earnshaw JJ. Prevention of infection in peripheral arterial reconstruction: A systematic review and meta-analysis, *J Vasc Surg* 2007; **46**(1):148–155.

Szilagyi DE, Hageman JH, Smith RF, Elliott JP. Spinal cord damage in surgery of the abdominal aorta, *Surgery* 1978; **83**:38.

Szilagyi DE, Smith RF, Elliott JP, Vrandecic MP. Infection in arterial reconstruction with synthetic grafts, *Am Surg* 1972; **176**:321–333.

Szilagyi DE, Smith RF, Elliott JP, Vrandecic MP. Infection in arterial reconstruction with synthetic grafts, *Ann Surg* 1972; **176**:321.

Tepel M, van der Giet M, Schwarzfeld C, *et al*. Prevention of radiographic-contrast-agent-induced reductions in renal function by acetylcysteine, *N Engl J Med* 2000; **343**:180.

Thompson MM, Smith J, Naylor AR, Nasim A, Sayers RD, Boyle JR, Tinkler K, Goodall S, Evans D, Bell PR. Ultrasound-based quantification of emboli during conventional and endovascular aneurysm repair, *J Endovasc Surg* 1997; **4**(1):33.

Timmers H, Wieling W, Karemaker J, Lenders J. Baroreflex failure: A neglected type of secondary hypertension, *Neth J Med* 2004; **62**:151–155.

Towne JB, Weiss DG, Hobson RW II. First-phase report of cooperative Veterans Administration asymptomatic carotid stenosis study: Operative morbidity and mortality, *J Vasc Surg* 1990; **11**:252–259.

Treiman RL, Cossman DV, Foran RF, *et al*. The influence of neutralizing heparin after carotid endarterectomy on postoperative stroke and wound hematoma, *J Vasc Surg* 1990; **12**:440–446.

Trimarchi S, Tsai T, Eagle KA, Isselbacher EM, Froehlich J, Cooper JV, Rampoldi V, Upchurch GR Jr. Acute abdominal aortic dissection: insight from the International Registry of Acute Aortic Dissection (IRAD). International Registry of Acute Aortic Dissection (IRAD) investigators, *J Vasc Surg* 2007; **46**(5):913–919.

Tsai S, Hollenbeck ST, Ryer EJ, Edlin R, Yamanouchi D, Kundi R, Wang C, Liu B, Kent KC. TGF-beta through Smad3 signaling stimulates vascular smooth muscle cell proliferation and neointimal formation, *Am J Physiol Heart Circ Physiol* 2009; **297**(2):H540–H549.

Tsai TT, Trimarchi S, Nienaber CA. Acute aortic dissection: perspectives from the International Registry of Acute Aortic Dissection (IRAD), *Eur J Vasc Endovasc Surg* 2009; **37**(2):149–159.

Turgut H, Sacar S, Kaleli I, Sacar M, Goksin I, Toprak S, Asan A, Cevahir N, Tekin K, Baltalarli A. Systemic and local antibiotic prophylaxis in the prevention of Staphylococcus epidermidis graft infection, *BMC Infect Dis* 2005; 5.

Van Damme H, Creemers E, Limet R. Ischaemic colitis following aortoiliac surgery, *Acta Chir Belg* 2000; **100**:21.

van Mook W, Rennenberg R, Schurink G, van Oostenbrugge R, Mess W, Hofman P, de Leeuw P. Cerebral hyperperfusion syndrome, *Lancet Neurol* 2005; **4**:877–888.

Vogel TR, Dombrovskiy VY, Carson JL, Haser PB, Lowry SF, Graham AM. Infectious complications after elective vascular surgical procedures, *J Vasc Surg* 2010; **51**(1):122–129.

Vogel TR, Symons R, Flum DR. The incidence and factors associated with graft infection after aortic aneurysm repair, *J Vasc Surg* 2008; **47**(2):264–269.

Vogten JM, Gerritsen WB, Ackerstaff RG, van Dongen EP, de Vries JP. Perioperative microemboli and platelet aggregation in patients undergoing carotid endarterectomy, *Vascular* 2008; **16**(3):154–160.

Walker J, Katzen J, Nabozny M, Young K, Glass C, Singh M, Illig K. Long-term results of endoscopic versus open saphenous vein harvest for lower extremity bypass, *J Vasc Surg* 2010, in press.

Ward HB, Moritz TE, Goldman S, Krupski WC, Littooy F, Pierpont G, Santilli S, Rapp J, Hattler B, Shunk K, Jaenicke C, Thottapurathu L, Ellis N, Reda DJ, Henderson WG. Coronary-artery revascularization before elective major vascular surgery, McFalls EO, *N Engl J Med* 2004; **351**(27):2795–2804.

Weinstein MH, Machleder HI, Sexual function after aorto-lliac surgery, *Ann Surg* 1975; **181**:787.

Welborn MB 3rd, Seeger JM. Prevention and management of sigmoid and pelvic ischemia associated with aortic surgery, *Semin Vasc Surg* 2001; **14**:255.

Wijewardena C, Yarham SI, Boyle JR, Gaunt ME. Postoperative arrhythmias in general surgical patients, Walsh SR, Tang T, Ann R, *Coll Surg Engl* 2007; **89**(2):91–95.

Xue FS, Li BW, Zhang GS, *et al*. The influence of surgical sites on early postoperative hypoxemia in adults undergoing elective surgery, *Anesth Analg* 1999; **88**:213.

Yang H, Raymer K, Butler R, Parlow J, Roberts R. The effects of perioperative beta-blockade: results of the Metoprolol after Vascular Surgery (MaVS) study, a randomized controlled trial, *Am Heart J* 2006; **152**(5):983–990.

Young B, Moore WS, Robertson JT, *et al*. An analysis of perioperative surgical mortality and morbidity in the asymptomatic carotid atherosclerosis study. ACAS Investigators. Asymptomatic Carotid Artheriosclerosis Study, *Stroke* 1996; **27**:2216–2224.

Youssef F, Jenkins MP, Dawson KJ, Berger L, Myint F, Hamilton G. The value of suction wound drain after carotid and femoral artery surgery: A randomised trial using duplex assessment of the volume of post-operative haematoma, *Eur J Vasc Endovasc Surg* 2005; **29**(2):162–166.

Zannetti S, Parente B, De Rango P, *et al*. Role of surgical techniques and operative findings in cranial and cervical nerve injuries during carotid endarterectomy, *Eur J Vasc Endovasc Surg* 1998; **15**:528–531.

[No authors listed]. Randomised trial of cholesterol lowering in 4444 patients with coronary heart disease: the Scandinavian Simvastatin Survival Study (4S), *Lancet* 1994; **344**(8934):1383–1389.

Index